THE HUMAN BRAIN
IN PHOTOGRAPHS
AND DIAGRAMS

THE HUMAN BRAIN IN PHOTOGRAPHS AND DIAGRAMS

THIRD EDITION

John Nolte, PhD

Professor of Cell Biology and Anatomy
The University of Arizona College of Medicine
Tucson, Arizona

Jay B. Angevine, Jr., PhD

Professor Emeritus of Cell Biology and Anatomy
The University of Arizona College of Medicine
Tucson, Arizona

with 650 *illustrations*

Cover photograph from a dissection by Grant Dahmer,
Department of Cell Biology and Anatomy,
University of Arizona College of Medicine

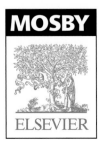

MOSBY

ELSEVIER

1600 John F. Kennedy Blvd.
Ste 1800
Philadelphia, PA 19103-2899

THE HUMAN BRAIN IN PHOTOGRAPHS AND DIAGRAMS   ISBN: 978-0-323-04573-5

Notice

Knowledge and best practice in this field are constantly changing. As new research and experience broaden our knowledge, changes in practice, treatment and drug therapy may become necessary or appropriate. Readers are advised to check the most current information provided (i) on procedures featured or (ii) by the manufacturer of each product to be administered, to verify the recommended dose or formula, the method and duration of administration, and contraindications. It is the responsibility of the practitioner, relying on their own experience and knowledge of the patient, to make diagnoses, to determine dosages and the best treatment for each individual patient, and to take all appropriate safety precautions. To the fullest extent of the law, neither the Publisher nor the Authors assume any liability for any injury and/or damage to persons or property arising out of or related to any use of the material contained in this book.

The Publisher

Library of Congress Cataloging-in-Publication Data
Nolte, John.
    The human brain in photographs and diagrams / John Nolte, Jay B. Angevine Jr.—3rd ed.
        p. ; cm.
    Includes index.
    ISBN 0-323-04573-1
    1. Brain—Atlases.   I. Angevine, Jay B.   II. Title.
    [DNLM: 1. Brain—anatomy & histology—Atlases. WL 17 N798h 2007]
    QM455.N65 2007
    611'.81—dc22

                                                                    2007000655

Acquisitions Editor: Madelene Hyde
Developmental Editor: Katie DeFrancesco
Publishing Services Manager: Linda Van Pelt
Project Manager: Francisco Morales
Design Direction: Gene Harris

Printed in China

Last digit is the print number: 9   8   7   6   5   4   3   2   1

To Our Students
whose enthusiasm maintains ours,
whose questions prod us to seek clarity and accuracy,
whose caring and curiosity make teaching fun;

and

To Paul Ivan Yakovlev
whose wisdom and foresight,
dignity, kindness, and generosity,
reverence for patients and joy in people,
enormous energy and personal youthfulness
created a world library of human and animal brains
and a world community of neurological scholars

Preface

Learning about the functional anatomy of the human central nervous system (CNS) is usually a daunting task. Structures that interdigitate and overlap in three dimensions contribute to the difficulty, as does a long list of intimidating names, many with origins in descriptive terminology derived from Latin and Greek. We have attempted in this book to make the task a little easier for students of the biological and health sciences by presenting systematic series of whole-brain sections in three different sets of planes, by relating these sections to three-dimensional reconstructions, and by trying to restrain ourselves when indicating structures.

We made a number of choices in organizing the materials for the first edition of this atlas and again in developing subsequent editions; in each instance we strove for simplicity. Unlabeled photographs are presented throughout the book, juxtaposed to faded-out versions of the same photographs with important structures outlined and labeled. This circumvents the common need to mentally superimpose a labeled drawing on a photograph. We pored over many hundreds of sections and chose what we believe to be comprehensive yet not excessive sets in each plane; sections illustrating major structures or major transitions are shown in greater detail and at a higher magnification. Every labeled structure is discussed briefly in a glossary at the end of the book. We made substantial improvements to this edition, as follows:

- Several additional views of gross brains (Chapter 1) were added.
- Enlarged views of parts of a few more levels of the spinal cord, brainstem, and axial and sagittal whole-brain sections (Chapters 2, 3, 6, and 7) were added.
- The "guided tours" at the beginning of Chapters 2, 3, 5, 6, and 7 were redone in color.
- Schematic illustrations of the CNS blood supply were included in Chapters 2, 3, 5, 6, and 7.
- The brief discussions of CNS pathways in Chapter 8 were thoroughly reworked to improve their

clarity, and an overview of corticobulbar pathways was added.
- A new and improved set of normal magnetic resonance images was used in Chapter 9, and more examples of the uses of clinical imaging to detect intracranial pathology were added.
- An extensive series of small photographs was used to illustrate the glossary.

The methods used in this book inevitably involve compromises. We labeled only structures that we believe are important for the knowledge base of undergraduate and professional students and omitted others dear to our hearts but perhaps not critical for these students. Hence, the fasciola cinerea so prominent in Figure 6–11 is not labeled, and the indusium griseum is mentioned only briefly in a footnote. In addition, explicitly outlining structures required some simplifications, and complex entities are sometimes indicated more simply as single structures. We think that the resulting pedagogical usefulness for students justifies these anatomical liberties.

Current technological methods allowed us to approach the construction of this atlas differently than we could have when it was first discussed. All the photographs of brains and sections used in the book were retouched digitally. Mounting medium, staining artifacts, and small cracks, folds, and scratches were removed from the digitized versions of the sections. The profiles of many small blood vessels were removed as well. The color balance was changed as appropriate to make the sections as uniform as possible. These procedures improved the illustrations aesthetically, while leaving their essential content unchanged. In addition, computer-based surface-reconstruction techniques made possible the beautiful three-dimensional images that appear in Chapter 4 and elsewhere in the book.

John Nolte
Jay B. Angevine, Jr.

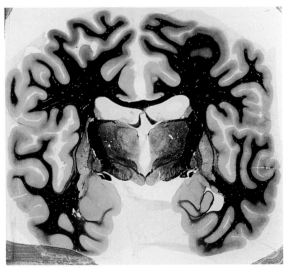

The section shown in Figure 5–7, before retouching.

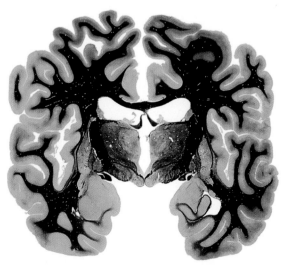

The section shown in Figure 5–7, retouched.

Acknowledgments

This book could never have happened without the help of many friends and colleagues. The photographic expertise of Nathan Nitzky, Jeb Zirato, and others in the Division of Biomedical Communications is evident throughout the book. Grant Dahmer and Dr. Norman Koelling prepared the prosections shown in Chapter 1. The sections shown in Chapter 2 were cut by Shelley Rowley, and those in Chapter 3 by John Nolte's colleague and friend, Pam Eller. John Sundsten produced the three-dimensional images shown in Chapter 4 and in some other parts of the book and shared in our excitement about this project. Paul Yakovlev, as detailed shortly, was the central figure in the production of the sections shown in Chapters 5 through 7. Drs. Ray Carmody, Robert Handy, Elena Plante, and Joe Seeger provided the images shown in Chapter 9 and helped with their interpretation. Jay's colleague and friend, Cheryl Cotman, produced the three-dimensional reconstructions of the limbic system shown in Chapter 8. Sasha Zill first described the strumus. Katie DeFrancesco was patient and always helpful. Kathy reappeared in JN's life and held it together. Midge cheered on JBA. We thank them all.

John Nolte
Jay B. Angevine, Jr.

A Note on the Whole-Brain Serial Sections and Their Origin

As crucial as computer technology is to our book, the whole-brain serial sections are its foundation. They were prepared during 1966 and 1967 in the Warren Anatomical Museum at Harvard Medical School. The work, in which I took part, was performed under the direction of Dr. Paul I. Yakovlev (1894–1983), who was curator of the museum from 1955 to 1961 and then Emeritus Clinical Professor of Neuropathology until 1969. Each brain, embedded whole in celloidin, was sectioned in coronal, horizontal, or sagittal planes on a giant microtome with a standing oblique 36-inch blade and a sliding brain holder. The sections, each 35 micrometers thick, were rolled and stored in test tubes in a console of 100 numbered receptacles. After processing pilot sections for suitability and quality, we stained every 20th section with Weigert's hematoxylin (Loyez method) for myelin and mounted it between sheets of window glass. Each preparation is thus about 4 mm thick, yet great depth and detail of cells and fibers are visible in it.

Such preparations illustrate the white matter and tracts of the brain by staining the myelin sheaths of axons black; gray matter and nuclei appear as more-or-less pale areas, depending on the number and caliber of myelinated fibers present. These sections, all from essentially normal brains, were added to an already huge collection representing more than 900 cerebra that Dr. Yakovlev had been building since 1930. Now a national resource known and available to neurological scholars worldwide, this priceless compilation, known as the Yakovlev Collection, is graciously housed by the Armed Forces Institute of Pathology in Washington, D.C. Today it comprises about 1600 specimens, normal and pathological, processed in a rigorously consistent manner from the start.

In mid-1967, with Dr. Yakovlev's blessing, I took with me to the University of Arizona some 1000 of the 8741 sections cut from the three normal brains used in Chapters 5 through 7 of this book. I had left Boston to join the faculty of the university's new College of Medicine in Tucson. Paul, my mentor from the time I came to Harvard in 1956, wanted to support me as I began teaching in a far-off land that he believed (perhaps correctly) to be a frontier: the "Wild West." As with everything else he did, it was thoughtful, kind, and generous. How he would have loved to see you studying the sections illustrated on these pages! And were he standing beside you, how much you would learn!

Unlike the fairly simple task of sectioning the brainstem, cutting perfect gapless whole-brain serial sections is difficult. The procedure was never more carefully undertaken or widely employed than by Paul, who used it at or in association with Harvard Medical School for 40 years. A central theme for him was this holistic method ("every part of the brain is there, nothing is left out . . ."), but no aspect of neuroanatomy or neuropathology failed to intrigue him. Although such sections had been made since the late 19th century (they are found in small numbers at many medical schools and in profusion at a few research institutes), Paul's are unique—in uniformity of preparation at every step from fixation to mounting and in unity of general neurological interest and comparability. Of this legacy (he called it "over 40 tons of glass"), Derek Denny-Brown, Emeritus Professor of Neurology at Harvard, wrote in 1972: "The perspective given by serial whole brain sections provides at once an arresting view of anatomical relationships in patterns of striking beauty. After working in the collection for years one still finds every occasion to view it illuminating and rewarding."

In 2000, artist/scientist Cheryl Cotman, anatomist Jay, and computer programmer Kevin Head traced and digitized structures from the serial sagittal sections shown in this atlas. They made a computer reconstruction and large hologram (3′ × 5′) of the human limbic system. We are indebted to Cheryl for her help in selecting images from her large collection of color-coded overall and regional views of the system. We are enlightened by her discovery that several limbic structures are quite differently shaped than traditionally believed. Like Jay, Paul would have found these results hard to accept. For example, Jay strongly contested her finding that the anterior commissure is more like a hangman's knot than the handlebars of a racing bicycle. But, again like Jay, Paul would have accepted her results with glee and laughter.

Jay B. Angevine, Jr.

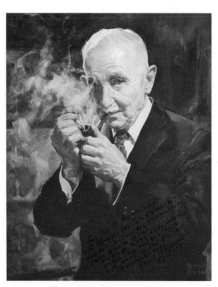

Paul I. Yakovlev, MD
1894–1983

An autographed copy of an oil portrait of Paul Yakovlev by Bettina Steinke. The original portrait was presented to the Warren Anatomical Museum at Harvard Medical School in 1978. (Courtesy of the Warren Museum in the Francis A. Countway Library of Medicine, Boston, Massachusetts.)

Contents

External Anatomy of the Brain

This atlas emphasizes views of the interior of the human central nervous system (CNS), sectioned in various planes. In Chapter 1, we lay some of the groundwork for understanding the arrangements of these interior structures by presenting the surface features with which they are continuous, and by giving a broad overview of the components of the CNS.

The CNS is composed of the spinal cord and the brain, the major components of which are indicated in Figure 1–1. The human brain is dominated by two very large cerebral hemispheres, separated from each other by a deep longitudinal fissure. Each hemisphere is convoluted externally in a fairly consistent pattern into a series of gyri, separated from each other by a series of sulci (an adaptation that makes more area available for the cortex that covers each cerebral hemisphere). Several prominent sulci are used as major landmarks to divide each hemisphere into five lobes*— frontal, parietal, occipital, temporal, and limbic—each of which contains a characteristic set of gyri (Figures 1–3 to 1–8). The two hemispheres are interconnected by a massive bundle of nerve fibers called the corpus callosum. Finally, certain areas of gray matter are embedded in the interior of each cerebral hemisphere. These include major components of the basal ganglia (or, more properly, basal nuclei) and limbic system (primarily the amygdala and hippocampus).

*In addition, the insula, an area of cerebral cortex buried deep in the lateral sulcus (see Fig.1–8C), is usually considered as a separate lobe.

They are apparent in the brain sections shown in Chapters 5 through 7.

The cerebral hemispheres of humans are so massive that they almost conceal the remaining major subdivisions of the brain—the diencephalon, brainstem, and cerebellum. Hemisecting a brain in the midsagittal plane, as in Figure 1–1B, reveals these components.

The diencephalon (literally the "in-between brain") is interposed between each cerebral hemisphere and the brainstem. The diencephalon contains the thalamus, a major way station for information seeking access to the cerebral cortex; the hypothalamus, a major control center for visceral and drive-related functions; and several other structures.

The brainstem, continuous caudally with the spinal cord, serves as a conduit for pathways traveling between the cerebellum or spinal cord and more rostral levels of the CNS. It also contains the neurons that receive or give rise to most of the cranial nerves.

The cerebellum (literally the "little brain") is even more intricately convoluted than the cerebral hemispheres to make room for an extensive covering of its own cortex. It plays a major role in the planning and coordination of movement. A deep transverse fissure (normally occupied over most of its extent by the tentorium cerebelli) separates the cerebellum from the overlying occipital and parietal lobes and continues deeper into the brain, partially separating the diencephalon from the cerebral hemispheres.

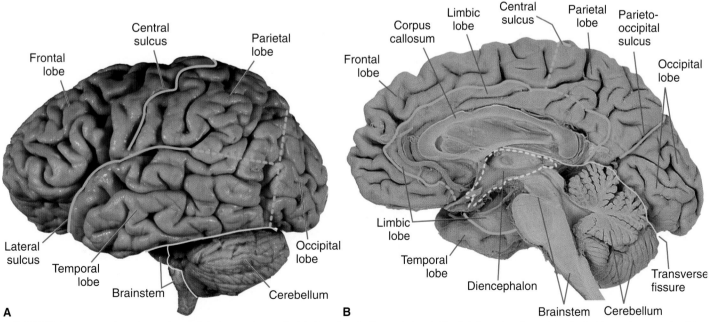

Figure 1–1 Lateral and medial surfaces of the brain, shown slightly less than half actual size. **A,** The left lateral surface of the brain (shown in more detail in Figs. 1–3, 1–5, and 1–8); anterior is to the left. **B,** The medial surface of the right half of the sagittally hemisected brain (shown in more detail in Fig. 1–7); anterior is to the left. *(Dissection by Grant Dahmer, Department of Cell Biology and Anatomy, University of Arizona College of Medicine.)*

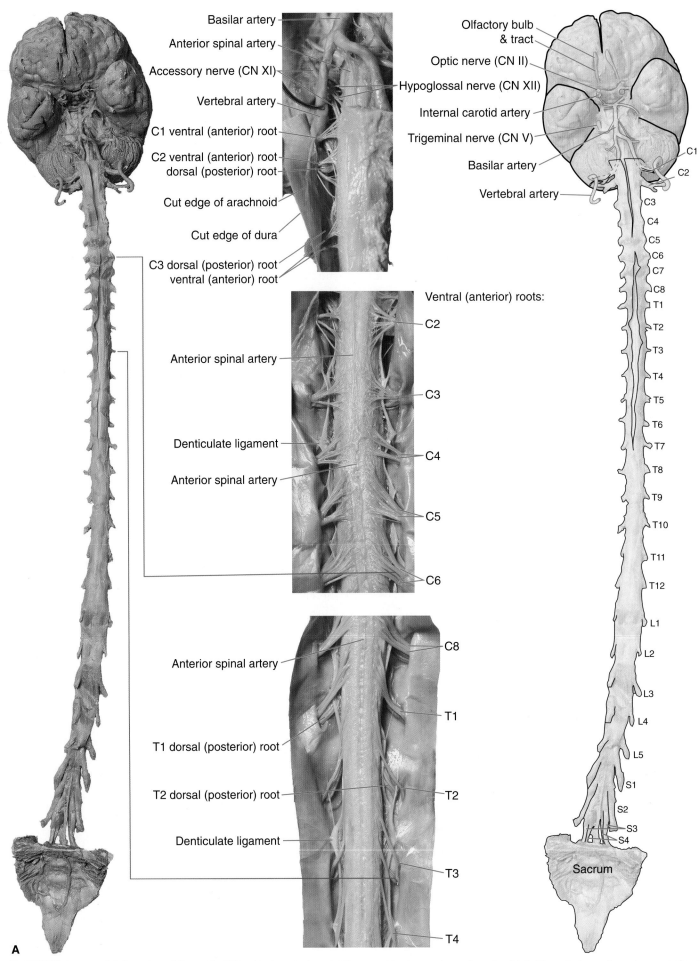

Figure 1–2   A masterful dissection of the entire CNS, with the spinal cord still encased in dura mater and arachnoid. **A,** The anterior surface, shown at about 0.3× actual size. Regions enlarged in the *insets,* after the dura mater and arachnoid were spread apart, are shown actual size.

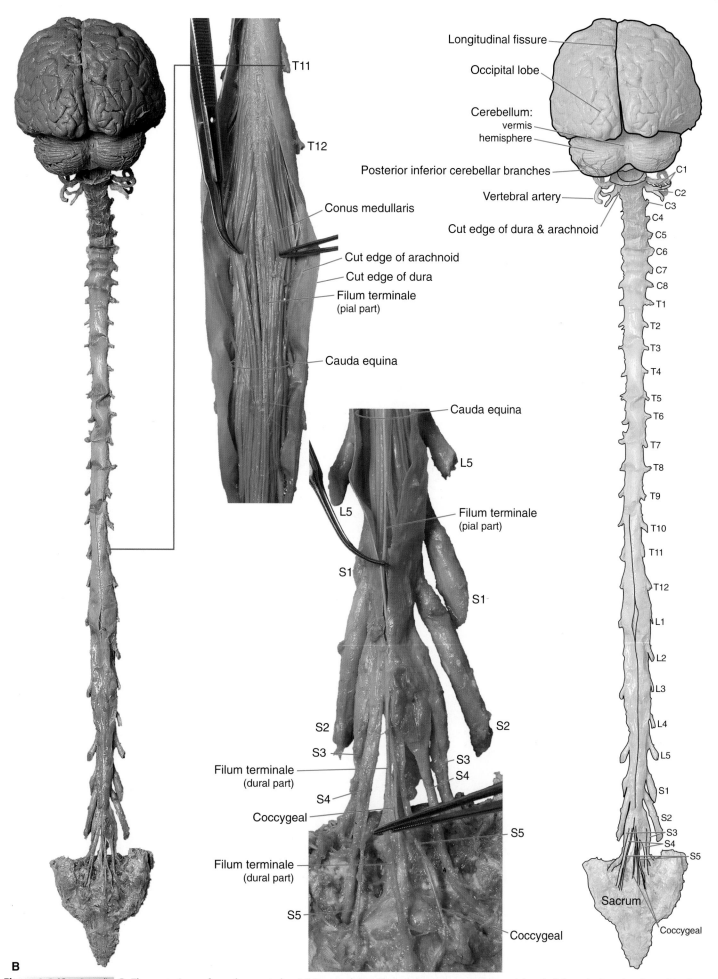

Longitudinal fissure

Occipital lobe

Cerebellum:
vermis
hemisphere

Posterior inferior cerebellar branches

Vertebral artery

Cut edge of dura & arachnoid

T11

T12

Conus medullaris

Cut edge of arachnoid

Cut edge of dura

Filum terminale (pial part)

Cauda equina

Cauda equina

L5

L5

Filum terminale (pial part)

S1

S1

S2

S2

S3

S3

S4

Filum terminale (dural part)

S4

Coccygeal

S5

Filum terminale (dural part)

S5

Coccygeal

C1
C2
C3
C4
C5
C6
C7
C8
T1
T2
T3
T4
T5
T6
T7
T8
T9
T10
T11
T12
L1
L2
L3
L4
L5
S1
S2
S3
S4
S5

Sacrum

Coccygeal

B

Figure 1–2 (Continued)   **B,** The posterior surface, shown at about 0.3× actual size. The cauda equina and the caudal end of the spinal cord, enlarged in the *insets* after the dura mater and arachnoid were spread apart, are shown actual size. *(Dissection by Dr. Norman Koelling, Department of Cell Biology and Anatomy, University of Arizona College of Medicine.)*

A

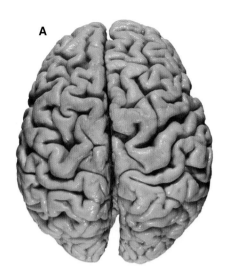

B

C

D

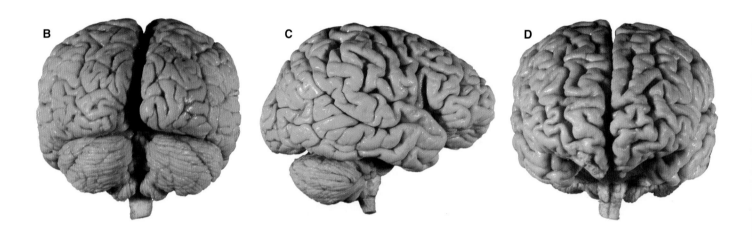

E

F

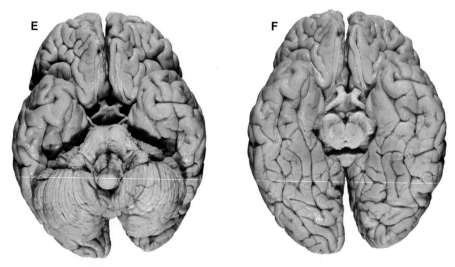

Figure 1–3   Multiple views of a brain, shown at about one third actual size. Only major structures are labeled here, but more details of the same brain can be seen in Figures 1–5, 1–8, and 1–9. **A,** The superior surface (anterior toward the top of the page). **B,** The posterior surface. **C,** The right lateral surface (anterior toward the right). **D,** The anterior surface. **E,** The inferior surface (anterior toward the top of the page).

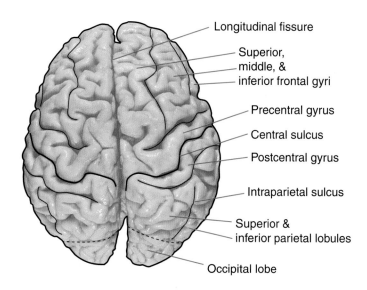

Longitudinal fissure

Superior, middle, & inferior frontal gyri

Precentral gyrus

Central sulcus

Postcentral gyrus

Intraparietal sulcus

Superior & inferior parietal lobules

Occipital lobe

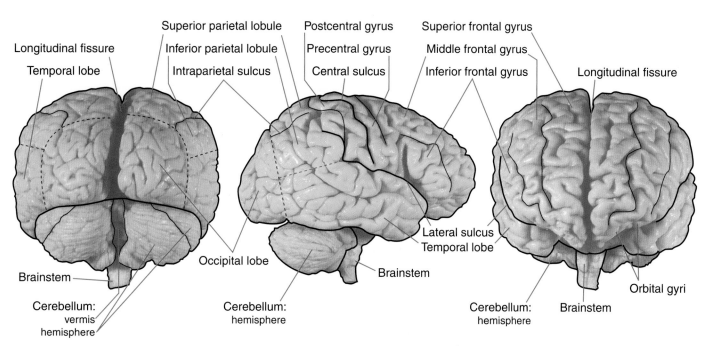

Superior parietal lobule

Inferior parietal lobule

Intraparietal sulcus

Longitudinal fissure

Temporal lobe

Postcentral gyrus

Precentral gyrus

Central sulcus

Superior frontal gyrus

Middle frontal gyrus

Inferior frontal gyrus

Longitudinal fissure

Brainstem

Cerebellum: vermis hemisphere

Occipital lobe

Cerebellum: hemisphere

Brainstem

Lateral sulcus

Temporal lobe

Cerebellum: hemisphere

Brainstem

Orbital gyri

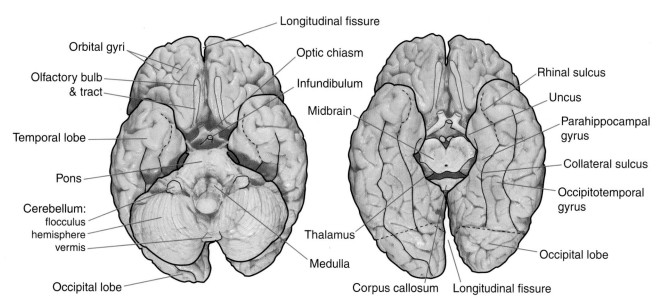

Longitudinal fissure

Orbital gyri

Olfactory bulb & tract

Temporal lobe

Pons

Cerebellum: flocculus hemisphere vermis

Occipital lobe

Optic chiasm

Infundibulum

Midbrain

Thalamus

Medulla

Rhinal sulcus

Uncus

Parahippocampal gyrus

Collateral sulcus

Occipitotemporal gyrus

Occipital lobe

Corpus callosum   Longitudinal fissure

Figure 1–3 (Continued)   **F,** The same inferior surface after removal of the cerebellum and most of the brainstem; the latter are shown in more detail in Figure 1–9. (The rhinal sulcus is drawn as a *dashed line* to indicate that it is separate from the collateral sulcus, even though in this particular brain the two are continuous.) *(Dissection by Grant Dahmer, Department of Cell Biology and Anatomy, University of Arizona College of Medicine.)*

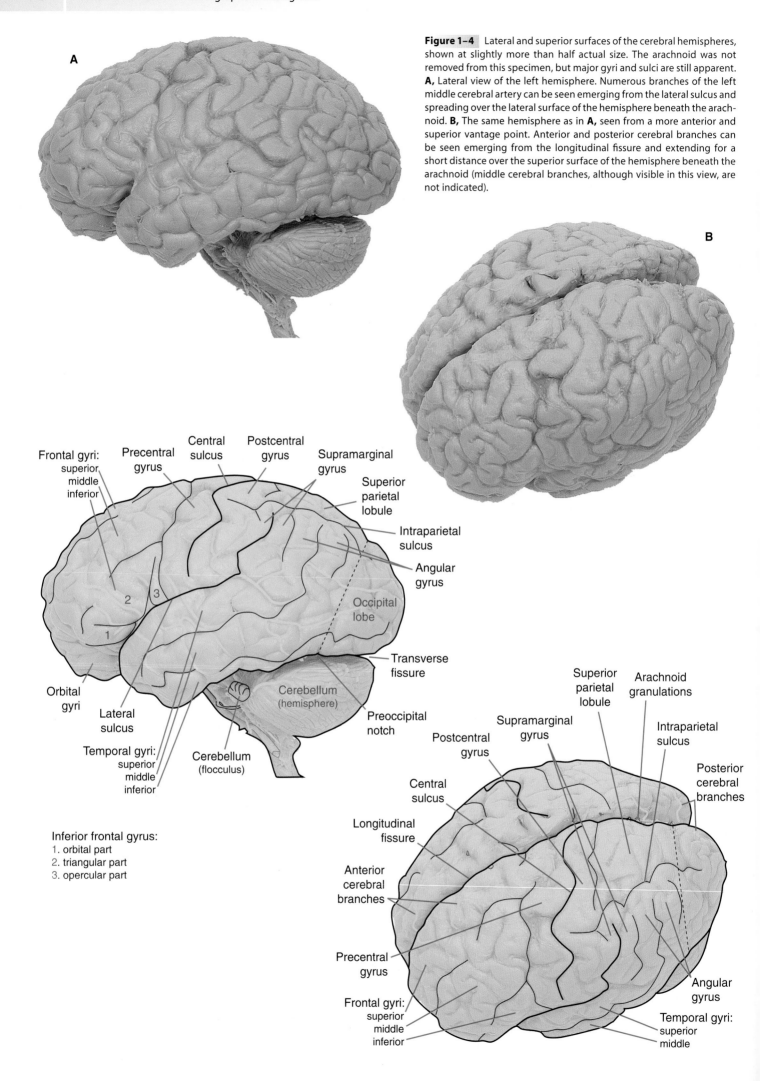

A

Figure 1-4 Lateral and superior surfaces of the cerebral hemispheres, shown at slightly more than half actual size. The arachnoid was not removed from this specimen, but major gyri and sulci are still apparent. **A,** Lateral view of the left hemisphere. Numerous branches of the left middle cerebral artery can be seen emerging from the lateral sulcus and spreading over the lateral surface of the hemisphere beneath the arachnoid. **B,** The same hemisphere as in **A,** seen from a more anterior and superior vantage point. Anterior and posterior cerebral branches can be seen emerging from the longitudinal fissure and extending for a short distance over the superior surface of the hemisphere beneath the arachnoid (middle cerebral branches, although visible in this view, are not indicated).

B

Frontal gyri:
superior
middle
inferior

Precentral gyrus

Central sulcus

Postcentral gyrus

Supramarginal gyrus

Superior parietal lobule

Intraparietal sulcus

Angular gyrus

Occipital lobe

Transverse fissure

Cerebellum (hemisphere)

Preoccipital notch

Orbital gyri

Lateral sulcus

Temporal gyri:
superior
middle
inferior

Cerebellum (flocculus)

Inferior frontal gyrus:
1. orbital part
2. triangular part
3. opercular part

Superior parietal lobule

Arachnoid granulations

Supramarginal gyrus

Intraparietal sulcus

Postcentral gyrus

Posterior cerebral branches

Central sulcus

Longitudinal fissure

Anterior cerebral branches

Precentral gyrus

Frontal gyri:
superior
middle
inferior

Angular gyrus

Temporal gyri:
superior
middle

C

Figure 1–4 (Continued)   **C,** Lateral view of the right hemisphere of the same brain shown in **A** and **B.** Numerous branches of the right middle cerebral artery can be seen emerging from the lateral sulcus and spreading over the lateral surface of the hemisphere beneath the arachnoid, and a few posterior cerebral branches emerge from the longitudinal fissure. Although the two cerebral hemispheres of human brains are approximately mirror images of each other, some slight asymmetries are common, particularly in certain language-related areas. Note in this specimen how much farther posteriorly the lateral sulcus extends in the left hemisphere **(A),** and how much larger the triangular part of the inferior frontal gyrus is on the left (see also Fig. 1–5). **D,** The same hemisphere as in **C,** seen from a more posterior and superior vantage point. Anterior and middle cerebral branches can be seen emerging from the longitudinal fissure and extending for a short distance over the superior surface of the hemisphere beneath the arachnoid (middle cerebral branches, although visible in this view, are not indicated). *(Dissection by Grant Dahmer, Department of Cell Biology and Anatomy, University of Arizona College of Medicine.)*

D

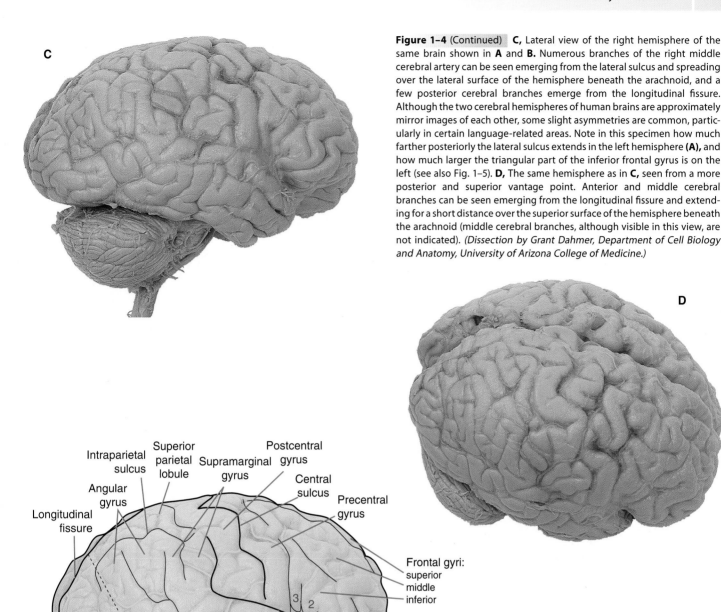

Inferior frontal gyrus:
1. orbital part
2. triangular part
3. opercular part

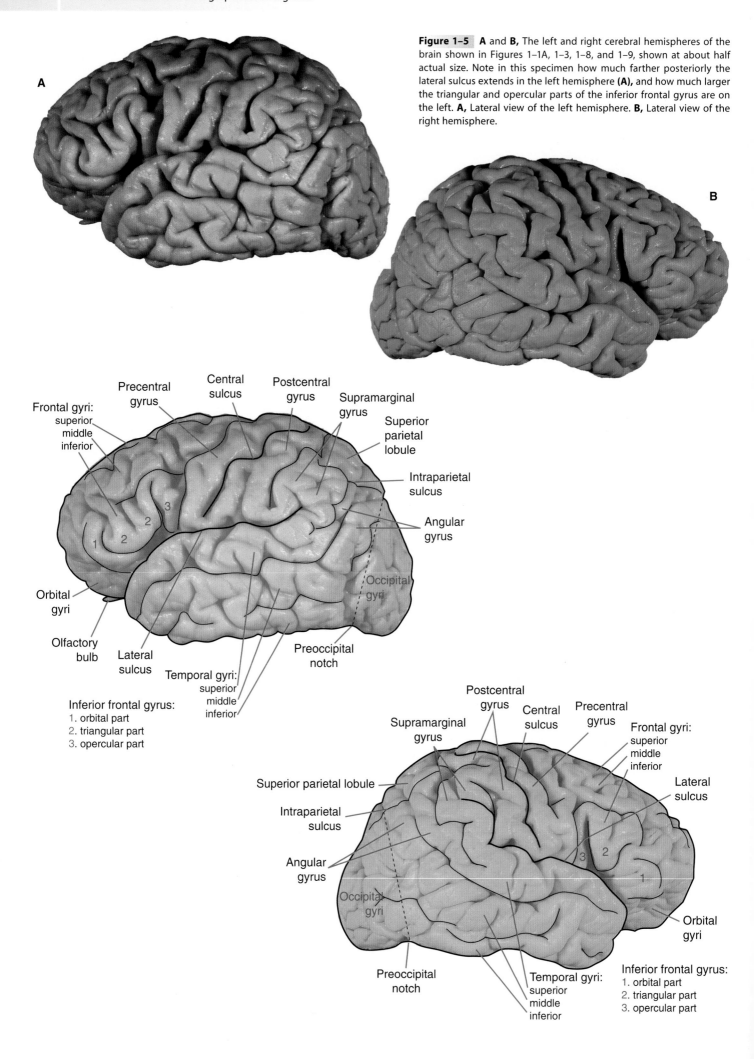

Figure 1-5 **A** and **B,** The left and right cerebral hemispheres of the brain shown in Figures 1-1A, 1-3, 1-8, and 1-9, shown at about half actual size. Note in this specimen how much farther posteriorly the lateral sulcus extends in the left hemisphere **(A),** and how much larger the triangular and opercular parts of the inferior frontal gyrus are on the left. **A,** Lateral view of the left hemisphere. **B,** Lateral view of the right hemisphere.

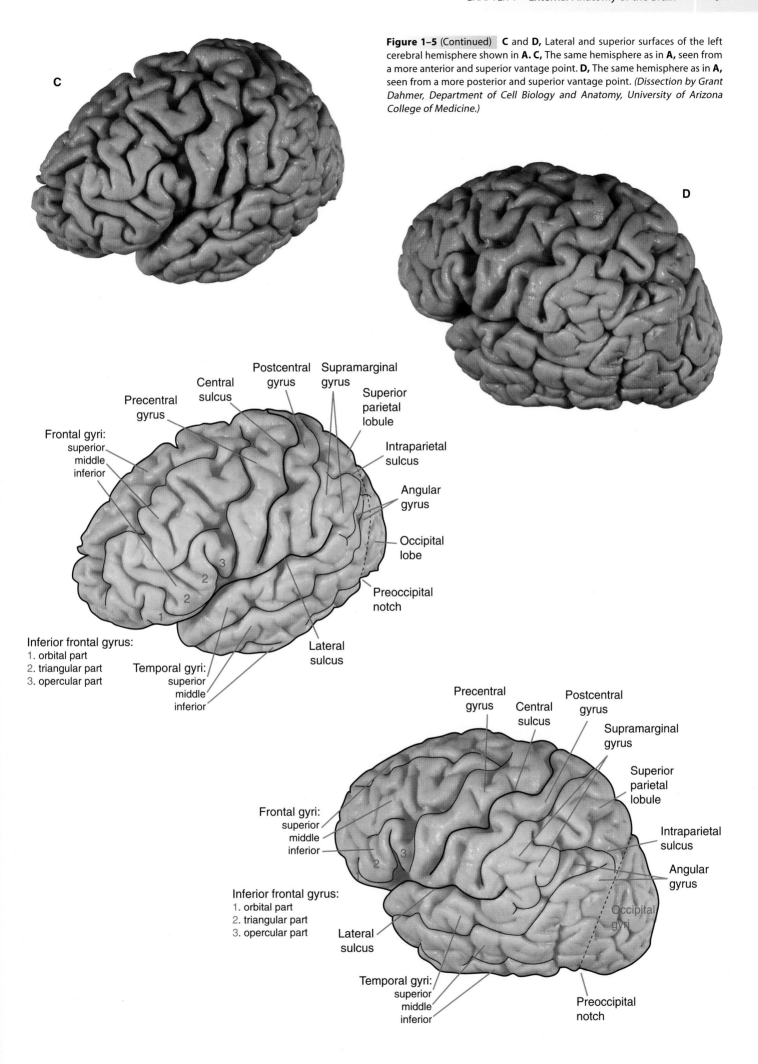

Figure 1–5 (Continued) **C** and **D,** Lateral and superior surfaces of the left cerebral hemisphere shown in **A. C,** The same hemisphere as in **A,** seen from a more anterior and superior vantage point. **D,** The same hemisphere as in **A,** seen from a more posterior and superior vantage point. *(Dissection by Grant Dahmer, Department of Cell Biology and Anatomy, University of Arizona College of Medicine.)*

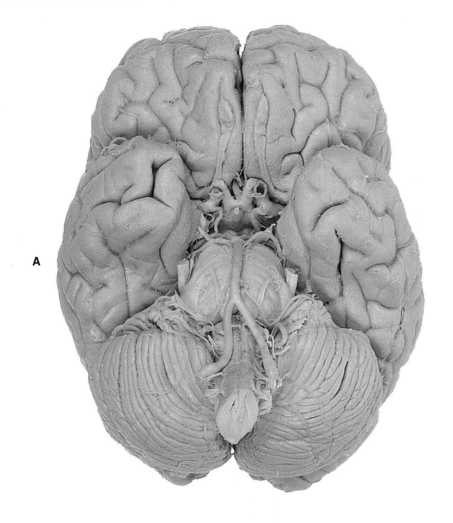

A

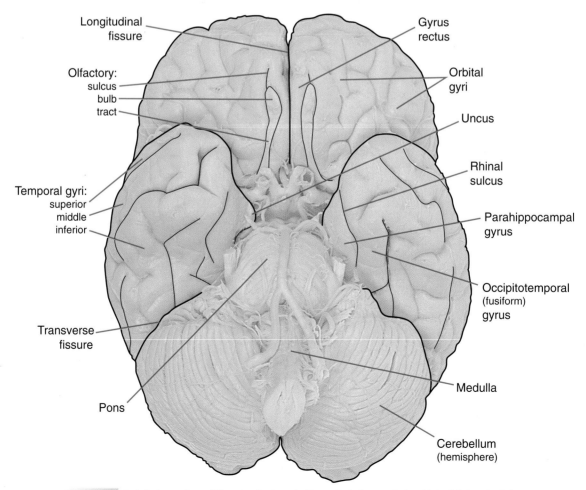

Longitudinal fissure

Gyrus rectus

Olfactory:
sulcus
bulb
tract

Orbital gyri

Uncus

Rhinal sulcus

Temporal gyri:
superior
middle
inferior

Parahippocampal gyrus

Occipitotemporal (fusiform) gyrus

Transverse fissure

Medulla

Pons

Cerebellum (hemisphere)

Figure 1–6   A, Inferior surface of the same brain as in Figure 1–4, shown at about two thirds actual size.

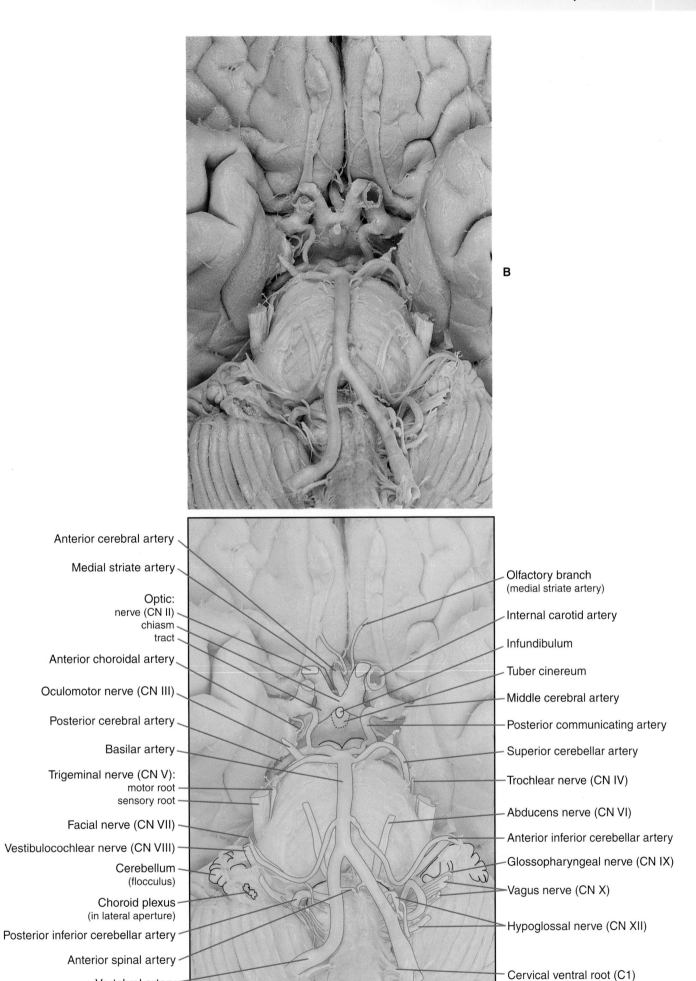

Anterior cerebral artery

Medial striate artery

Optic:
nerve (CN II)
chiasm
tract

Anterior choroidal artery

Oculomotor nerve (CN III)

Posterior cerebral artery

Basilar artery

Trigeminal nerve (CN V):
motor root
sensory root

Facial nerve (CN VII)

Vestibulocochlear nerve (CN VIII)

Cerebellum
(flocculus)

Choroid plexus
(in lateral aperture)

Posterior inferior cerebellar artery

Anterior spinal artery

Vertebral artery

Olfactory branch
(medial striate artery)

Internal carotid artery

Infundibulum

Tuber cinereum

Middle cerebral artery

Posterior communicating artery

Superior cerebellar artery

Trochlear nerve (CN IV)

Abducens nerve (CN VI)

Anterior inferior cerebellar artery

Glossopharyngeal nerve (CN IX)

Vagus nerve (CN X)

Hypoglossal nerve (CN XII)

Cervical ventral root (C1)

B

Figure 1–6 (Continued) **B,** The brainstem and the base of the forebrain, shown at about 1.2× actual size. (The large left posterior communicating artery is a commonly seen variant of the circle of Willis.) *(Dissection by Grant Dahmer, Department of Cell Biology and Anatomy, University of Arizona College of Medicine.)*

A

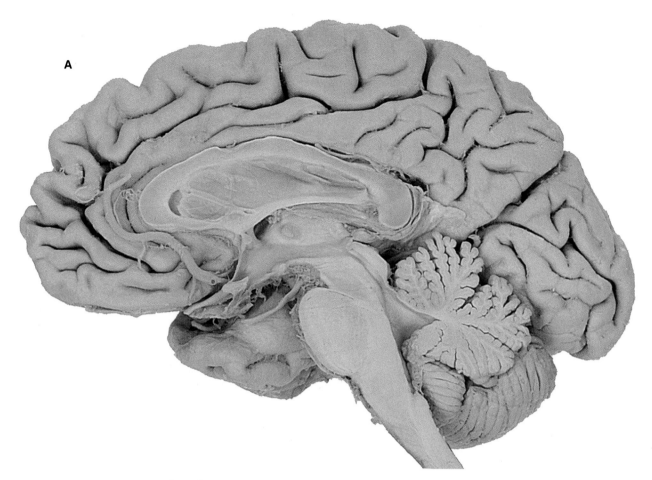

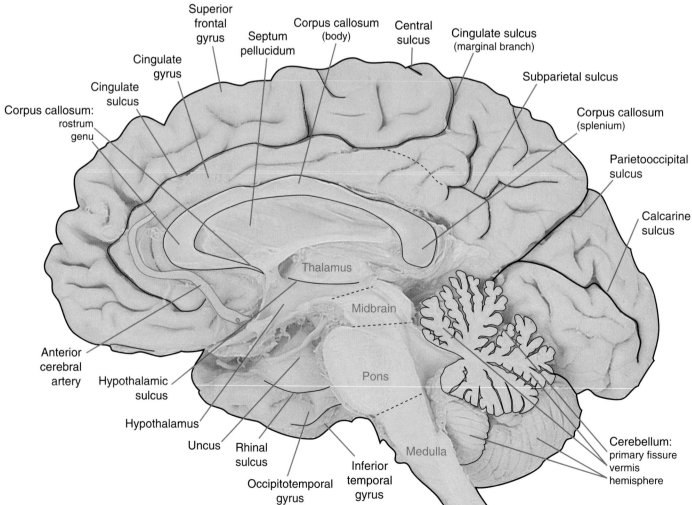

Figure 1–7   A, Medial surface of the right half of a sagittally hemisected brain, shown actual size. The *dashed line* interconnecting the cingulate and subparietal sulci is meant to indicate that in some brains these two sulci are continuous.

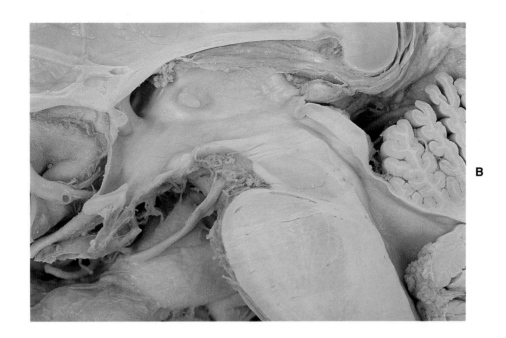

B

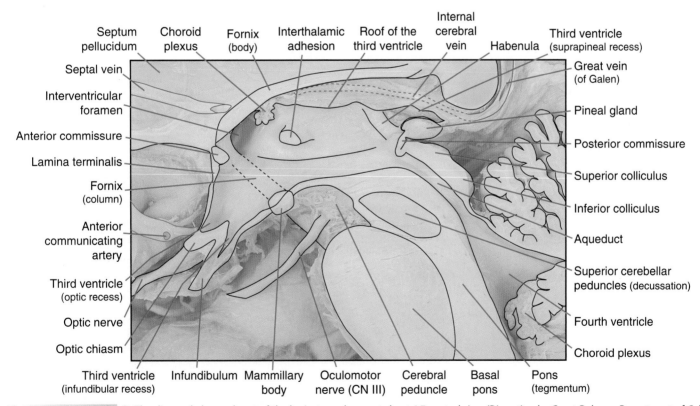

Figure 1–7 (Continued)   **B,** The diencephalon and part of the brainstem, shown at about 1.7× actual size. *(Dissection by Grant Dahmer, Department of Cell Biology and Anatomy, University of Arizona College of Medicine.)*

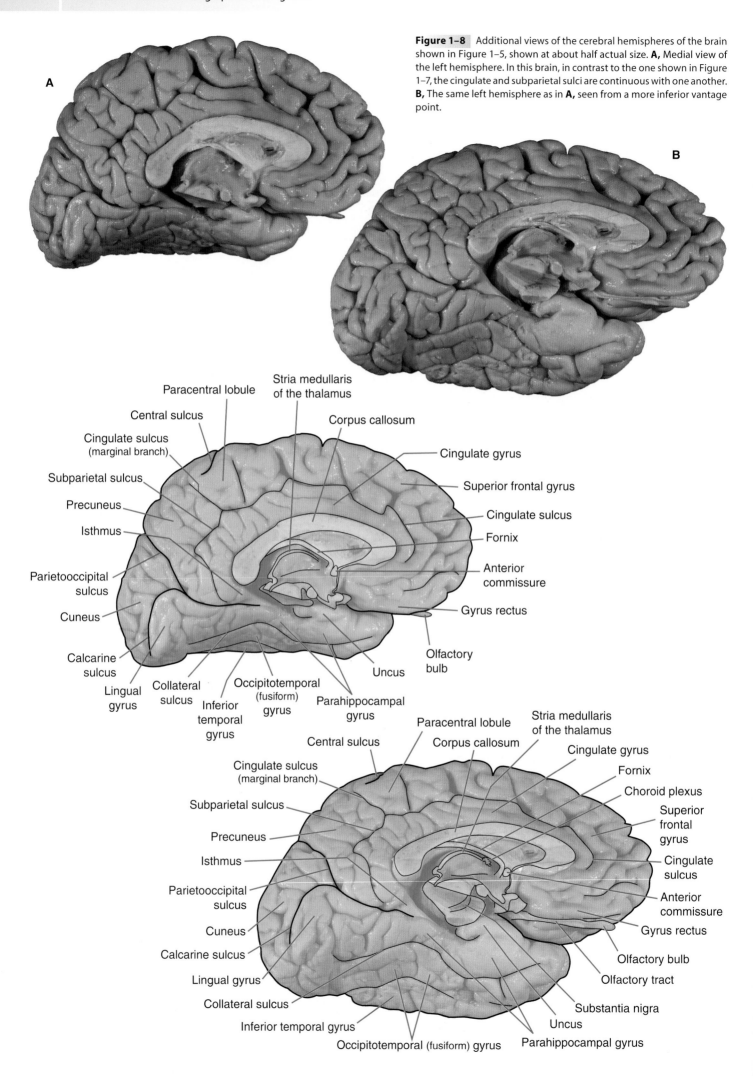

Figure 1–8 Additional views of the cerebral hemispheres of the brain shown in Figure 1–5, shown at about half actual size. **A,** Medial view of the left hemisphere. In this brain, in contrast to the one shown in Figure 1–7, the cingulate and subparietal sulci are continuous with one another. **B,** The same left hemisphere as in **A,** seen from a more inferior vantage point.

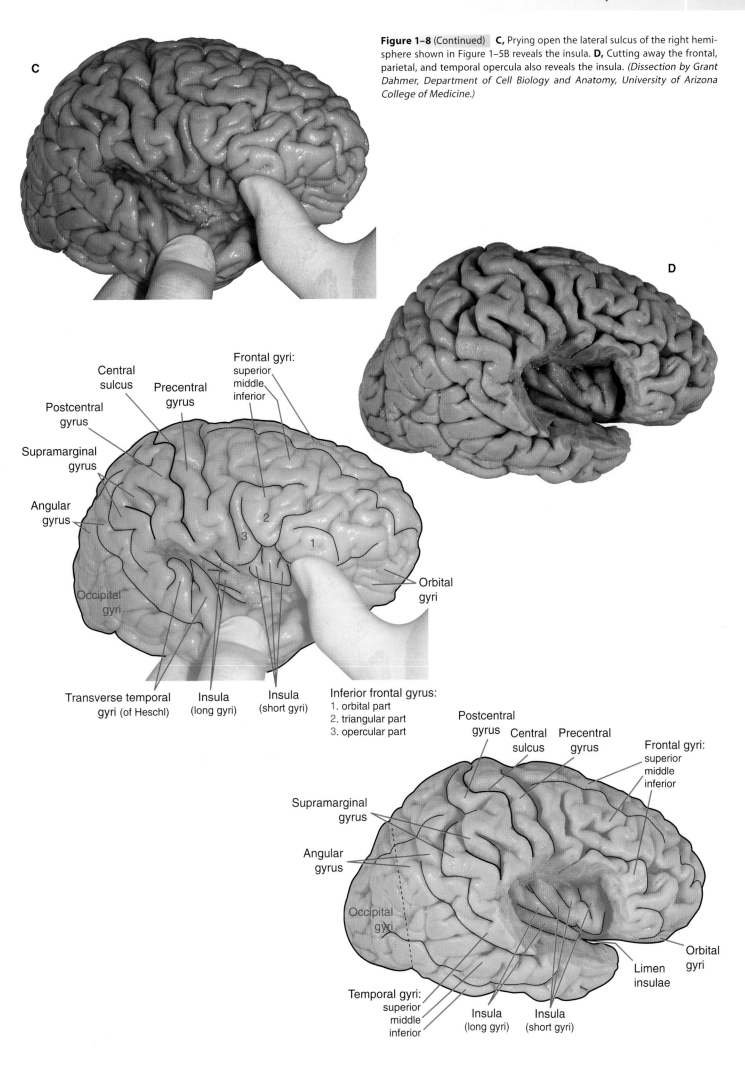

Figure 1–8 (Continued)   **C,** Prying open the lateral sulcus of the right hemisphere shown in Figure 1–5B reveals the insula. **D,** Cutting away the frontal, parietal, and temporal opercula also reveals the insula. *(Dissection by Grant Dahmer, Department of Cell Biology and Anatomy, University of Arizona College of Medicine.)*

C

D

Central sulcus
Precentral gyrus
Frontal gyri:
superior
middle
inferior
Postcentral gyrus
Supramarginal gyrus
Angular gyrus
Occipital gyri
2
3
1
Orbital gyri
Transverse temporal gyri (of Heschl)
Insula (long gyri)
Insula (short gyri)
Inferior frontal gyrus:
1. orbital part
2. triangular part
3. opercular part

Postcentral gyrus
Central sulcus
Precentral gyrus
Frontal gyri:
superior
middle
inferior
Supramarginal gyrus
Angular gyrus
Occipital gyri
Orbital gyri
Limen insulae
Temporal gyri:
superior
middle
inferior
Insula (long gyri)
Insula (short gyri)

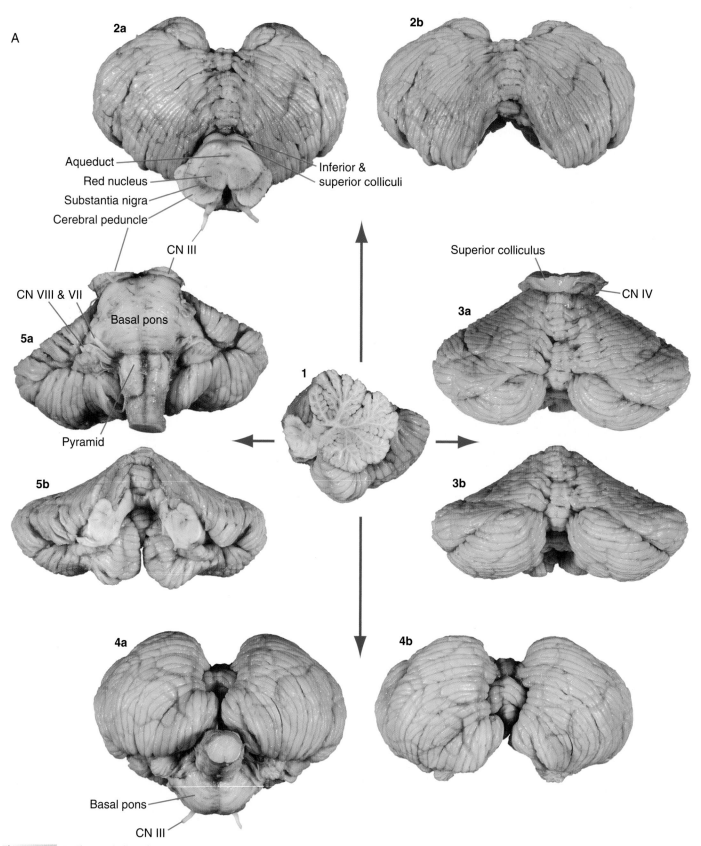

Figure 1–9 A, The cerebellum from the same brain as in Figure 1–3, shown at about 0.6× actual size. Views of the superior *(2)*, posterior *(3)*, inferior *(4)*, and anterior *(5)* surfaces are shown, before and after the brainstem was removed.

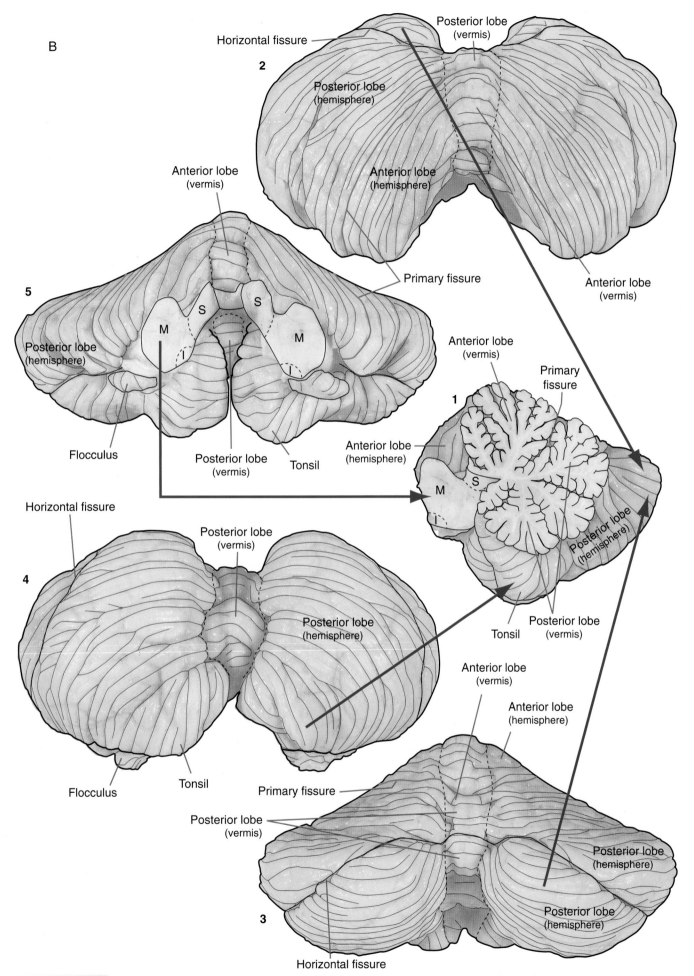

Figure 1–9 (Continued)   **B,** Major structures of the same cerebellum, shown actual size. *I, M,* and *S* indicate the inferior, middle, and superior cerebellar peduncles. *(Dissection by Grant Dahmer, Department of Cell Biology and Anatomy, University of Arizona College of Medicine.)*

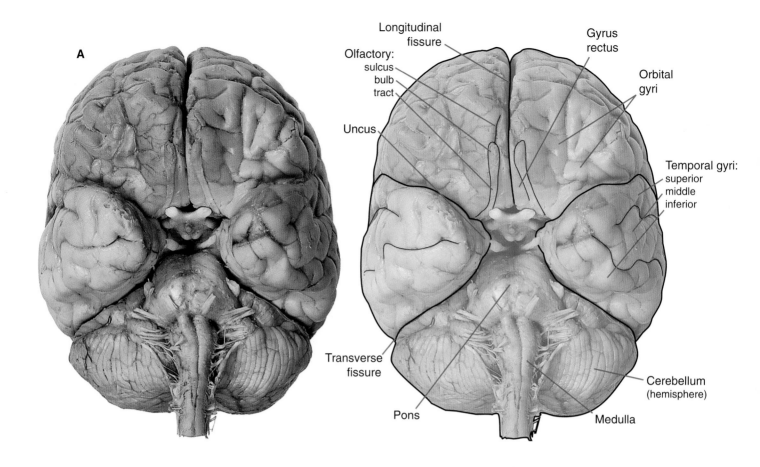

A

Longitudinal fissure

Olfactory:
sulcus
bulb
tract

Uncus

Transverse fissure

Pons

Gyrus rectus

Orbital gyri

Temporal gyri:
superior
middle
inferior

Cerebellum (hemisphere)

Medulla

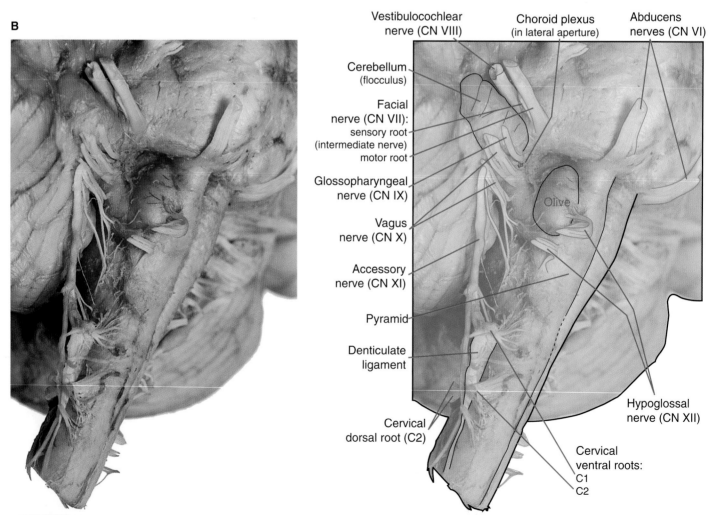

B

Vestibulocochlear nerve (CN VIII)

Cerebellum (flocculus)

Facial nerve (CN VII):
sensory root (intermediate nerve)
motor root

Glossopharyngeal nerve (CN IX)

Vagus nerve (CN X)

Accessory nerve (CN XI)

Pyramid

Denticulate ligament

Cervical dorsal root (C2)

Choroid plexus (in lateral aperture)

Abducens nerves (CN VI)

Olive

Hypoglossal nerve (CN XII)

Cervical ventral roots:
C1
C2

Figure 1–10 Inferior and lateral views of the cerebrum and brainstem, demonstrating the cranial nerves. **A,** Inferior view, shown at about two thirds actual size. **B,** Lateral and inferior view, shown at about 2.7× actual size.

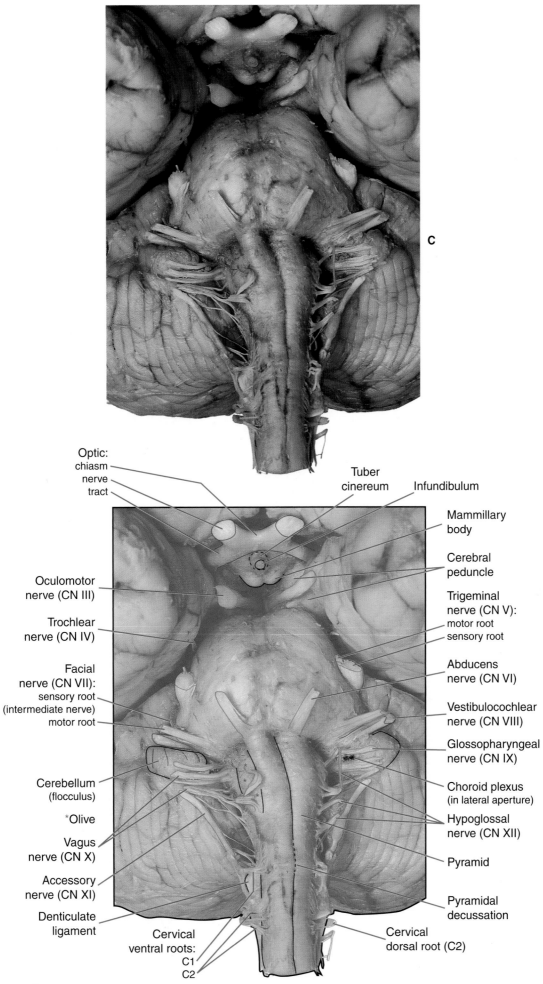

C

Optic:
chiasm
nerve
tract

Tuber
cinereum

Infundibulum

Mammillary
body

Cerebral
peduncle

Oculomotor
nerve (CN III)

Trigeminal
nerve (CN V):
motor root
sensory root

Trochlear
nerve (CN IV)

Abducens
nerve (CN VI)

Facial
nerve (CN VII):
sensory root
(intermediate nerve)
motor root

Vestibulocochlear
nerve (CN VIII)

Glossopharyngeal
nerve (CN IX)

Cerebellum
(flocculus)

Choroid plexus
(in lateral aperture)

*Olive

Hypoglossal
nerve (CN XII)

Vagus
nerve (CN X)

Pyramid

Accessory
nerve (CN XI)

Pyramidal
decussation

Denticulate
ligament

Cervical
ventral roots:
C1
C2

Cervical
dorsal root (C2)

Figure 1–10 (Continued)   **C,** Inferior view, shown at about 1.4× actual size. *(Dissection by Dr. Norman Koelling, Department of Cell Biology and Anatomy, University of Arizona College of Medicine.)*

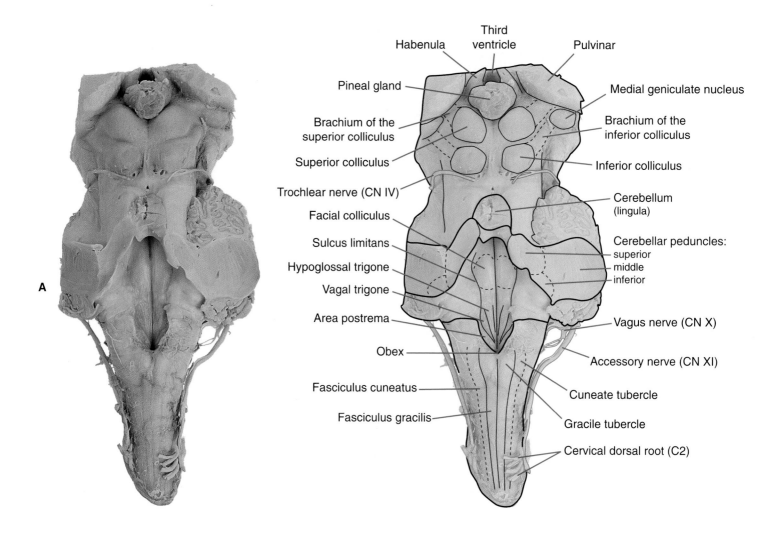

Third
ventricle
Habenula
Pulvinar

Pineal gland
Medial geniculate nucleus

Brachium of the
superior colliculus
Brachium of the
inferior colliculus

Superior colliculus
Inferior colliculus

Trochlear nerve (CN IV)
Cerebellum
(lingula)

Facial colliculus
Cerebellar peduncles:
superior
middle
inferior

Sulcus limitans

Hypoglossal trigone

Vagal trigone

Area postrema
Vagus nerve (CN X)

Obex
Accessory nerve (CN XI)

Fasciculus cuneatus
Cuneate tubercle

Fasciculus gracilis
Gracile tubercle

Cervical dorsal root (C2)

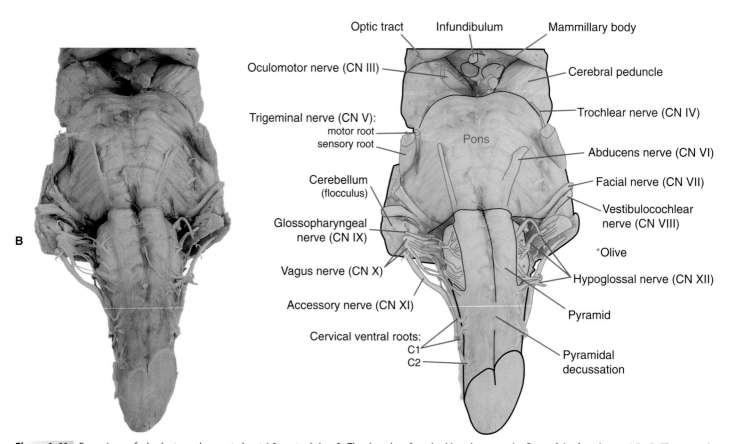

Optic tract   Infundibulum   Mammillary body

Oculomotor nerve (CN III)
Cerebral peduncle

Trigeminal nerve (CN V):
Trochlear nerve (CN IV)
motor root
sensory root   Pons
Abducens nerve (CN VI)

Facial nerve (CN VII)

Cerebellum
(flocculus)
Vestibulocochlear
nerve (CN VIII)

Glossopharyngeal
nerve (CN IX)
*Olive

Vagus nerve (CN X)
Hypoglossal nerve (CN XII)

Accessory nerve (CN XI)
Pyramid

Cervical ventral roots:
C1
C2
Pyramidal
decussation

Figure 1–11   Four views of a brainstem, shown at about 1.3× actual size. **A,** The dorsal surface, looking down on the floor of the fourth ventricle. **B,** The ventral surface.

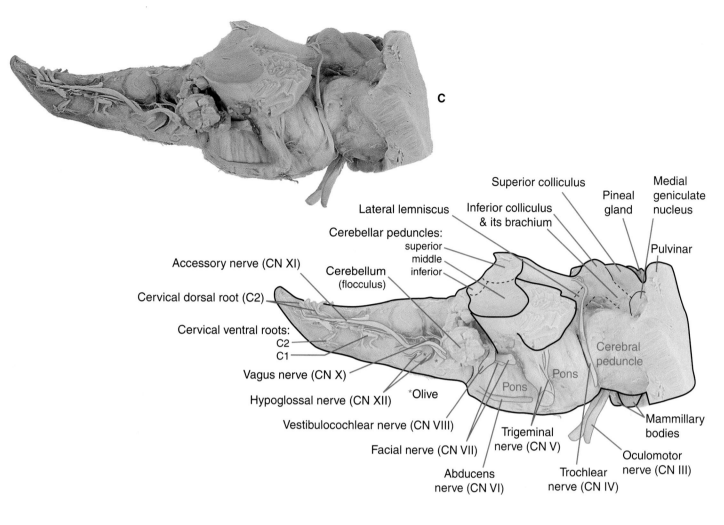

C

Superior colliculus
Medial geniculate nucleus
Pineal gland
Lateral lemniscus
Inferior colliculus & its brachium
Cerebellar peduncles:
superior
middle
inferior
Pulvinar
Accessory nerve (CN XI)
Cerebellum (flocculus)
Cervical dorsal root (C2)
Cervical ventral roots:
C2
C1
Cerebral peduncle
Vagus nerve (CN X)
Hypoglossal nerve (CN XII)
Pons
Pons
*Olive
Pons
Mammillary bodies
Vestibulocochlear nerve (CN VIII)
Trigeminal nerve (CN V)
Oculomotor nerve (CN III)
Facial nerve (CN VII)
Abducens nerve (CN VI)
Trochlear nerve (CN IV)

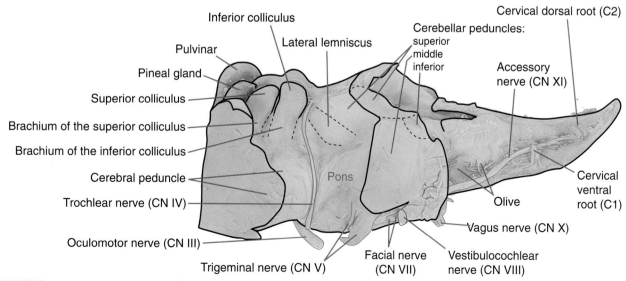

D

Cervical dorsal root (C2)
Inferior colliculus
Cerebellar peduncles:
superior
middle
inferior
Accessory nerve (CN XI)
Pulvinar
Lateral lemniscus
Pineal gland
Superior colliculus
Brachium of the superior colliculus
Brachium of the inferior colliculus
Cerebral peduncle
Pons
Cervical ventral root (C1)
Trochlear nerve (CN IV)
Olive
Oculomotor nerve (CN III)
Vagus nerve (CN X)
Trigeminal nerve (CN V)
Facial nerve (CN VII)
Vestibulocochlear nerve (CN VIII)

Figure 1–11 (Continued)   Four views of a brainstem. **C,** Right side. **D,** Left side. *(Dissection by Grant Dahmer, Department of Anatomy, University of Arizona College of Medicine.)*

Transverse Sections of the Spinal Cord

The spinal cord is perhaps the most simply arranged part of the CNS. Its basic structure, indicated in a schematic drawing of the eighth cervical segment (Figure 2–1), is the same at every level—a butterfly-shaped core of gray matter surrounded by white matter. An often indistinct central canal in the middle of the butterfly is the remnant of the lumen of the embryonic neural tube.

The extensions of the gray matter posteriorly and anteriorly are termed the posterior and anterior (dorsal and ventral) horns. The zone where the two horns meet is the intermediate gray. At every level, the posterior horn is capped by a zone of closely packed small neurons, the substantia gelatinosa. Beyond this, there are level-to-level variations in the configuration of the spinal gray (Figure 2–2). For example, the motor neurons that innervate skeletal muscle are located in the anterior horns, so these horns expand laterally in lumbar and lower cervical segments to accommodate the many motor neurons required for the muscles of the lower and upper extremities. Other examples are indicated in Figure 2–2. When studied in detail, the spinal gray matter can be partitioned into a series of 10 layers (Rexed's laminae), as indicated on the right side of Figure 2–1. Some of these laminae have clear functional significance. For example, lamina II corresponds to the substantia gelatinosa, which plays an important role in regulating painful and thermal sensations.

Spinal white matter contains pathways ascending to or descending from higher levels of the nervous system, as well as nerve fibers interconnecting different levels of the spinal cord. The horns of the gray matter divide the white matter into posterior, lateral, and anterior funiculi. In contrast to the level-to-level variations in the gray matter, the total amount of white matter increases steadily at progressively higher spinal levels. Moving rostrally, the ascending pathways enlarge as progressively more fibers are added to them; the descending pathways do the same because fewer fibers have left them.

Information travels to and from the spinal gray matter in the dorsal and ventral roots. The dorsal roots convey the central processes of afferents with cell bodies in dorsal root ganglia. As the roots approach the spinal cord, they break up into filaments, each of which sorts itself into a medial division, containing the large-diameter afferents, and a lateral division, containing the small-diameter afferents. This is the beginning of two great streams of somatosensory information that travel rostrally in the CNS. The large fibers, primarily carrying information about touch and position, send branches into multiple levels of the gray matter and may send a branch rostrally in the posterior funiculus. The small fibers, primarily carrying information about pain and temperature, traverse a distinctive area of the white matter (Lissauer's tract) and end more superficially in the posterior horn. Subsequent connections of both classes of afferents are reviewed in Chapter 8.

In this chapter (as in all chapters in this atlas), only the largest and best-known spinal structures and pathways are indicated. Many others are either known to exist in humans or inferred from animal studies. In many cases, however, their functional significance is not well understood.

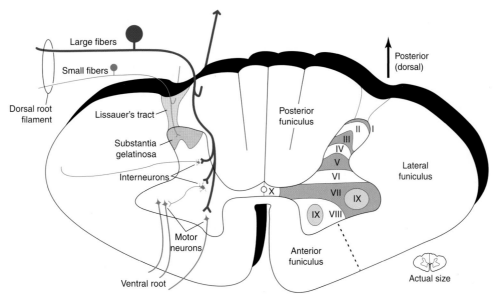

Figure 2–1 Schematic drawing of the spinal cord at the level of the eighth cervical segment. *(Modified from Nolte J: The human brain, ed 5, St. Louis, 2002, Mosby.)*

Figure 2-2   A–H, Cross sections of a spinal cord at eight different levels.

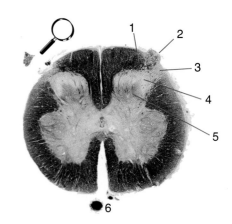

A, The fourth sacral segment (S4). Several features common to all spinal levels can be seen. The substantia gelatinosa (4) caps the posterior horn (5). Also, afferent fibers entering through dorsal rootlets (2) sort themselves into small-diameter fibers that move laterally and enter Lissauer's tract (3) and large-diameter fibers that enter more medially (1) at the edge of the posterior funiculus. (This sorting occurs at all spinal levels and can be seen in all of the sections in this series.) Little white matter is present in any of the funiculi because most fibers either have already left descending pathways or have not yet entered ascending pathways. The anterior spinal artery (6) is cut in cross section as it runs longitudinally near the anterior median fissure of the cord. Shown enlarged in Figure 2–3.

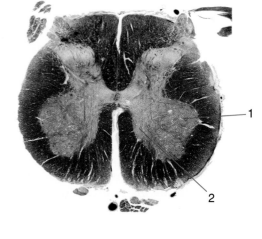

B, The fifth lumbar segment (L5). This segment is in the lumbar enlargement (which extends from about L2 to S3) and has anterior horns that are enlarged, primarily in their lateral aspects (1), to accommodate motor neurons for leg and foot muscles. Motor neurons located more medially (2) in the anterior horn innervate more proximal muscles, in this case hip muscles.

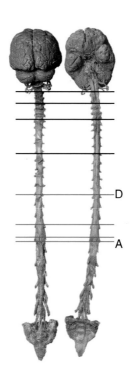

C, The second lumbar segment (L2). The posterior funiculus (1) is larger because ascending fibers carrying touch and position information from the lower limb have been added. The lateral funiculus is also larger, reflecting increased numbers of descending fibers in the lateral corticospinal tract (2) and ascending fibers in the spinothalamic tract (4). This section is at the rostral end of the lumbar enlargement, so the anterior horn (5) no longer is enlarged laterally. Clarke's nucleus (3), which extends from about T1 to L3 and contains the cells of origin of the posterior spinocerebellar tract, makes its appearance. The anterior white commissure (6), a route through which axons can cross the midline, is present at this and all other spinal levels. Shown enlarged in Figure 2–4.

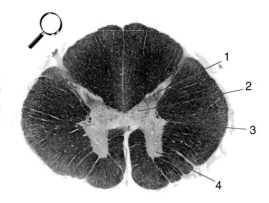

D, The tenth thoracic segment (T10). The posterior (1) and anterior (4) horns are slender, corresponding to the relative dearth of sensory information arriving at this level and the relatively small number of motor neurons needed. Sympathetic preganglionic neurons form a lateral horn (3) containing the intermediolateral cell column, a characteristic feature of thoracic segments. Clarke's nucleus (2) is still apparent. Shown enlarged in Figure 2–5.

Figure 2–2 (Continued)   Cross sections of a spinal cord.

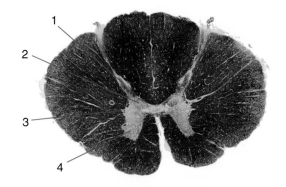

E, The fifth thoracic segment (T5). The posterior *(1)* and anterior *(4)* horns are even more slender, reflecting the relative paucity of sensory information arriving from the trunk and the relatively small number of motor neurons required by trunk muscles. Clarke's nucleus *(2),* although smaller, is still present, as is the lateral horn *(3).*

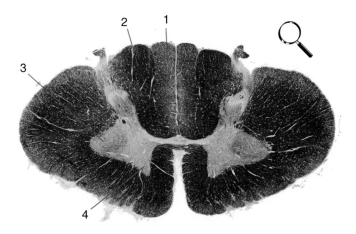

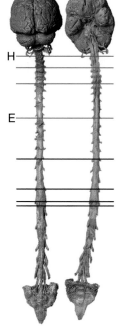

F, The eighth cervical segment (C8), near the caudal end of the cervical enlargement (C5 to T1). The posterior funiculus is subdivided by a partial glial partition into fasciculus gracilis *(1),* conveying touch and position information from the lower limb, and fasciculus cuneatus *(2),* conveying touch and position information from the upper limb. The anterior horn is enlarged, primarily in its lateral aspect *(3),* to accommodate motor neurons for hand and forearm muscles. Motor neurons in more medial parts of the anterior horn *(4)* innervate more proximal muscles, such as the triceps. Shown enlarged in Figure 2–6.

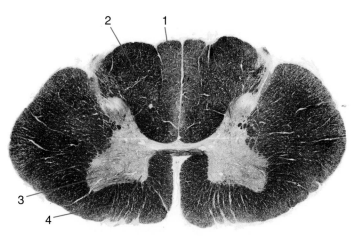

G, The fifth cervical segment (C5), still in the cervical enlargement. As in the previous section, the posterior funiculus is subdivided into fasciculus gracilis *(1)* and fasciculus cuneatus *(2),* and the anterior horn includes an expanded lateral region *(3)* (here containing motor neurons for forearm muscles) and the more medial area *(4)* that is present at all spinal levels (and at this level innervates shoulder muscles).

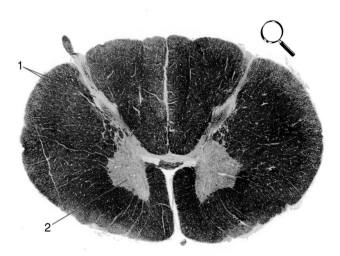

H, The third cervical segment (C3), rostral to the cervical enlargement. The posterior horn *(1)* is more slender, reflecting the smaller amount of afferent input arriving from the neck. The anterior horn *(2)* is no longer enlarged laterally. The area of white matter is larger, however, than in any other section in this series, reflecting the near-maximal size of ascending and descending pathways. Shown enlarged in Figure 2–7.

Figure 2–3   Fourth sacral segment (S4).

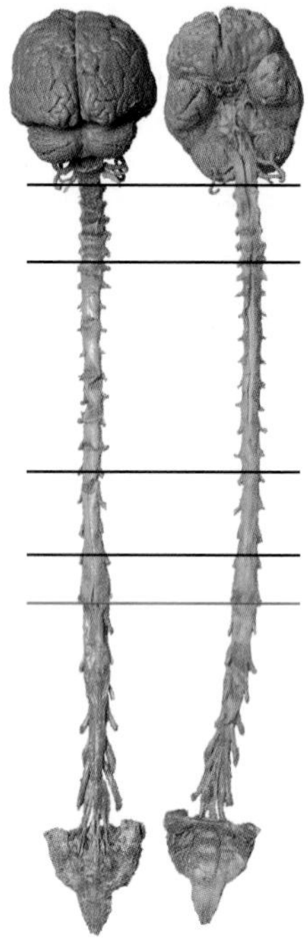

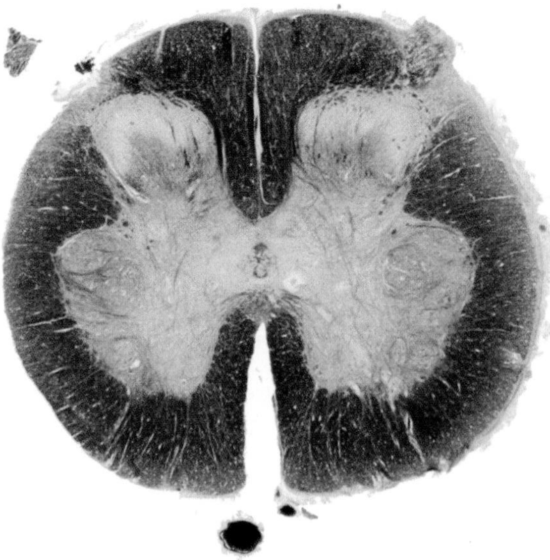

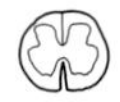

Actual Size

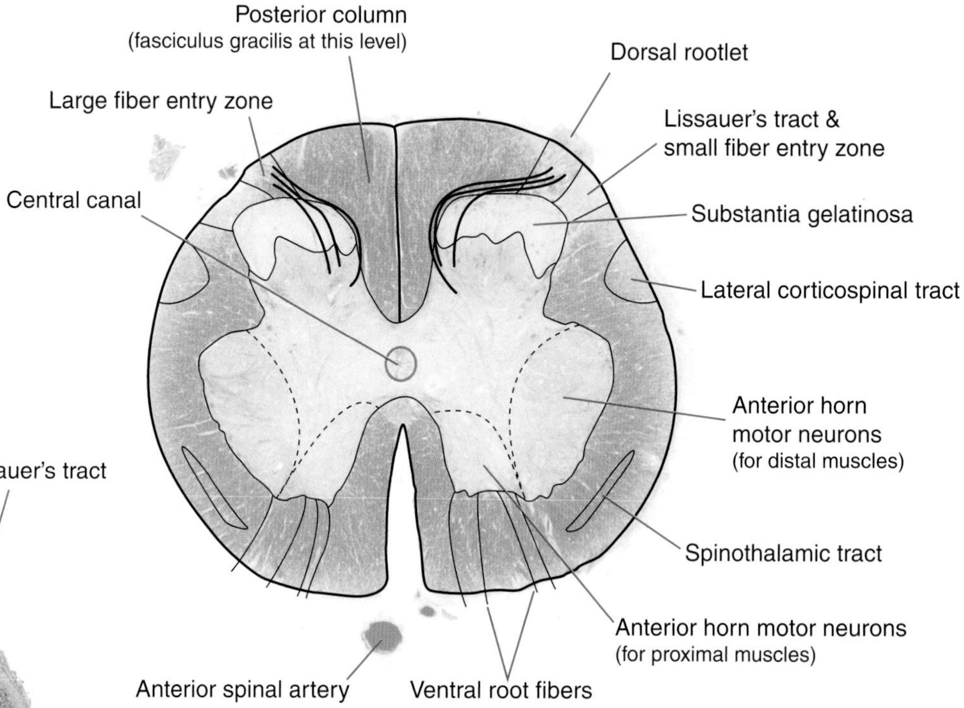

Posterior column
(fasciculus gracilis at this level)

Large fiber entry zone

Central canal

Dorsal rootlet

Lissauer's tract &
small fiber entry zone

Substantia gelatinosa

Lateral corticospinal tract

Anterior horn
motor neurons
(for distal muscles)

Spinothalamic tract

Anterior horn motor neurons
(for proximal muscles)

Anterior spinal artery

Ventral root fibers

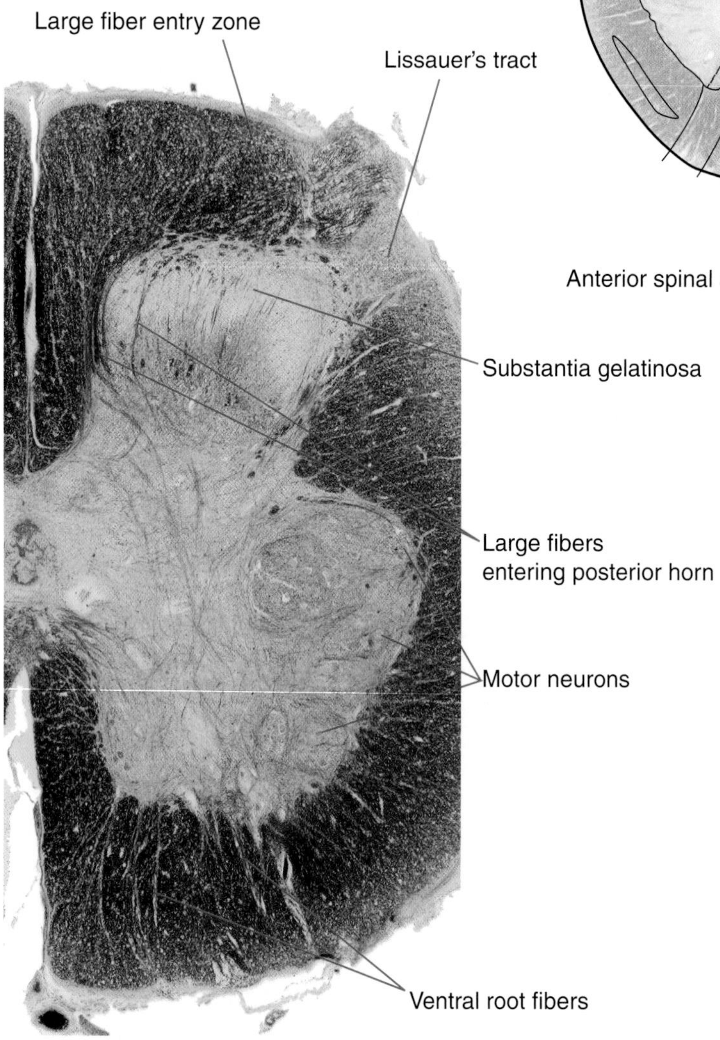

Large fiber entry zone

Lissauer's tract

Substantia gelatinosa

Large fibers
entering posterior horn

Motor neurons

Ventral root fibers

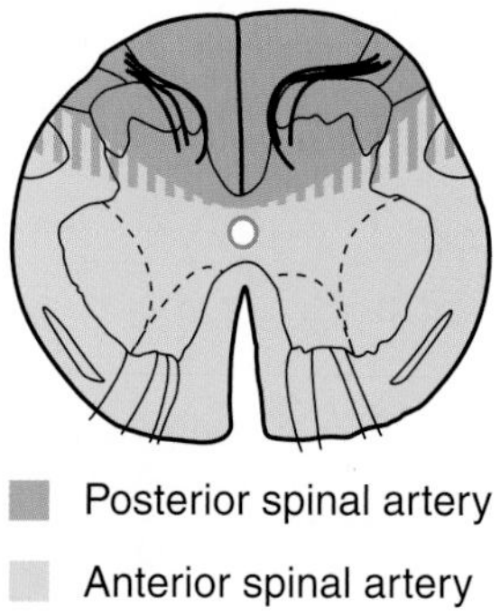

Posterior spinal artery

Anterior spinal artery

Figure 2–4   Second lumbar segment (L2).

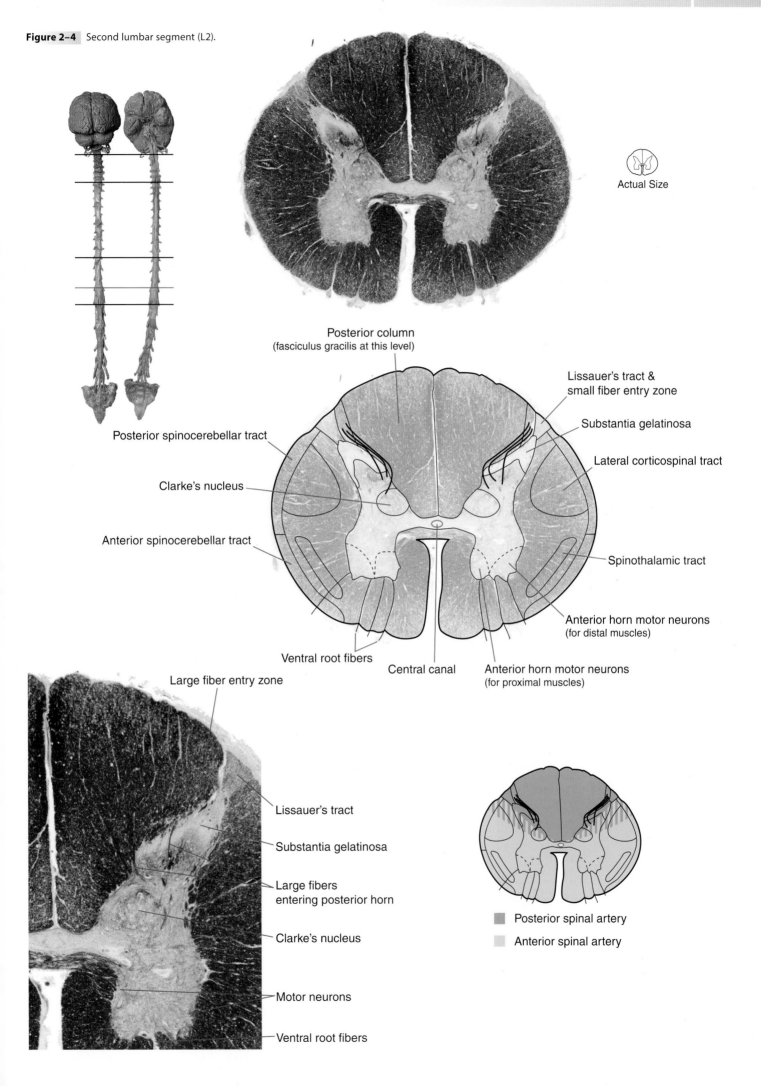

Actual Size

Posterior column
(fasciculus gracilis at this level)

Lissauer's tract &
small fiber entry zone

Substantia gelatinosa

Lateral corticospinal tract

Posterior spinocerebellar tract

Clarke's nucleus

Anterior spinocerebellar tract

Spinothalamic tract

Anterior horn motor neurons
(for distal muscles)

Ventral root fibers

Central canal

Anterior horn motor neurons
(for proximal muscles)

Large fiber entry zone

Lissauer's tract

Substantia gelatinosa

Large fibers
entering posterior horn

Clarke's nucleus

Motor neurons

Ventral root fibers

Posterior spinal artery

Anterior spinal artery

Figure 2–5   Tenth thoracic segment (T10).

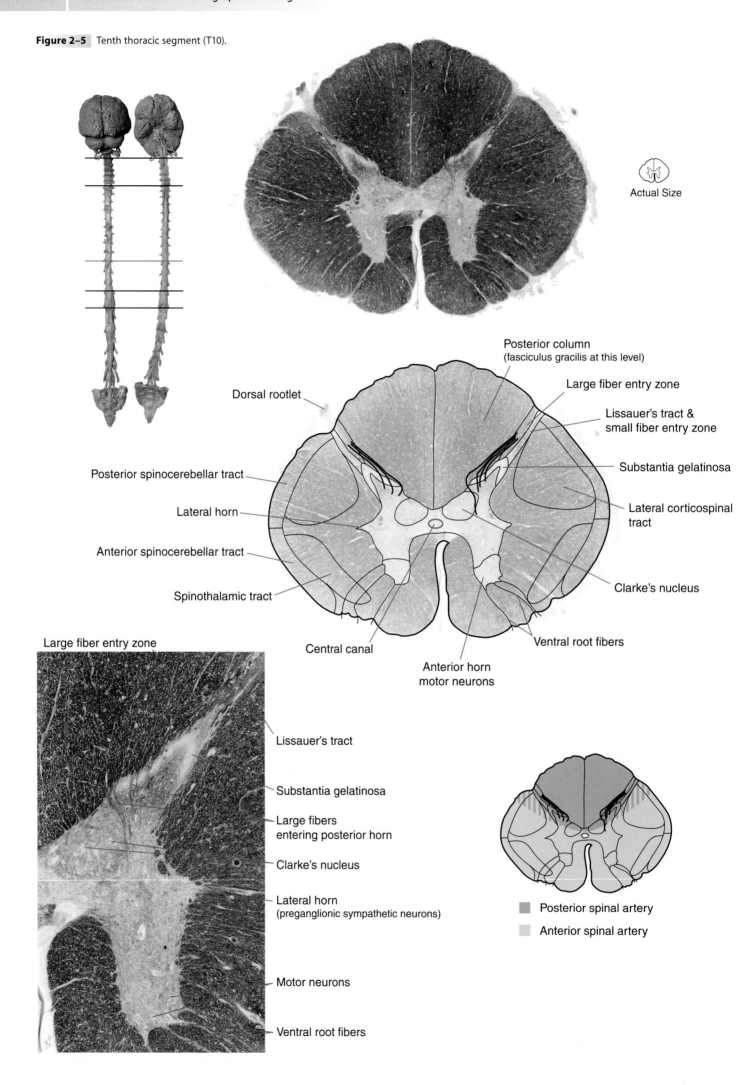

Actual Size

Posterior column
(fasciculus gracilis at this level)

Dorsal rootlet

Large fiber entry zone

Lissauer's tract &
small fiber entry zone

Posterior spinocerebellar tract

Substantia gelatinosa

Lateral horn

Lateral corticospinal
tract

Anterior spinocerebellar tract

Clarke's nucleus

Spinothalamic tract

Ventral root fibers

Central canal

Anterior horn
motor neurons

Large fiber entry zone

Lissauer's tract

Substantia gelatinosa

Large fibers
entering posterior horn

Clarke's nucleus

Lateral horn
(preganglionic sympathetic neurons)

Motor neurons

Ventral root fibers

Posterior spinal artery

Anterior spinal artery

Figure 2-6   Eighth cervical segment (C8).

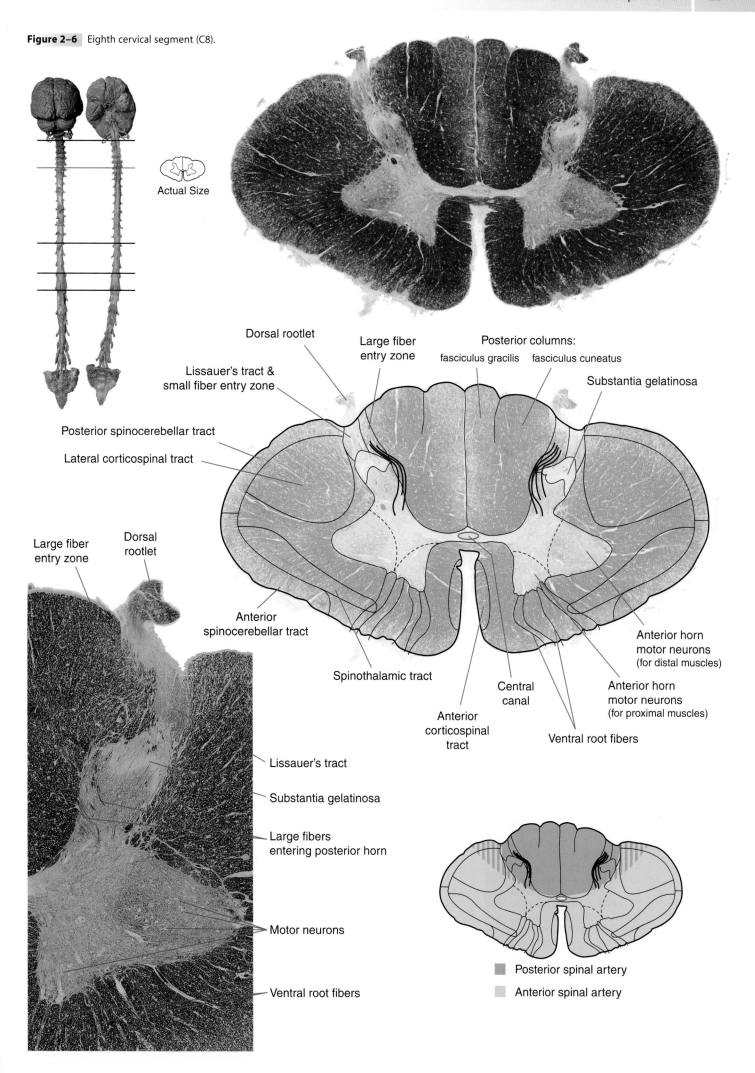

Actual Size

Dorsal rootlet

Large fiber entry zone

Posterior columns:
fasciculus gracilis   fasciculus cuneatus

Lissauer's tract & small fiber entry zone

Substantia gelatinosa

Posterior spinocerebellar tract

Lateral corticospinal tract

Large fiber entry zone

Dorsal rootlet

Anterior spinocerebellar tract

Anterior horn motor neurons (for distal muscles)

Spinothalamic tract

Central canal

Anterior horn motor neurons (for proximal muscles)

Anterior corticospinal tract

Ventral root fibers

Lissauer's tract

Substantia gelatinosa

Large fibers entering posterior horn

Motor neurons

Ventral root fibers

Posterior spinal artery

Anterior spinal artery

Figure 2–7 Third cervical segment (C3).

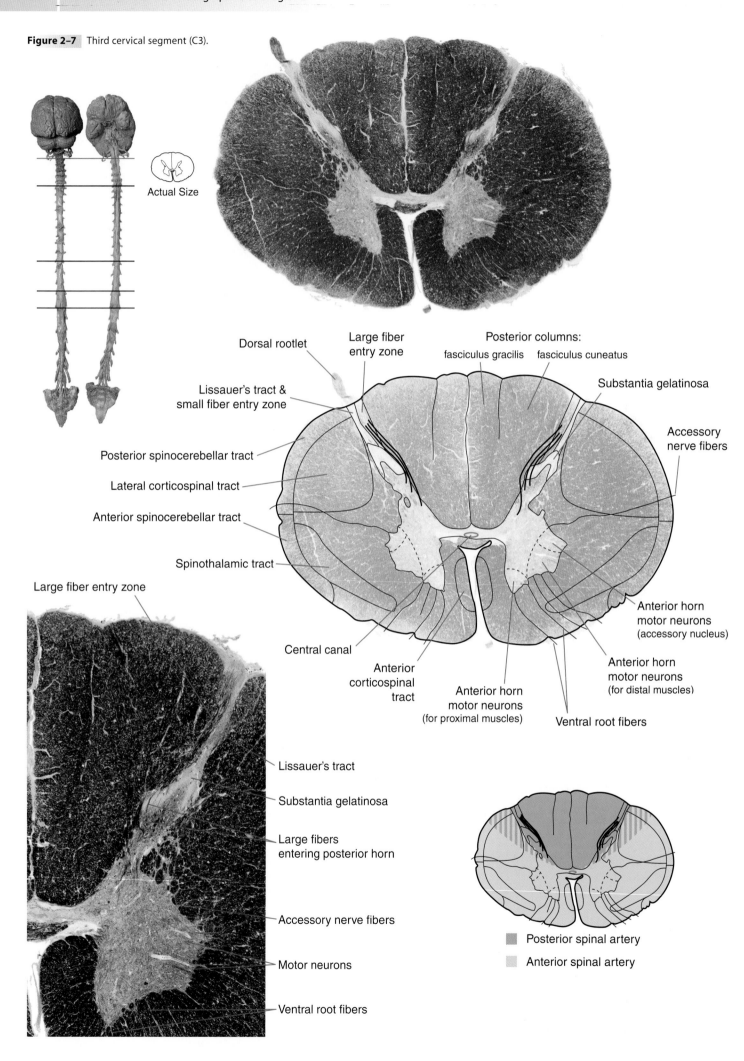

Actual Size

Dorsal rootlet

Large fiber entry zone

Posterior columns: fasciculus gracilis   fasciculus cuneatus

Lissauer's tract & small fiber entry zone

Substantia gelatinosa

Posterior spinocerebellar tract

Accessory nerve fibers

Lateral corticospinal tract

Anterior spinocerebellar tract

Spinothalamic tract

Large fiber entry zone

Anterior horn motor neurons (accessory nucleus)

Central canal

Anterior corticospinal tract

Anterior horn motor neurons (for distal muscles)

Anterior horn motor neurons (for proximal muscles)

Ventral root fibers

Lissauer's tract

Substantia gelatinosa

Large fibers entering posterior horn

Accessory nerve fibers

Motor neurons

Ventral root fibers

Posterior spinal artery

Anterior spinal artery

3

Transverse Sections of the Brainstem

The brainstem contains the continuations of the long tracts seen in the spinal cord, together with nuclei and tracts associated with cranial nerves and the cerebellum. These various tracts and nuclei surround, traverse, or are embedded in the reticular formation (named for its anatomical appearance—the Latin word *reticulum* means "network"), which forms a central core at all brainstem levels.

This chapter considers the level-to-level arrangements of structures as seen in transverse sections of the brainstem; many of the same structures are revisited in Chapter 8 as parts of functional systems. The sections were made by Pam Eller and stained, similar to the spinal cord sections in the previous chapter, by the Klüver-Barrera method, using luxol fast blue for myelin and a neutral red counterstain (which, despite its name, is a basic stain with an affinity for nucleic acids). The result is blue-violet staining of white matter and red staining of large neurons with prominent Nissl substance (e.g., hypoglossal motor neurons in Figure 3–10) and of areas tightly packed with small neurons (e.g., the granular layer of cerebellar cortex in Figure 3–10). A parasagittal section of the brainstem (Figure 3–1) is used as a reference view throughout the chapter. It includes some of the features characteristic of each brainstem level (Figure 3–2), such as the superior and inferior colliculi of the midbrain, the basal pons, and the medullary pyramids.

The three major longitudinal pathways (lateral corticospinal tract, posterior columns, and spinothalamic tract) that were followed through the spinal cord in Chapter 2 extend into the brainstem in consistent ways, as indicated in Figure 3–3. Corticospinal fibers travel in the most ventral part of the brainstem, traversing the cerebral peduncle, basal pons, and medullary pyramid. At the spinomedullary junction, most of the fibers in each pyramid cross the midline (in the pyramidal decussation) and form the lateral corticospinal tract. The posterior columns terminate in the posterior column nuclei (nucleus gracilis and nucleus cuneatus) of the medulla. Efferent fibers from these nuclei decussate in the medulla to form the medial lemniscus, which reaches the thalamus. The medial lemniscus starts out near the midline and moves progressively more laterally as it proceeds through the brainstem (Figure 3–4), rotating nearly 180 degrees in the process. The spinothalamic tract at all levels of the brainstem is at or near the lateral edge of the reticular formation. Cranial nerve nuclei also are arranged in reasonably consistent ways, as indicated schematically in Figure 3–3 and in more detail in subsequent figures.

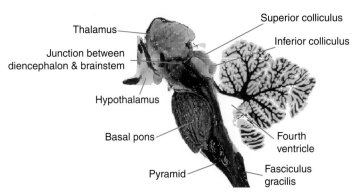

Figure 3–1 Parasagittal section of the brainstem and diencephalon.

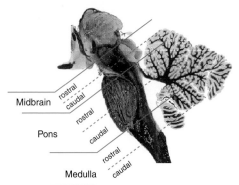

Figure 3–2 Levels of the brainstem.

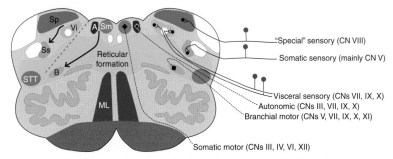

Figure 3–3 Arrangement of cranial nerve nuclei in the rostral medulla. The left side of the figure indicates how visceral sensory (*Vi*), somatic sensory *(Ss)*, and "special" sensory *(Sp)* (e.g., vestibular) nuclei are located lateral to the nuclei containing preganglionic autonomic neurons *(A)*, somatic motor neurons *(Sm)*, and motor neurons for muscles of branchial arch origin *(B)* (e.g., muscles of the larynx and pharynx). The cranial nerves containing each of these components are indicated on the right. (Not all of the nerves indicated actually emerge from the rostral medulla; they are included here for summary purposes.) CST, corticospinal tract; ML, medial lemniscus; STT, spinothalamic tract. *(Modified from Nolte J: The human brain, ed 5, St. Louis, 2002, Mosby.)*

Figure 3–4   Schematic views of six transverse sections of the brainstem, each enlarged about three times, indicating major long tracts and cranial nerve nuclei. These are the same sections shown photographically in Figures 3–9, 3–10, 3–12, 3–13, 3–15, and 3–16, and they correspond to planes of section indicated in Figure 3–6. Abbreviations are as in Figure 3–6.

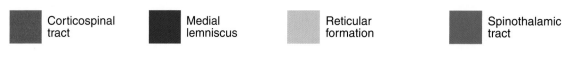

Corticospinal tract   Medial lemniscus   Reticular formation   Spinothalamic tract

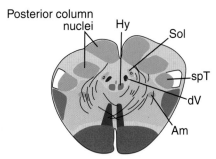

A, Caudal medulla (see Fig. 3–9).

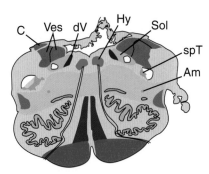

B, Rostral medulla (see Fig. 3–10).

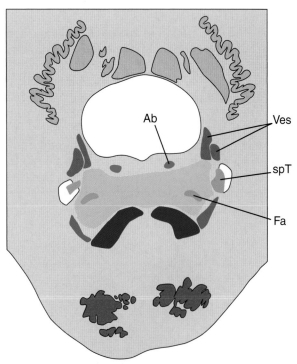

C, Caudal pons (see Fig. 3–12).

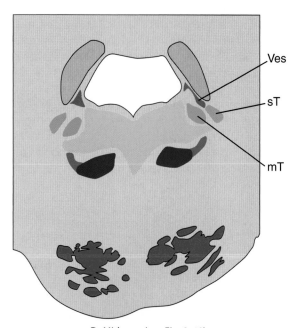

D, Midpons (see Fig. 3–13).

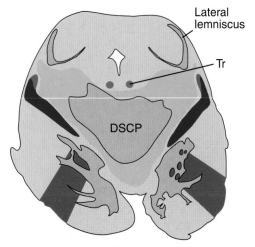

E, Caudal midbrain (see Fig. 3–15).

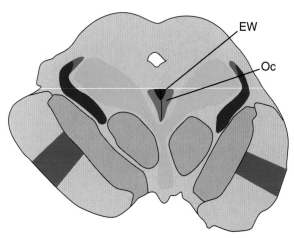

F, Rostral midbrain (see Fig. 3–16).

Figure 3–5 Schematic views of six transverse sections of the brainstem, each enlarged about 3×, indicating areas of arterial supply. These are the same sections shown photographically in Figures 3–9, 3–10, 3–12, and 3–14 through 3–16, and they correspond to planes of section indicated in Figure 3–6. At each level, the brainstem supply is a series of wedge-shaped territories, with anterolateral areas fed by midline arteries (e.g., vertebral, basilar) and posterolateral areas fed by circumferential branches (e.g., posterior inferior cerebellar artery, posterior cerebral artery).

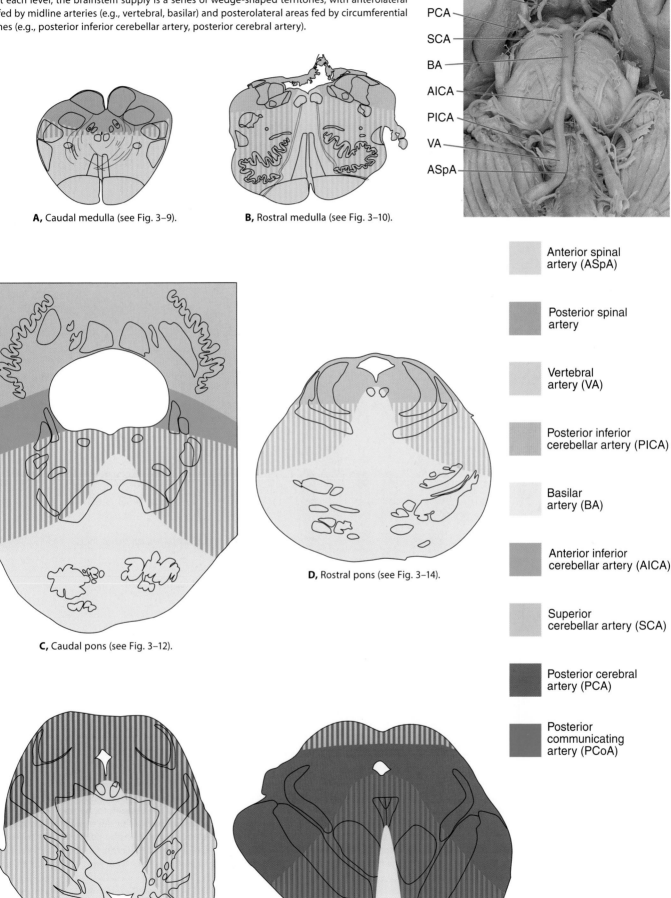

PCoA

PCA

SCA

BA

AICA

PICA

VA

ASpA

A, Caudal medulla (see Fig. 3–9).

B, Rostral medulla (see Fig. 3–10).

Anterior spinal artery (ASpA)

Posterior spinal artery

Vertebral artery (VA)

Posterior inferior cerebellar artery (PICA)

Basilar artery (BA)

Anterior inferior cerebellar artery (AICA)

Superior cerebellar artery (SCA)

Posterior cerebral artery (PCA)

Posterior communicating artery (PCoA)

C, Caudal pons (see Fig. 3–12).

D, Rostral pons (see Fig. 3–14).

E, Caudal midbrain (see Fig. 3–15).

F, Rostral midbrain (see Fig. 3–16).

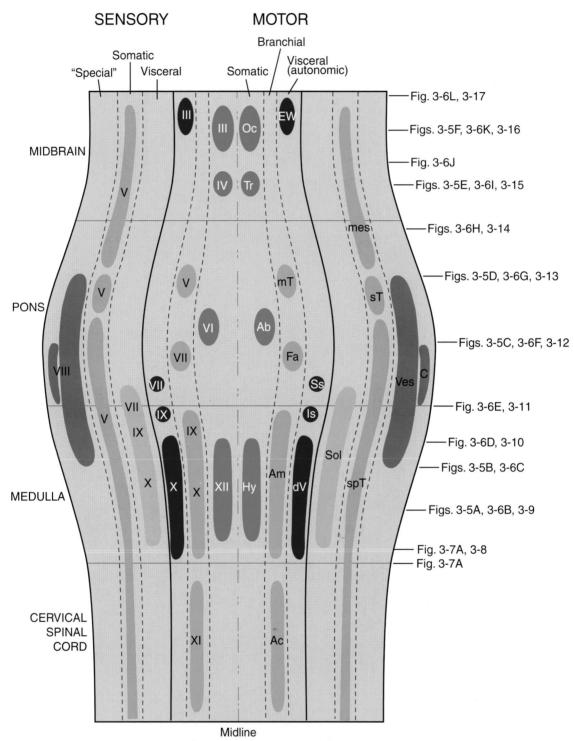

Figure 3–6 The longitudinal arrangement of functional types of cranial nerve nuclei in the brainstem. The cranial nerves involved with each type of function are indicated on the left side of the diagram, and the actual nuclei are indicated on the right side. Ab, abducens nucleus; Ac, accessory nucleus; Am, nucleus ambiguus; C, cochlear nuclei; dV, dorsal motor nucleus of the vagus; EW, Edinger-Westphal nucleus (a subdivision of the oculomotor nucleus); Fa, facial nucleus; Hy, hypoglossal nucleus; Is, inferior salivatory nucleus; mes, mesencephalic nucleus of the trigeminal; mT, motor nucleus of the trigeminal; Oc, oculomotor nucleus; Sol, nucleus of the solitary tract; spT, spinal nucleus of the trigeminal; Ss, superior salivatory nucleus; sT, main sensory nucleus of the trigeminal; Tr, trochlear nucleus; Ves, vestibular nuclei. All of these nuclei (except the salivatory nuclei) are indicated in one or more of the cross sections indicated along the right side of the figure. *(Modified from Nieuwenhuys R, et al: The human central nervous system: a synopsis and atlas, ed 3, New York, 1988, Springer-Verlag.)*

Figure 3-7   Cross sections of a brainstem at 13 different levels.

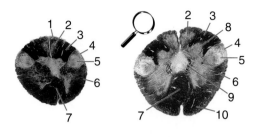

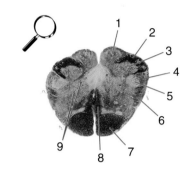

A, Spinomedullary junction. Fasciculus cuneatus (3) proceeds rostrally toward nucleus cuneatus (8, not yet present in the section on the left), and fasciculus gracilis (1) begins to terminate in nucleus gracilis (2). In the more rostral section on the right, internal arcuate fibers (9) leave the posterior column nuclei to cross the midline and form the medial lemniscus. The spinal trigeminal tract (4), at this level containing trigeminal pain and temperature afferents, and the spinal trigeminal nucleus (5), where these afferents terminate, replace Lissauer's tract and the posterior horn of the spinal cord. The spinothalamic tract (6) is located ventrolaterally, much as it was in the spinal cord. Corticospinal fibers that descended through the internal capsule, cerebral peduncle, basal pons, and medullary pyramid (10) now cross the midline in the pyramidal decussation (7). The section on the right is shown enlarged in Figure 3-8.

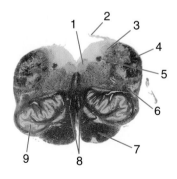

B, Caudal medulla. Fasciculus gracilis has ended in the nucleus gracilis (1), and fasciculus cuneatus (2) ends in the nucleus cuneatus (3). Efferents from these posterior column nuclei (9) arc across the midline and form the medial lemniscus (8). The spinothalamic tract (6) is in its typical location in the lateral part of the reticular formation, and the corticospinal tract traverses the pyramids (7). Trigeminal primary afferent fibers descend through the spinal trigeminal tract (4) to termination sites in the spinal trigeminal nucleus (5). Shown enlarged in Figure 3-9.

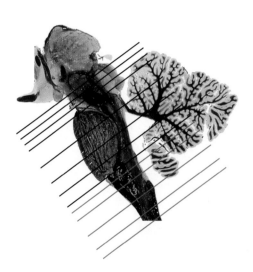

C, Rostral medulla. The central canal of the spinal cord and caudal medulla has given way to the fourth ventricle; part of its roof can be seen (2). Structures associated with cranial nerves appear in the floor of the fourth ventricle, including the hypoglossal nucleus (1), vestibular nuclei (3), and the solitary tract (5) surrounded by its nucleus. Efferents from the inferior olivary nucleus (9) arc across the midline and join the contralateral inferior cerebellar peduncle (4). The locations of the spinothalamic tract (6), medial lemniscus (8), and corticospinal tract (7) are unchanged. Shown enlarged in Figure 3-8.

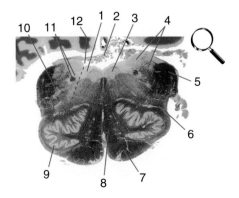

D, Rostral medulla. A plane (dashed line) descending from the sulcus limitans (12) separates cranial nerve nuclei into a more medial group of motor nuclei and a more lateral group of sensory nuclei. Motor nuclei at this level include the hypoglossal nucleus (3) and the dorsal motor nucleus of the vagus (1, adjacent to the sulcus limitans). More laterally are the vestibular nuclei (4), spinal trigeminal nucleus (10), and the solitary tract and its nucleus (11, adjacent to the sulcus limitans). The locations of the medial lemniscus (8), spinothalamic tract (6), and corticospinal tract (7, in the pyramid) are unchanged. The inferior cerebellar peduncle (5) is substantially larger because efferents from the contralateral inferior olivary nucleus (9) have accumulated in it. Choroid plexus (2) can be seen in the roof of the fourth ventricle. Shown enlarged in Figure 3-10.

Illustration continued on following page

Figure 3–7 (Continued)   Cross sections of a brainstem at 13 different levels.

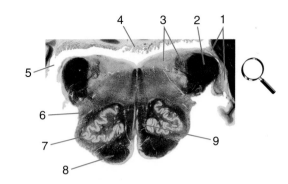

E, Pontomedullary junction. The fourth ventricle extends laterally, leading off into the lateral recess (5); choroid plexus (4) is visible in the roof of the ventricle. Vestibular (3) and cochlear (1) nuclei occupy the ventricular floor. The inferior cerebellar peduncle (2) has reached maximum size and is about to enter the cerebellum. The positions of the spinothalamic tract (6), inferior olivary nucleus (7), medial lemniscus (9), and corticospinal tract (8) are unchanged. Shown enlarged in Figure 3–11.

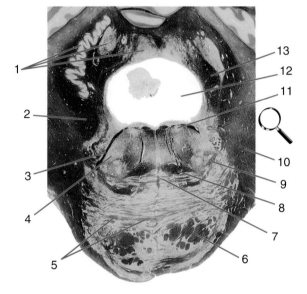

F, Caudal pons. The floor of the fourth ventricle (12) is occupied by the abducens nucleus (11), together with facial nerve fibers that emerge from the facial nucleus (4), hook around the abducens nucleus as the genu of the facial nerve, and leave the brainstem as the root of the facial nerve (3). The spinothalamic tract (9) is still located laterally in the reticular formation. The medial lemniscus (8) begins to move laterally and is traversed by crossing auditory fibers (7) of the trapezoid body. The corticospinal tract (6) is dispersed in the basal pons, surrounded by pontine nuclei and their transversely oriented efferents (5), which cross the midline and form the middle cerebellar peduncle (10). Deep cerebellar nuclei (1) appear in the roof of the fourth ventricle, and the superior cerebellar peduncle (13) begins to form adjacent to them. The inferior cerebellar peduncle (2) enters the cerebellum. Shown enlarged in Figure 3–12.

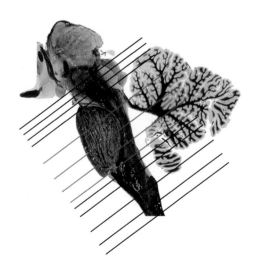

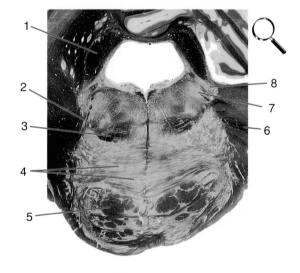

G, Midpons, at the level of entry of the trigeminal nerve (6). Many trigeminal fibers end in the main sensory nucleus of the trigeminal (8) or arise in the trigeminal motor nucleus (7). The superior cerebellar peduncle (1), carrying most of the output of the cerebellum, begins to enter the brainstem. The spinothalamic tract (2) is still located laterally in the reticular formation, the medial lemniscus (3) continues to move laterally, and the corticospinal tract (5) is still dispersed in the basal pons (4). Shown enlarged in Figure 3–13.

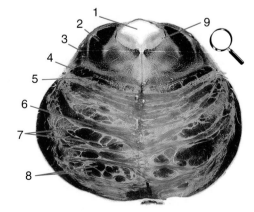

H, Rostral pons, near the pons-midbrain junction. The fourth ventricle (1) narrows as it approaches the aqueduct. The superior cerebellar peduncle (2) moves deeper into the brainstem just before beginning to decussate. The medial lemniscus (5) is a flattened band of fibers with the spinothalamic tract (4) laterally adjacent to it. The lateral lemniscus (3) conveys ascending auditory fibers to the midbrain. The corticospinal tract (8) is surrounded by pontine nuclei (7) and their transversely oriented efferents (6). The locus ceruleus (9) is a small collection of pigmented neurons that provide most of the noradrenergic innervation of the CNS (see Fig. 8–36). Shown enlarged in Figure 3–14.

Figure 3–7 (Continued)   Cross sections of a brainstem at 13 different levels.

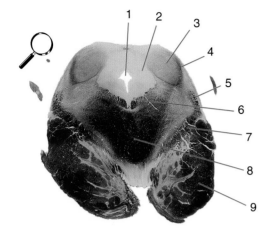

I, Caudal midbrain. The lateral lemniscus (4) ends in the inferior colliculus (3). The spinothalamic tract (5) and medial lemniscus (7) form a continuous band of fibers. The massive decussation of the superior cerebellar peduncles (8) occupies the center of the reticular formation. The basal pons gives way to a cerebral peduncle (9) on each side. The tiny trochlear nucleus (6) appears. At all midbrain levels, the cerebral aqueduct (1) is surrounded by periaqueductal gray matter (2). Shown enlarged in Figure 3–15.

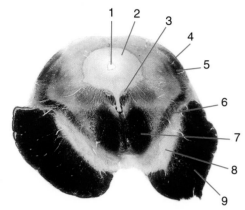

J, Mid-midbrain. Characteristic midbrain features such as the aqueduct (1) and periaqueductal gray (2) can be seen, but no colliculi are present. The brachium of the inferior colliculus (4), spinothalamic tract (5), medial lemniscus (6), and now-crossed superior cerebellar peduncle (7) all are on their way to the thalamus. The oculomotor nucleus (3), substantia nigra (8), and cerebral peduncle (9) appear—all harbingers of the rostral midbrain.

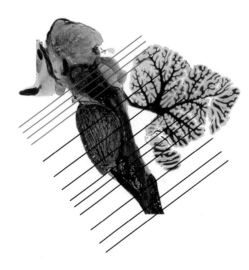

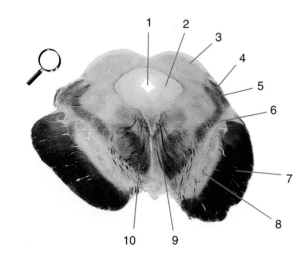

K, Rostral midbrain. The superior colliculus (3) appears, and the oculomotor nucleus (9) is fully formed. The auditory pathway continues in the brachium of the inferior colliculus (4). The positions and appearance of the cerebral aqueduct (1), periaqueductal gray (2), spinothalamic tract (5), medial lemniscus (6), and cerebral peduncle (7) are little changed. Cerebellar efferents that reached the midbrain in the superior cerebellar peduncle (10) begin to pass through or around the red nucleus. The substantia nigra (8) is more prominent. Shown enlarged in Figure 3–16.

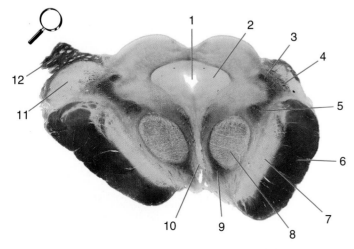

L, Rostral midbrain, near the level of the midbrain-diencephalon junction. The cerebral aqueduct (1), periaqueductal gray (2), spinothalamic tract (3), medial lemniscus (5), cerebral peduncle (6), and substantia nigra (7) are still evident. The brachium of the inferior colliculus (4) ends in the medial geniculate nucleus (11), the first thalamic nucleus to appear in this plane of section. Cerebellar efferents (9) pass through and around the red nucleus (8) on their way to the thalamus. The ventral tegmental area (10) is a medial collection of neurons that provide the dopaminergic innervation of frontal cortex and limbic structures (see Fig. 8–37). Efferents from some retinal ganglion cells and visual cortex traverse the brachium of the superior colliculus (12) on their way to the superior colliculus. Shown enlarged in Figure 3–17.

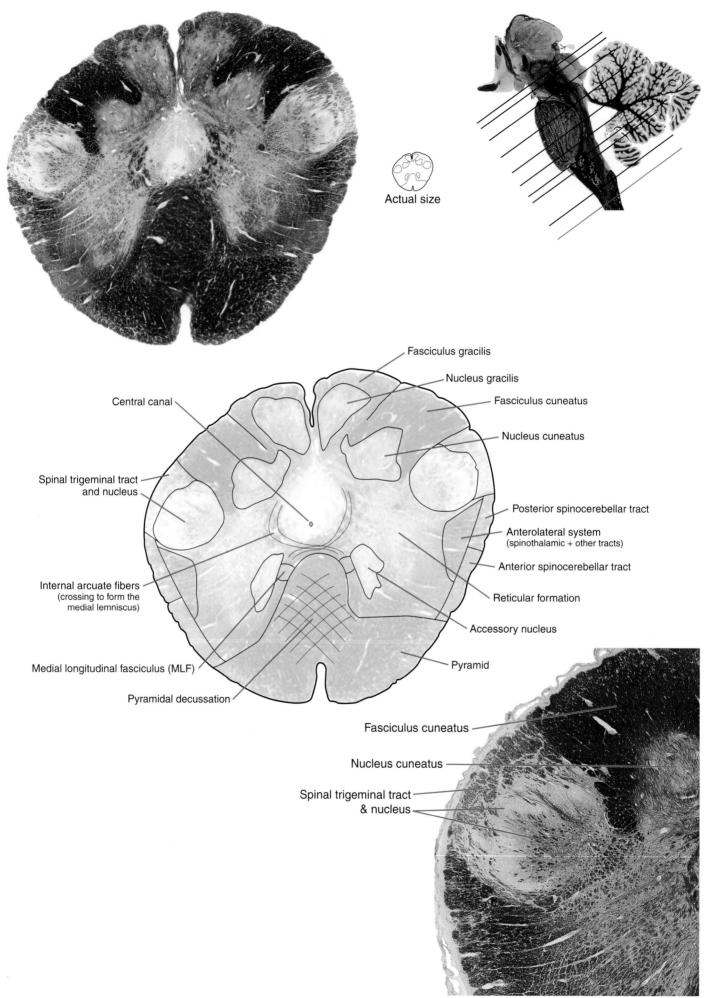

Actual size

Fasciculus gracilis

Nucleus gracilis

Fasciculus cuneatus

Nucleus cuneatus

Central canal

Spinal trigeminal tract
and nucleus

Posterior spinocerebellar tract

Anterolateral system
(spinothalamic + other tracts)

Anterior spinocerebellar tract

Internal arcuate fibers
(crossing to form the
medial lemniscus)

Reticular formation

Accessory nucleus

Medial longitudinal fasciculus (MLF)

Pyramid

Pyramidal decussation

Fasciculus cuneatus

Nucleus cuneatus

Spinal trigeminal tract
& nucleus

Figure 3–8   Caudal medulla, near the spinomedullary junction.

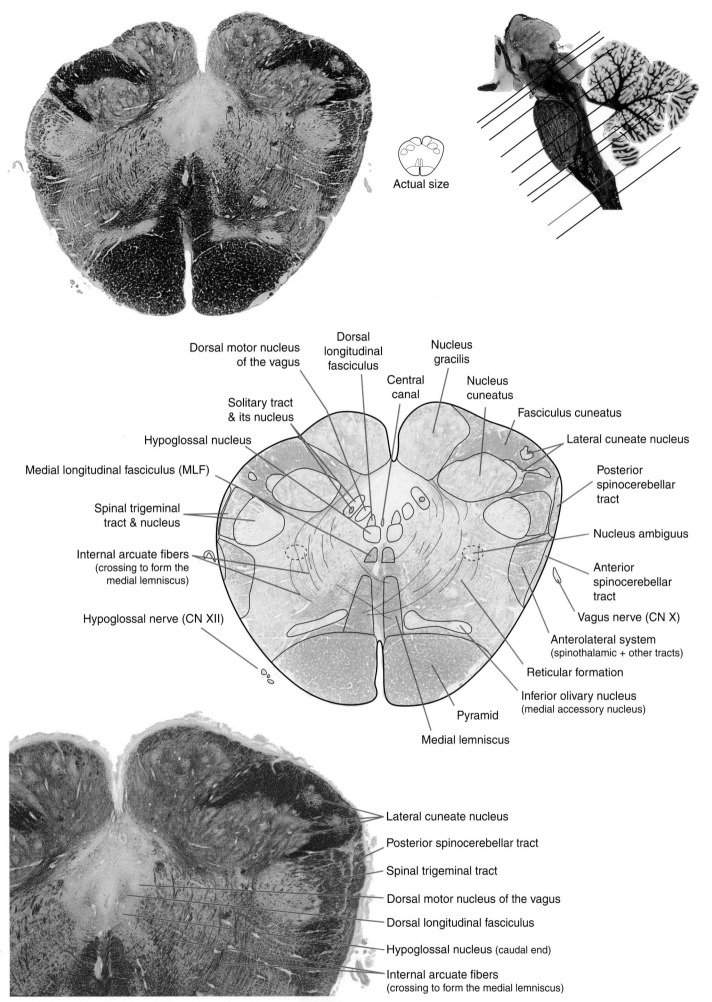

Actual size

Dorsal motor nucleus of the vagus

Dorsal longitudinal fasciculus

Nucleus gracilis

Central canal

Nucleus cuneatus

Solitary tract & its nucleus

Fasciculus cuneatus

Hypoglossal nucleus

Lateral cuneate nucleus

Medial longitudinal fasciculus (MLF)

Posterior spinocerebellar tract

Spinal trigeminal tract & nucleus

Nucleus ambiguus

Internal arcuate fibers (crossing to form the medial lemniscus)

Anterior spinocerebellar tract

Hypoglossal nerve (CN XII)

Vagus nerve (CN X)

Anterolateral system (spinothalamic + other tracts)

Reticular formation

Inferior olivary nucleus (medial accessory nucleus)

Pyramid

Medial lemniscus

Lateral cuneate nucleus

Posterior spinocerebellar tract

Spinal trigeminal tract

Dorsal motor nucleus of the vagus

Dorsal longitudinal fasciculus

Hypoglossal nucleus (caudal end)

Internal arcuate fibers (crossing to form the medial lemniscus)

Figure 3–9 Caudal medulla.

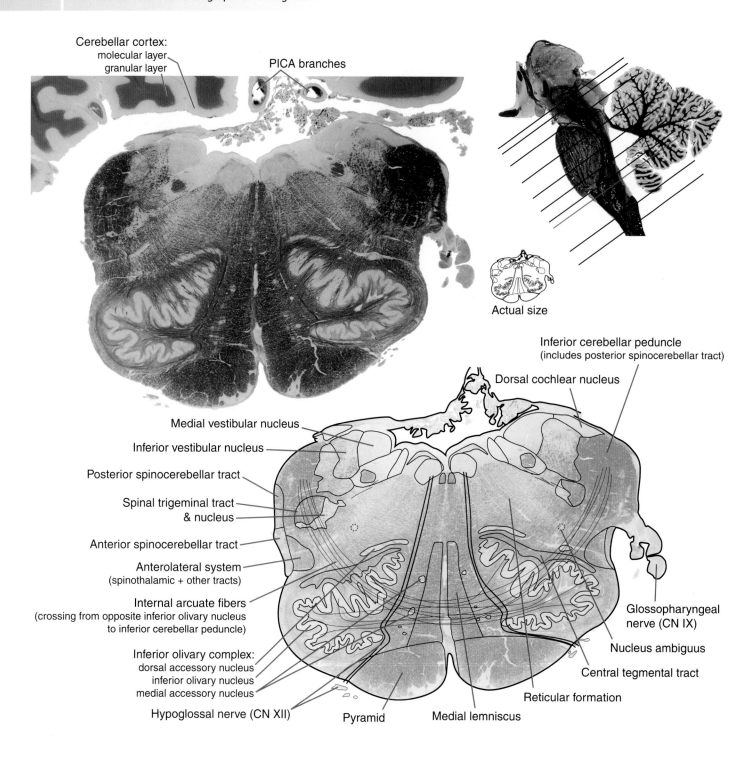

Cerebellar cortex:
  molecular layer
  granular layer

PICA branches

Actual size

Inferior cerebellar peduncle
(includes posterior spinocerebellar tract)

Dorsal cochlear nucleus

Medial vestibular nucleus

Inferior vestibular nucleus

Posterior spinocerebellar tract

Spinal trigeminal tract
& nucleus

Anterior spinocerebellar tract

Anterolateral system
(spinothalamic + other tracts)

Internal arcuate fibers
(crossing from opposite inferior olivary nucleus
to inferior cerebellar peduncle)

Inferior olivary complex:
  dorsal accessory nucleus
  inferior olivary nucleus
  medial accessory nucleus

Hypoglossal nerve (CN XII)

Pyramid

Medial lemniscus

Reticular formation

Central tegmental tract

Nucleus ambiguus

Glossopharyngeal
nerve (CN IX)

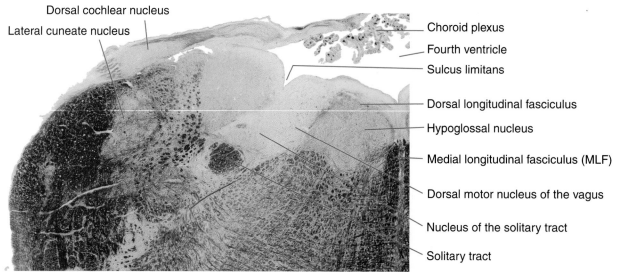

Dorsal cochlear nucleus

Lateral cuneate nucleus

Choroid plexus

Fourth ventricle

Sulcus limitans

Dorsal longitudinal fasciculus

Hypoglossal nucleus

Medial longitudinal fasciculus (MLF)

Dorsal motor nucleus of the vagus

Nucleus of the solitary tract

Solitary tract

Figure 3-10   Rostral medulla. PICA, posterior inferior cerebellar artery.

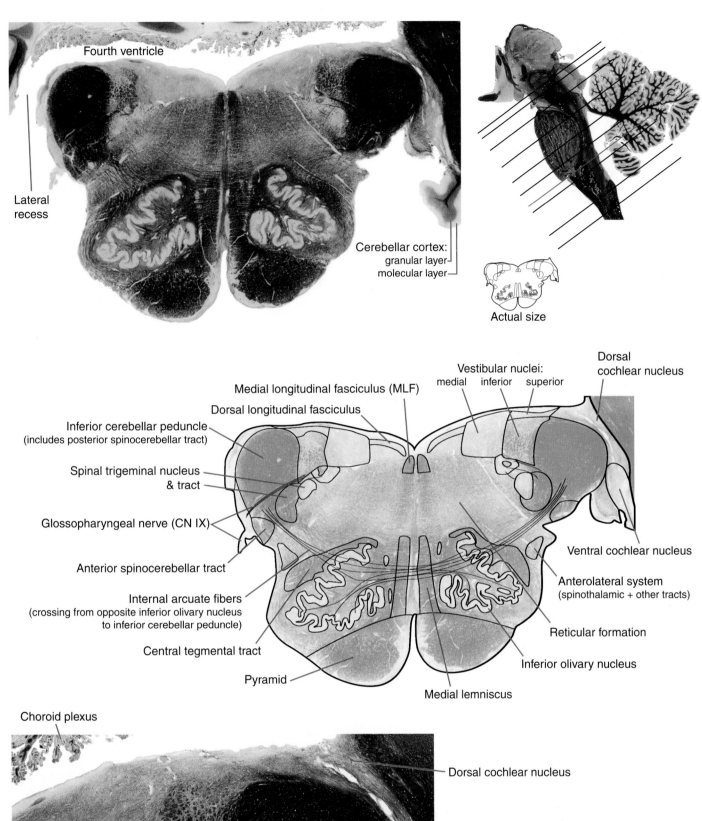

Fourth ventricle

Lateral recess

Cerebellar cortex:
granular layer
molecular layer

Actual size

Vestibular nuclei:
medial   inferior   superior

Dorsal cochlear nucleus

Medial longitudinal fasciculus (MLF)

Dorsal longitudinal fasciculus

Inferior cerebellar peduncle
(includes posterior spinocerebellar tract)

Spinal trigeminal nucleus & tract

Glossopharyngeal nerve (CN IX)

Anterior spinocerebellar tract

Internal arcuate fibers
(crossing from opposite inferior olivary nucleus
to inferior cerebellar peduncle)

Central tegmental tract

Pyramid

Medial lemniscus

Ventral cochlear nucleus

Anterolateral system
(spinothalamic + other tracts)

Reticular formation

Inferior olivary nucleus

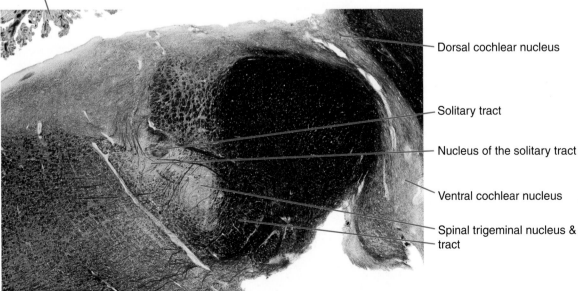

Choroid plexus

Dorsal cochlear nucleus

Solitary tract

Nucleus of the solitary tract

Ventral cochlear nucleus

Spinal trigeminal nucleus & tract

Figure 3–11 Pontomedullary junction.

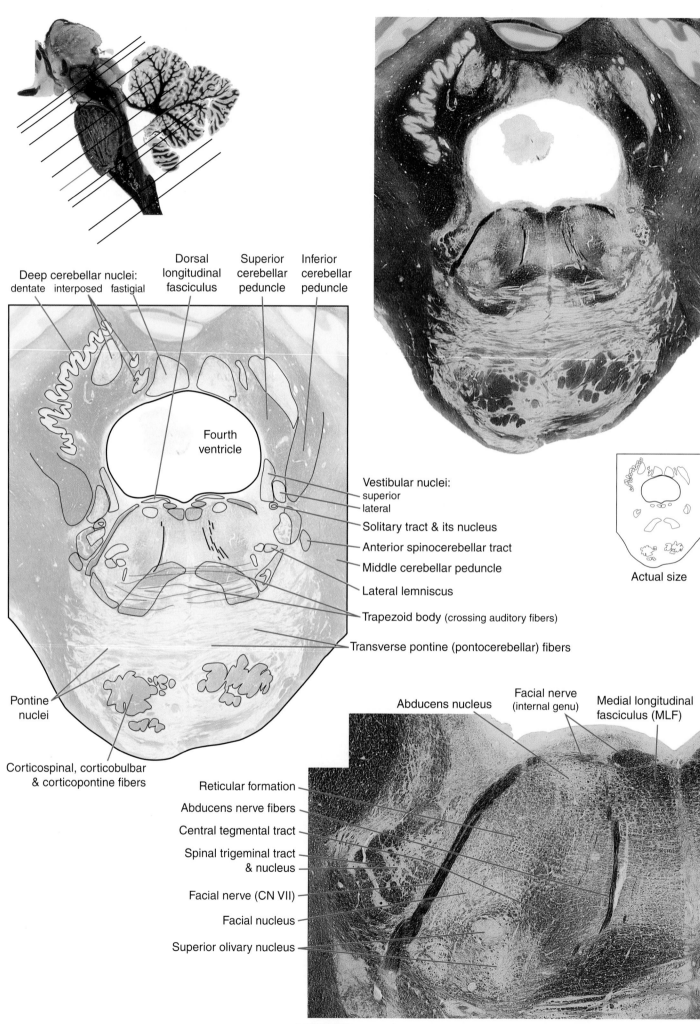

Deep cerebellar nuclei:
dentate interposed fastigial

Dorsal
longitudinal
fasciculus

Superior
cerebellar
peduncle

Inferior
cerebellar
peduncle

Fourth
ventricle

Vestibular nuclei:
superior
lateral

Solitary tract & its nucleus

Anterior spinocerebellar tract

Middle cerebellar peduncle

Lateral lemniscus

Trapezoid body (crossing auditory fibers)

Transverse pontine (pontocerebellar) fibers

Pontine
nuclei

Corticospinal, corticobulbar
& corticopontine fibers

Actual size

Abducens nucleus

Facial nerve
(internal genu)

Medial longitudinal
fasciculus (MLF)

Reticular formation

Abducens nerve fibers

Central tegmental tract

Spinal trigeminal tract
& nucleus

Facial nerve (CN VII)

Facial nucleus

Superior olivary nucleus

Figure 3–12   Caudal pons.

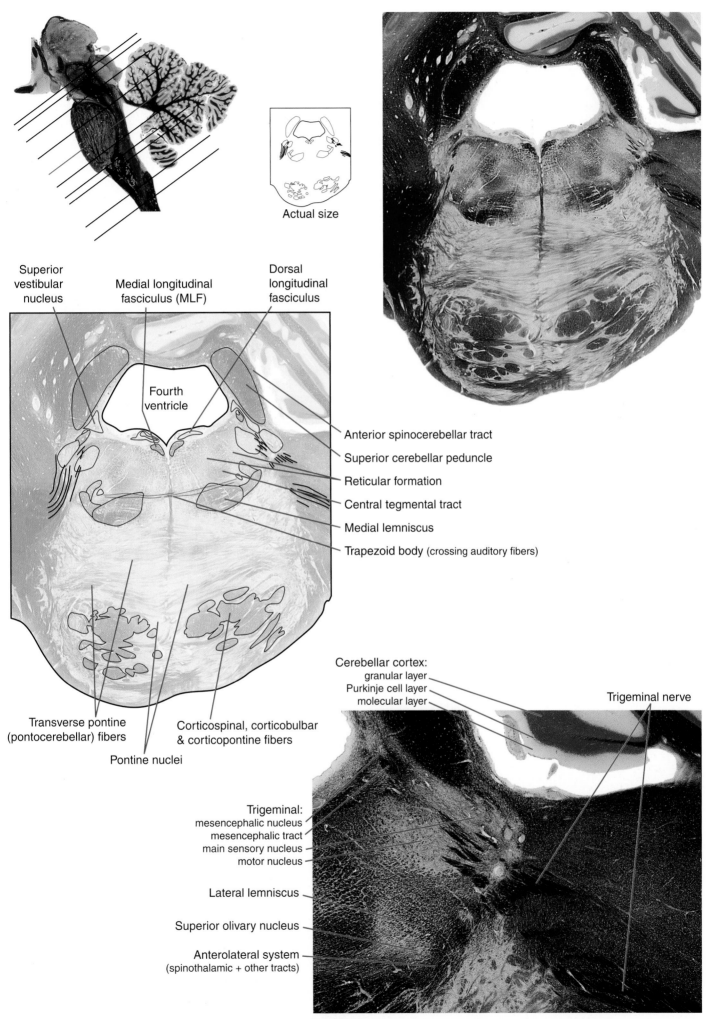

Actual size

Superior vestibular nucleus

Medial longitudinal fasciculus (MLF)

Dorsal longitudinal fasciculus

Fourth ventricle

Anterior spinocerebellar tract

Superior cerebellar peduncle

Reticular formation

Central tegmental tract

Medial lemniscus

Trapezoid body (crossing auditory fibers)

Transverse pontine (pontocerebellar) fibers

Corticospinal, corticobulbar & corticopontine fibers

Pontine nuclei

Cerebellar cortex:
granular layer
Purkinje cell layer
molecular layer

Trigeminal nerve

Trigeminal:
mesencephalic nucleus
mesencephalic tract
main sensory nucleus
motor nucleus

Lateral lemniscus

Superior olivary nucleus

Anterolateral system (spinothalamic + other tracts)

Figure 3–13 Midpons.

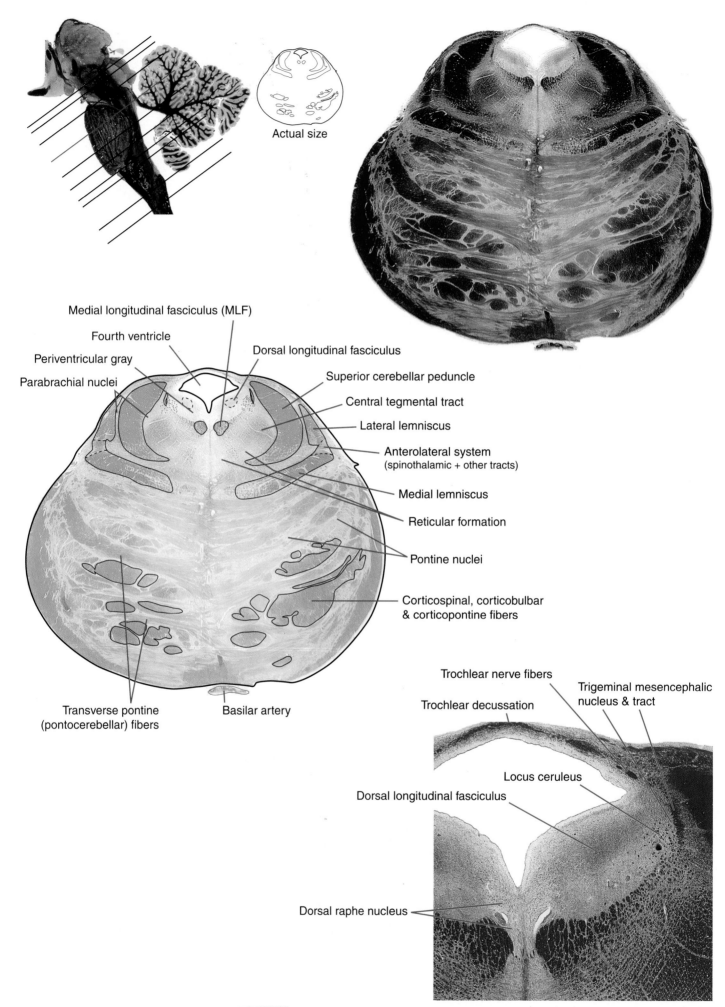

Actual size

Medial longitudinal fasciculus (MLF)

Fourth ventricle

Periventricular gray

Parabrachial nuclei

Dorsal longitudinal fasciculus

Superior cerebellar peduncle

Central tegmental tract

Lateral lemniscus

Anterolateral system
(spinothalamic + other tracts)

Medial lemniscus

Reticular formation

Pontine nuclei

Corticospinal, corticobulbar
& corticopontine fibers

Transverse pontine
(pontocerebellar) fibers

Basilar artery

Trochlear nerve fibers

Trochlear decussation

Trigeminal mesencephalic
nucleus & tract

Locus ceruleus

Dorsal longitudinal fasciculus

Dorsal raphe nucleus

Figure 3–14   Rostral pons, near the pons-midbrain junction.

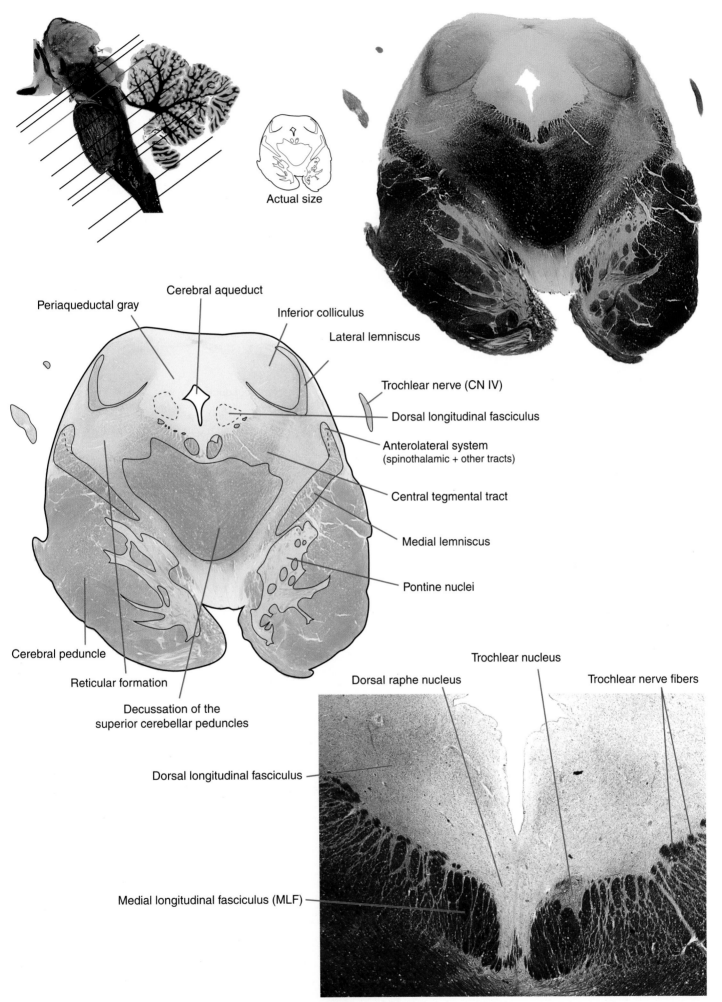

Actual size

Periaqueductal gray

Cerebral aqueduct

Inferior colliculus

Lateral lemniscus

Trochlear nerve (CN IV)

Dorsal longitudinal fasciculus

Anterolateral system
(spinothalamic + other tracts)

Central tegmental tract

Medial lemniscus

Pontine nuclei

Cerebral peduncle

Reticular formation

Decussation of the
superior cerebellar peduncles

Dorsal raphe nucleus

Trochlear nucleus

Trochlear nerve fibers

Dorsal longitudinal fasciculus

Medial longitudinal fasciculus (MLF)

Figure 3–15 Caudal midbrain.

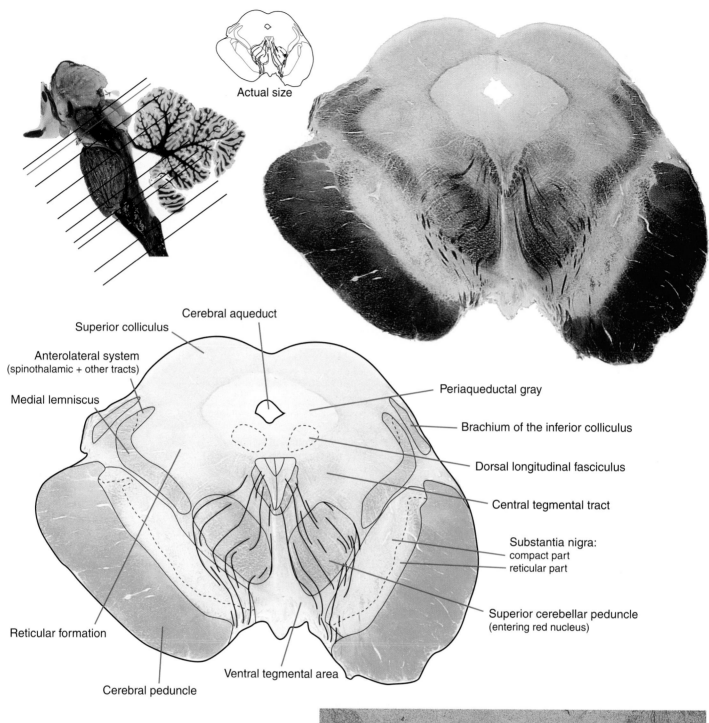

Actual size

Superior colliculus

Cerebral aqueduct

Anterolateral system
(spinothalamic + other tracts)

Medial lemniscus

Periaqueductal gray

Brachium of the inferior colliculus

Dorsal longitudinal fasciculus

Central tegmental tract

Substantia nigra:
compact part
reticular part

Superior cerebellar peduncle
(entering red nucleus)

Reticular formation

Ventral tegmental area

Cerebral peduncle

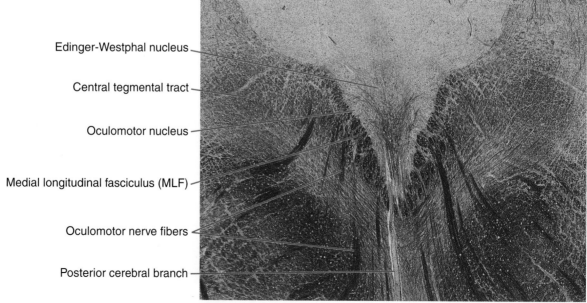

Edinger-Westphal nucleus

Central tegmental tract

Oculomotor nucleus

Medial longitudinal fasciculus (MLF)

Oculomotor nerve fibers

Posterior cerebral branch

Figure 3–16   Rostral midbrain.

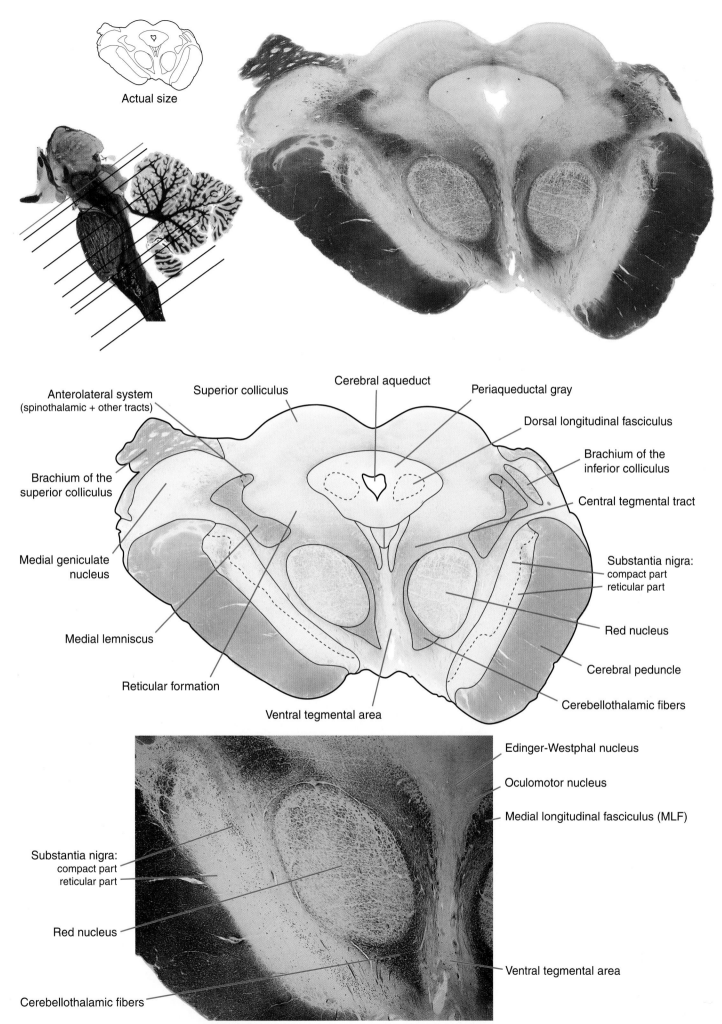

Actual size

Anterolateral system
(spinothalamic + other tracts)

Superior colliculus

Cerebral aqueduct

Periaqueductal gray

Dorsal longitudinal fasciculus

Brachium of the
superior colliculus

Brachium of the
inferior colliculus

Central tegmental tract

Medial geniculate
nucleus

Substantia nigra:
compact part
reticular part

Medial lemniscus

Red nucleus

Cerebral peduncle

Reticular formation

Cerebellothalamic fibers

Ventral tegmental area

Edinger-Westphal nucleus

Oculomotor nucleus

Medial longitudinal fasciculus (MLF)

Substantia nigra:
compact part
reticular part

Red nucleus

Ventral tegmental area

Cerebellothalamic fibers

Figure 3–17   Rostral midbrain, near the midbrain-diencephalon junction.

4

Building a Brain: Three-Dimensional Reconstructions

The interior of the cerebrum is occupied by a series of structures that fit neatly together in three-dimensional space. As a consequence of the embryological development of the brain, some cerebral structures (e.g., lateral ventricle, caudate nucleus) curve around in a great C-shaped arch (Figure 4–1), whereas others are more centrally located. One of the greatest impediments to understanding the interrelationships of cerebral structures in three dimensions is the typical presentation of the nervous system in a series of two-dimensional sections cut in various planes (as it is presented in much of this book).

As a partial solution to this dilemma, this chapter presents an overview of the arrangement of cerebral structures in the form of a series of computer-generated reconstructions (provided by Dr. John W. Sundsten and his colleagues, Department of Biological Structure, University of Washington School of Medicine). The images were made by cutting serial sections of a single human brain, digitizing outlines of structures of interest, and using these outlines to reconstruct (by computer) individual structures or groups of structures. Beginning with the reconstruction of the brainstem, cerebellum, and diencephalon shown in Figure 4–2, major structures of the cerebral hemispheres are added sequentially in Figure 4–3. Similar three-dimensional reconstructions are used in Chapters 5 through 7 to indicate the planes of sections through the forebrain.

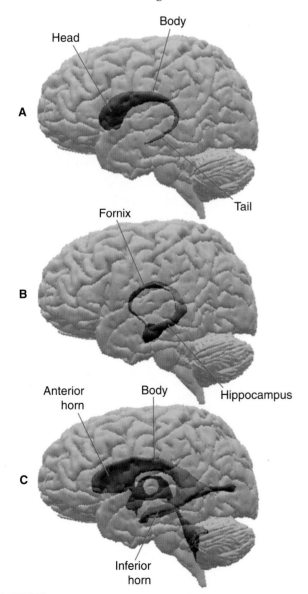

Figure 4–1 Three examples of C-shaped telencephalic structures: the caudate nucleus **(A),** hippocampus/fornix system **(B),** and lateral ventricle **(C).** (*Modified from Nolte J: The human brain, ed 5, St. Louis, 2002, Mosby.*)

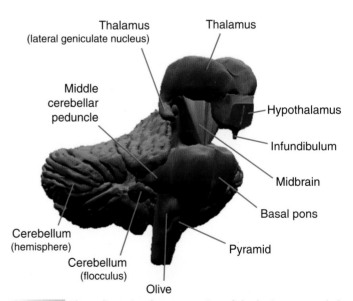

Figure 4–2 Three-dimensional reconstruction of the brainstem, cerebellum, and diencephalon. In an intact brain, the hypothalamus is continuous anteriorly with the preoptic and septal areas; in this reconstruction, the hypothalamus is shown ending abruptly at its approximate border with these structures. The midbrain is configured with a flattened anterior surface because the cerebral peduncle is not yet present; it is added in Figure 4–3E.

Figure 4–3   A–H, Building a brain.

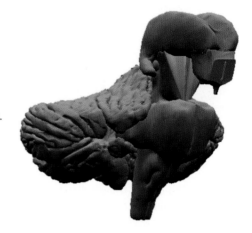

A, The reconstruction of the brainstem, cerebellum, and diencephalon shown in Figure 4–2.

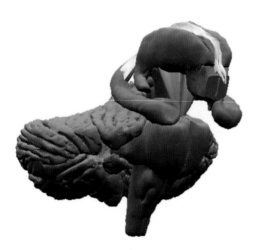

B, The hippocampus *(purple)* is a special cortical area folded into the medial part of the temporal lobe, adjacent to the inferior horn of the lateral ventricle. The fornix *(white)* is a major output pathway from the hippocampus. It curves around in a C-shaped course (the Latin word *fornix* means "arch") and terminates primarily in the hypothalamus and septal area.

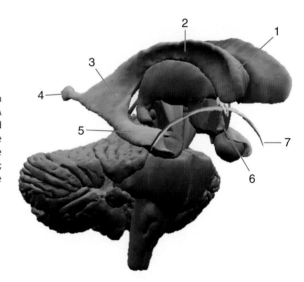

C, The lateral ventricle is another C-shaped structure, curving from an anterior horn *(1)* in the frontal lobe, through a body *(2)*, and into an inferior horn *(5)* in the temporal lobe. A posterior horn *(4)* extends backward into the occipital lobe. The body, posterior horn, and inferior horn meet in the atrium *(3)* of the lateral ventricle. The body and anterior horn have a concave lateral surface; in reality, parts of the caudate nucleus occupy this depression (see Fig. 4–3D). The third ventricle *(6)* extends anteriorly beyond the truncated hypothalamus; in an intact brain, this anterior extension would be bordered by the preoptic area. The anterior commissure *(7)* contains fibers interconnecting the temporal lobes.

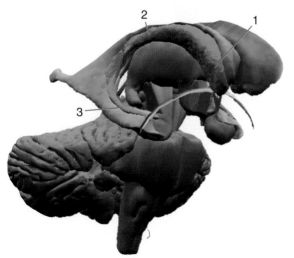

D, The caudate nucleus, another C-shaped structure, curves through the hemisphere adjacent to the lateral ventricle. Its enlarged head *(1)* and body *(2)* account for the indented lateral wall of the anterior horn and body of the ventricle (see Fig. 4–3C). The attenuated tail *(3)* of the caudate nucleus forms part of the wall of the inferior horn of the ventricle.

Figure 4–3 (Continued)   Building a brain.

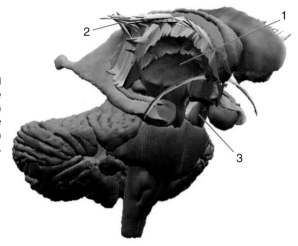

E, The internal capsule *(1)* is a thick band of fibers that covers the lateral aspect of the head of the caudate nucleus and the thalamus. It contains most of the fibers interconnecting the cerebral cortex and subcortical sites. Above the internal capsule, these fibers fan out within the cerebral hemisphere as the corona radiata *(2)*. Many of the cortical efferent fibers in the internal capsule funnel down into the cerebral peduncle *(3)*. The internal capsule also has a concave lateral surface; in this case, the lenticular nucleus occupies the depression (see Fig. 4–3F).

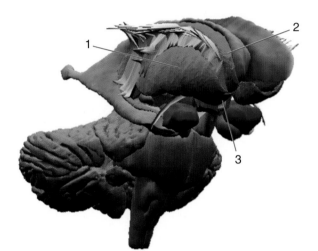

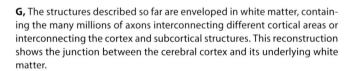

F, The lenticular nucleus *(1)*, itself a combination of the putamen and the globus pallidus, occupies the depression in the internal capsule (see Fig. 4–3E). The putamen (the more lateral of the two) and the caudate nucleus *(2)* are actually continuous masses of gray matter. The area of continuity is called the nucleus accumbens *(3)*. The amygdala *(red)* is a collection of nuclei underlying the medial surface of the temporal lobe at the anterior end of the hippocampus.

G, The structures described so far are enveloped in white matter, containing the many millions of axons interconnecting different cortical areas or interconnecting the cortex and subcortical structures. This reconstruction shows the junction between the cerebral cortex and its underlying white matter.

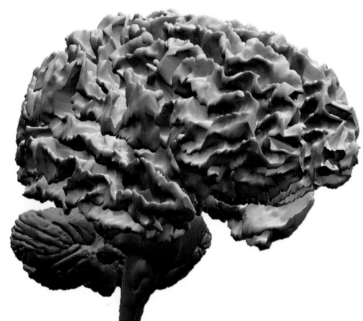

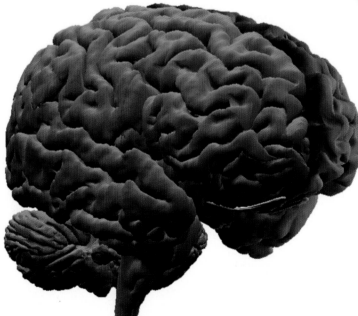

H, Finally, a thin (1.5 to 4.5 mm) layer of cerebral cortex covers each hemisphere.

Coronal Sections

This is the first of three chapters showing sections of entire human brains, in this case illustrating approximately coronal planes. Forebrain structures are emphasized, but parts of the brainstem and cerebellum are indicated as well. The organization of various functional systems in the forebrain (e.g., thalamus, hippocampus) is presented in Chapter 8.

Drawings showing typical areas of arterial supply in each section also are provided in this chapter and the next two chapters. We have simplified these in two major ways. First, arterial territories are shown as sharply demarcated from each other, when in reality there is significant interdigitation and overlap. Second, penetrating arteries arise from all the vessels of the circle of Willis; however, we have incorporated those from the anterior and posterior communicating arteries with those from the anterior and posterior cerebral arteries.

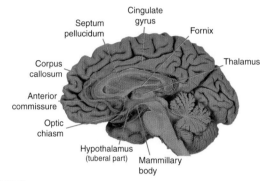

Figure 5–1 The hemisected brain from Figure 1–6, used in much of this chapter to indicate planes of section.

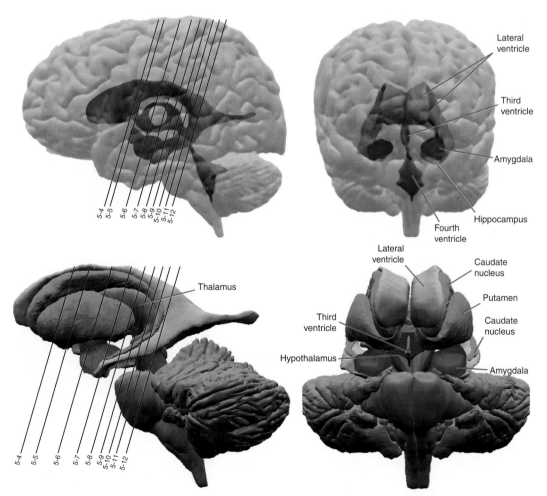

Figure 5–2 The planes of section shown in this chapter, indicated on three-dimensional reconstructions. *(Courtesy of Dr. John W. Sundsten, Department of Biological Structure, University of Washington School of Medicine.)*

Figure 5–3   A–X, Twenty-four coronal sections of a brain, arranged in an anterior-to-posterior sequence from the anterior edge of the corpus callosum to the middle of the occipital lobe.

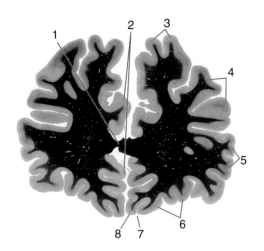

A, Anterior end of the genu of the corpus callosum *(1)*. Convolutions that comprise most of the frontal lobe are the superior *(3)*, middle *(4)*, and inferior *(5)* frontal gyri; orbital gyri *(6)*; and gyrus rectus *(8)*. The cingulate gyrus *(2)* is cut twice, once above and once below the genu of the corpus callosum. The olfactory sulcus *(7)*, which is occupied by the olfactory tract at a slightly more posterior level, lies just lateral to the gyrus rectus.

B, The anterior horn of the lateral ventricle *(3)* appears. A septum pellucidum *(2)* forms the medial wall of each lateral ventricle. The corpus callosum is now cut in two places, once through its body *(1)* above the septum pellucidum and once *(4)* as the genu begins to taper into the rostrum below the septum pellucidum.

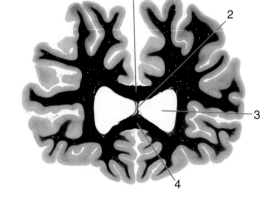

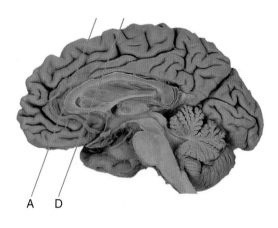

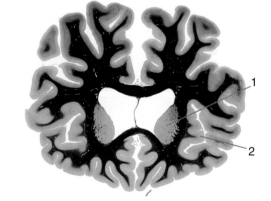

C, The head of the caudate nucleus *(1)* appears in the lateral wall of the lateral ventricle. The anterior region of the insula *(2)* also is visible at this level, overlying the caudate nucleus.

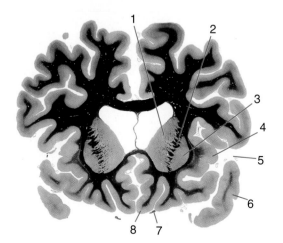

D, The rostral end of the putamen *(3)* is separated from the head of the caudate nucleus *(1)* by the anterior limb of the internal capsule *(2)*. The putamen, the larger of the two parts of the lenticular nucleus, is overlaid for its entire extent by the insula *(4)*. The olfactory tract *(7)* lies in the olfactory sulcus, just lateral to gyrus rectus *(8)*. The section passes through the tip of the temporal lobe *(6)*, separated from the frontal lobe by the lateral sulcus *(5)*.

Figure 5–3 (Continued)   Coronal sections.

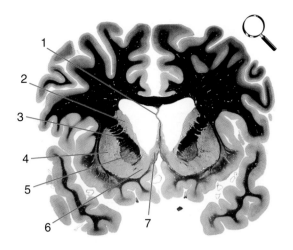

E, The globus pallidus *(5)* makes its appearance medial to the putamen *(4)*; the two together comprise the lenticular nucleus. Nucleus accumbens *(6)*, the region of continuity between the putamen and the head of the caudate nucleus, also is apparent. The septum pellucidum *(1)* is continuous with the septal nuclei *(7)*. (The proximity of the nucleus accumbens to the septal nuclei was reflected in its earlier but now outmoded name—nucleus accumbens septi, "the nucleus leaning against the septum.") The anterior limb of the internal capsule *(3)* still occupies the cleft between the lenticular nucleus and the head of the caudate nucleus *(2)*. Shown enlarged in Figure 5–4.

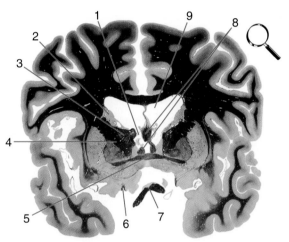

F, The level of the interventricular foramen *(1)* and anterior commissure *(5)* is a transition point for many structures, for example, from the head to the body of the caudate nucleus *(2)* and from the anterior horn to the body of the lateral ventricle *(9)*. This section shaves off the anterior end of the thalamus *(3)*, passes through the genu of the internal capsule *(4)*, and cuts the fornix twice *(8)* as it curves ventrally toward the hypothalamus. The olfactory tract *(6)* joins the base of the forebrain, and the optic chiasm *(7)* appears. Shown enlarged in Figure 5–5.

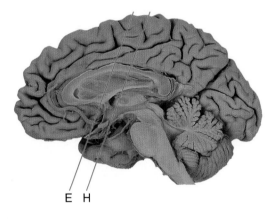

G, Anterior diencephalon. Characteristic diencephalic features include the third ventricle *(11)*, hypothalamus *(7)*, and thalamic nuclei—anterior *(1)* and ventral anterior *(2)*. The external *(3)* and internal *(4)* segments of the globus pallidus are apparent, as is the anterior end of the amygdala *(8)*. Fibers that cross in the anterior commissure *(5)* accumulate beneath the lenticular nucleus. The fornix is cut twice, through the body *(12)* and column *(9)*. The optic tract *(6)* and posterior limb of the internal capsule *(10)* also are present.

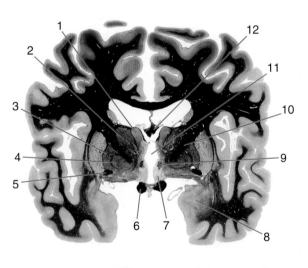

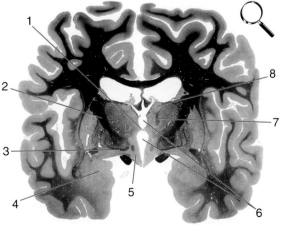

H, The mammillothalamic tract *(7)* enters the anterior nucleus *(8)* of the thalamus. The two thalami fuse at the interthalamic adhesion *(1)* or massa intermedia, which bridges the third ventricle *(6)*. The ansa lenticularis *(3,* literally the "handle of the lenticular nucleus") emerges from the inferior surface of the globus pallidus and hooks around the posterior limb of the internal capsule *(2)*. The amygdala *(4)* is larger, and the middle of the three zones of the hypothalamus (the tuberal zone, *5)* is present. Shown enlarged in Figure 5–6.

Illustration continued on following page

Figure 5–3 (Continued)   Coronal sections.

I, Additional efferents from the globus pallidus penetrate the posterior limb of the internal capsule (2) as the lenticular fasciculus and collect on the other side (1) before entering the thalamus. The column of the fornix (4) continues through the hypothalamus, where it soon ends in the mammillary body. The surface of the temporal lobe includes the superior (3), middle (5), and inferior (6) temporal gyri and the occipitotemporal (7) and parahippocampal (8) gyri. The amygdala (9) has reached nearly maximal size.

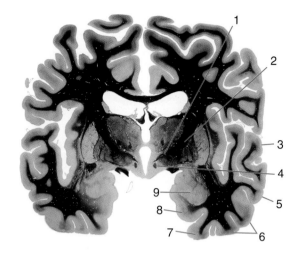

J, Midthalamus. The dorsomedial (2) and ventrolateral (3) nuclei are prominent at this level. The optic tract (6) proceeds posteriorly toward its thalamic termination in the lateral geniculate nucleus. The column of the fornix ends in the mammillary body (10), which gives rise to the mammillothalamic tract (9). The lateral ventricle is another in a series of forebrain structures to be cut twice, here through the body (1) and through the inferior horn (8), which has appeared adjacent to the amygdala (7). The putamen (4) and the globus pallidus (5) begin to get smaller.

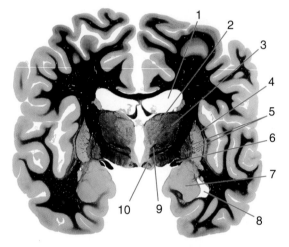

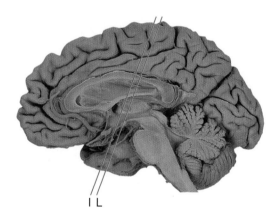

I L

K, Level of the mammillary bodies (6). Efferents from the globus pallidus and cerebellum collect beneath the thalamus in the thalamic fasciculus (2) before moving dorsally into the ventral lateral (1) and ventral anterior (see Fig. 5–3G) nuclei. The appropriately named subthalamic nucleus (3) appears beneath the thalamus. The amygdala (4) begins to get smaller, and the hippocampus (5) assumes a position adjacent to the inferior horn of the lateral ventricle. Shown enlarged in Figure 5–7.

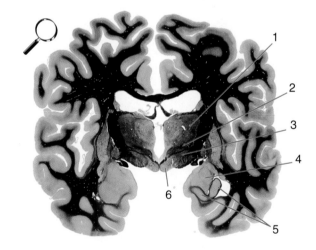

L, Brainstem structures begin to appear. The rostral end of the substantia nigra (8) is adjacent to the subthalamic nucleus (9). Many fibers in the posterior limb of the internal capsule (3) continue into the cerebral peduncle (7). Several structures are now cut twice, such as the body (1) and inferior horn (6) of the lateral ventricle and the body (2) and tail (4) of the caudate nucleus. The hippocampus (5) has almost completely replaced the amygdala on the right side of the section; the fornix (10), the principal output bundle of the hippocampus, proceeds anteriorly in its characteristic trajectory medial to the lateral ventricle.

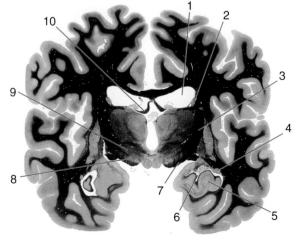

Figure 5–3 (Continued) Coronal sections.

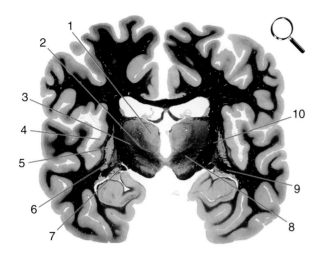

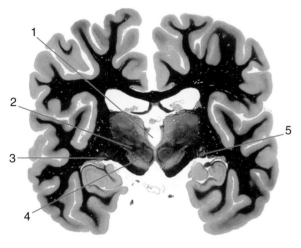

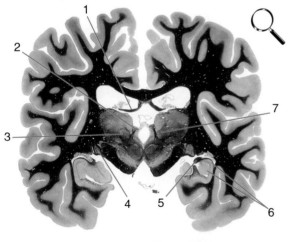

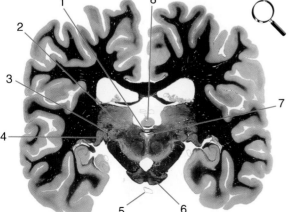

M, The dorsomedial *(1)*, ventral posteromedial *(2)*, and ventral posterolateral *(3)* nuclei now account for most of the thalamus. The putamen *(5)* and globus pallidus *(6)* continue to get smaller, as does the overlying insula *(4)*. Cerebellar efferents *(8)* proceed rostrally toward the ventral lateral nucleus of the thalamus (see Fig. 5–3K), and the optic tract *(7)* continues posteriorly toward the lateral geniculate nucleus. The posterior limb *(10)* and sublenticular part *(9)* of the internal capsule partially surround the lenticular nucleus. Shown enlarged in Figure 5–8.

N, Posterior to the lenticular nucleus, the third ventricle *(1)* is smaller as the plane of section gets closer to the cerebral aqueduct. Cerebellar efferents *(2)* that have passed through or around the red nucleus *(4)* collect beneath the thalamus. The optic tract *(3)* begins to terminate in the lateral geniculate nucleus *(5)* on the right side of the section.

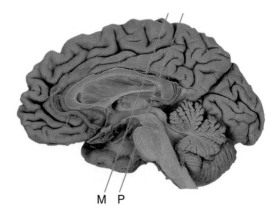

M P

O, Near the diencephalon-midbrain junction, the lateral geniculate nucleus *(4)* is present on both sides, and the largest of the thalamic intralaminar nuclei, the centromedian nucleus *(3)*, is apparent. The habenula *(2)* gives rise to the habenulointerpeduncular tract *(7)*. Fornix fibers are again cut twice, this time where they are suspended from the corpus callosum as the posterior part of the body *(1)*, and where they are still attached to the hippocampus *(6)* as the fimbria *(5)*. Shown enlarged in Figure 5–9.

P, Posterior commissure *(1)*, at the diencephalon-midbrain junction. The third ventricle has been replaced by the cerebral aqueduct *(7)*, and a bit of the basal pons *(6)* appears, accompanied by the basilar artery *(5)*. The only parts of the thalamus left are the pulvinar *(2)* and the medial *(3)* and lateral *(4)* geniculate nuclei. The pineal gland *(8)* is in the midline just above the posterior commissure. Shown enlarged in Figure 5–10.

Illustration continued on following page

Figure 5–3 (Continued)   Coronal sections.

Q, Posterior thalamus. Only the pulvinar *(6)* and the medial geniculate nucleus *(9)* remain. The plane of section approaches the posterior edge of C-shaped telencephalic structures, so the two parts of twice-cut structures draw closer together—the crus *(13)* and fimbria *(12)*, the body *(5)* and tail *(7)* of the caudate nucleus, the body *(4)* and inferior horn *(8)* of the lateral ventricle. Several brainstem structures are apparent, including the aqueduct *(2)* surrounded by periaqueductal gray *(3)*, the medial lemniscus *(10)*, and the crossed superior cerebellar peduncle *(11)*. The pineal gland *(1)* is still present above the most rostral part of the midbrain (the pretectal area). Shown enlarged in Figure 5–11.

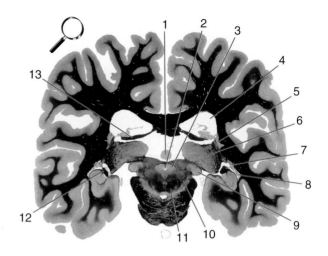

R, Splenium of the corpus callosum *(1)*. The section passes tangentially through the posterior edge of the caudate nucleus *(8)*, through fibers of the fornix as they pass from the fimbria *(5)* into the crus *(3)*, and through the lateral ventricle as the body *(4)* joins the inferior horn *(6)*. The superior colliculus *(9)* and the decussation of the superior cerebellar peduncles *(7)* can be seen in the brainstem. A little piece of the pulvinar *(2)* is all that remains of the thalamus. Shown enlarged in Figure 5–12.

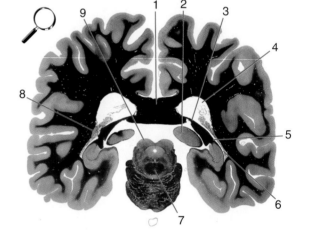

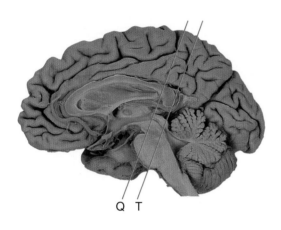

S, The section passes tangentially through the posterior end of the hippocampus *(3)* as it curves up underneath the splenium of the corpus callosum *(1)* and through the crus *(2)* of the fornix, the atrium *(5)* of the lateral ventricle, and the decussation of the superior cerebellar peduncles *(4)*.

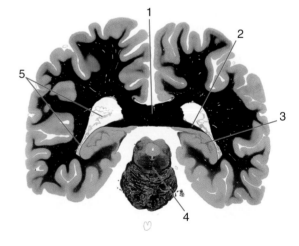

T, Posterior edge of the splenium of the corpus callosum *(1)*. The section passes through an enlarged mass of choroid plexus (the glomus, *7*) projecting back into the posterior horn of the lateral ventricle and through remnants of the hippocampus *(2)*. The cerebellar hemispheres *(4)* begin to appear, the lateral lemniscus *(3)* ends in the inferior colliculus *(6)*, and the trigeminal nerve *(5)* is attached to the pons.

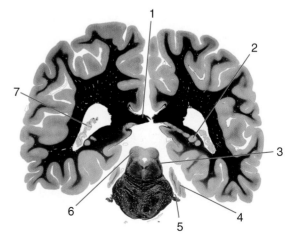

Figure 5–3 (Continued) Coronal sections.

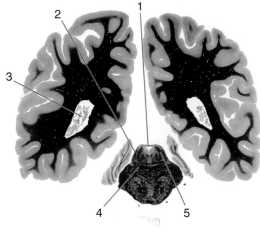

U, Choroid plexus *(3)* still protrudes into the posterior horn of the lateral ventricle. The aqueduct *(1)* begins to enlarge into the rostral part of the fourth ventricle. The lateral *(2)* and medial *(4)* lemnisci and the superior cerebellar peduncle *(5)* are apparent in the pons.

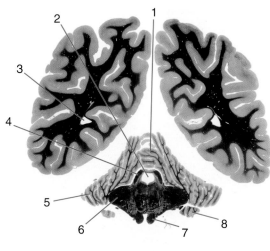

V, Last bit of the posterior horn of the lateral ventricle *(3)*. The cerebellar vermis *(1)*, hemispheres *(5)*, and flocculus *(8)* can be distinguished. The aqueduct has opened into the fourth ventricle *(2)*, and the superior *(4)* and middle *(6)* cerebellar peduncles and the pyramid *(7)* are present.

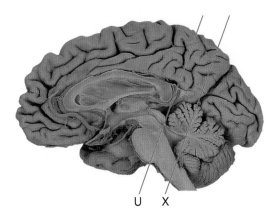

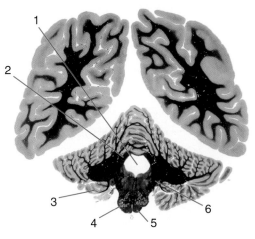

W, Pons and medulla. The fourth ventricle *(1)* is large, the pyramid *(5)* is massive, and the inferior olivary nucleus *(4)* is now present. The superior cerebellar peduncle *(2)* leaves the cerebellum, and the inferior cerebellar peduncle *(6)* enters. The cerebellar flocculus *(3)* is still located adjacent to the pontomedullary junction.

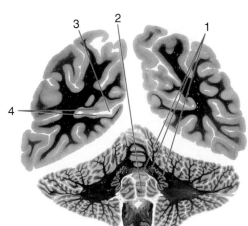

X, Deep cerebellar nuclei *(1)* and nodulus *(2)*. The calcarine sulcus *(3)*, with visual cortex in its upper and lower banks *(4)*, deeply indents the medial surface of the occipital lobe.

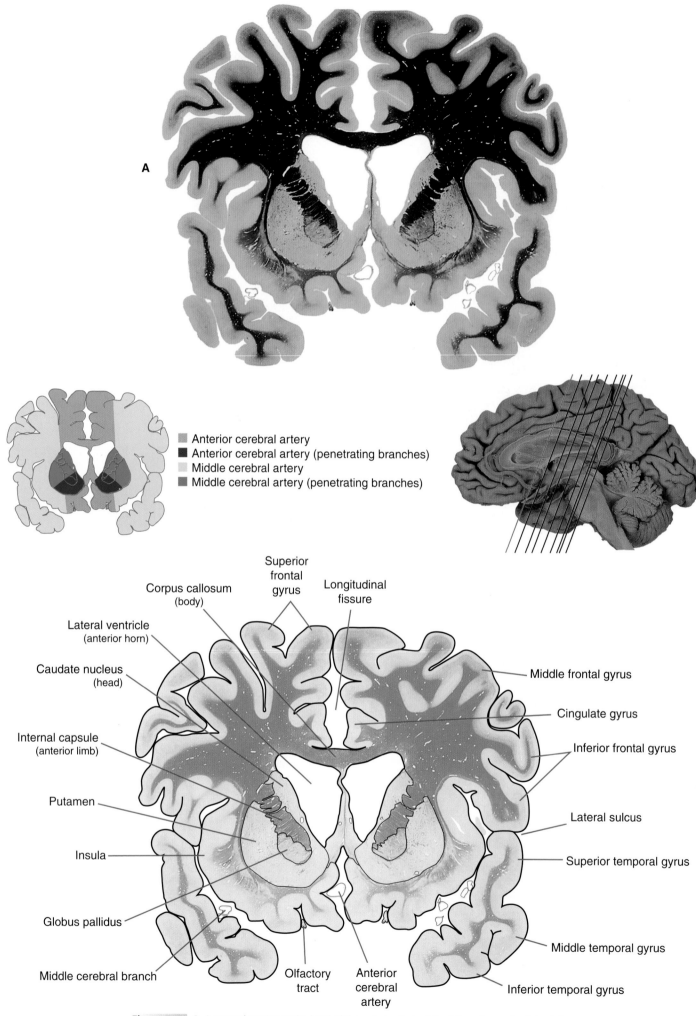

A

Anterior cerebral artery
Anterior cerebral artery (penetrating branches)
Middle cerebral artery
Middle cerebral artery (penetrating branches)

Corpus callosum (body)

Superior frontal gyrus

Longitudinal fissure

Lateral ventricle (anterior horn)

Caudate nucleus (head)

Internal capsule (anterior limb)

Putamen

Insula

Globus pallidus

Middle cerebral branch

Olfactory tract

Anterior cerebral artery

Middle frontal gyrus

Cingulate gyrus

Inferior frontal gyrus

Lateral sulcus

Superior temporal gyrus

Middle temporal gyrus

Inferior temporal gyrus

Figure 5–4   A, A coronal section at the level of the anterior limb of the internal capsule. Actual size.

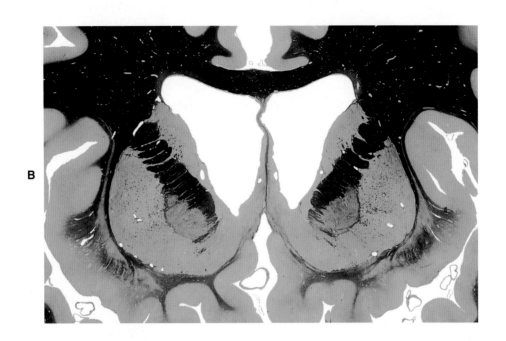

B

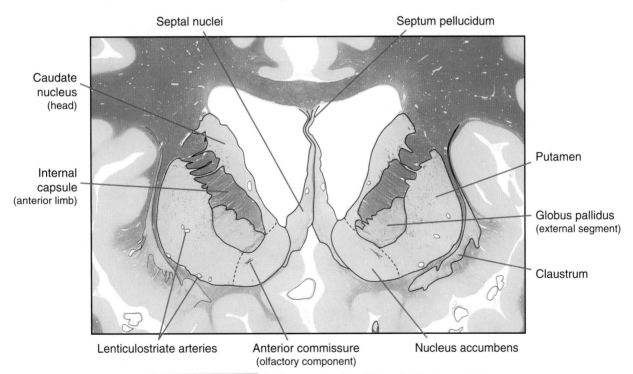

Septal nuclei   Septum pellucidum

Caudate
nucleus
(head)

Internal
capsule
(anterior limb)

Putamen

Globus pallidus
(external segment)

Claustrum

Lenticulostriate arteries   Anterior commissure   Nucleus accumbens
                                 (olfactory component)

Figure 5–4 (Continued)   **B,** The central region of Figure 5–4A, enlarged 1.5×.

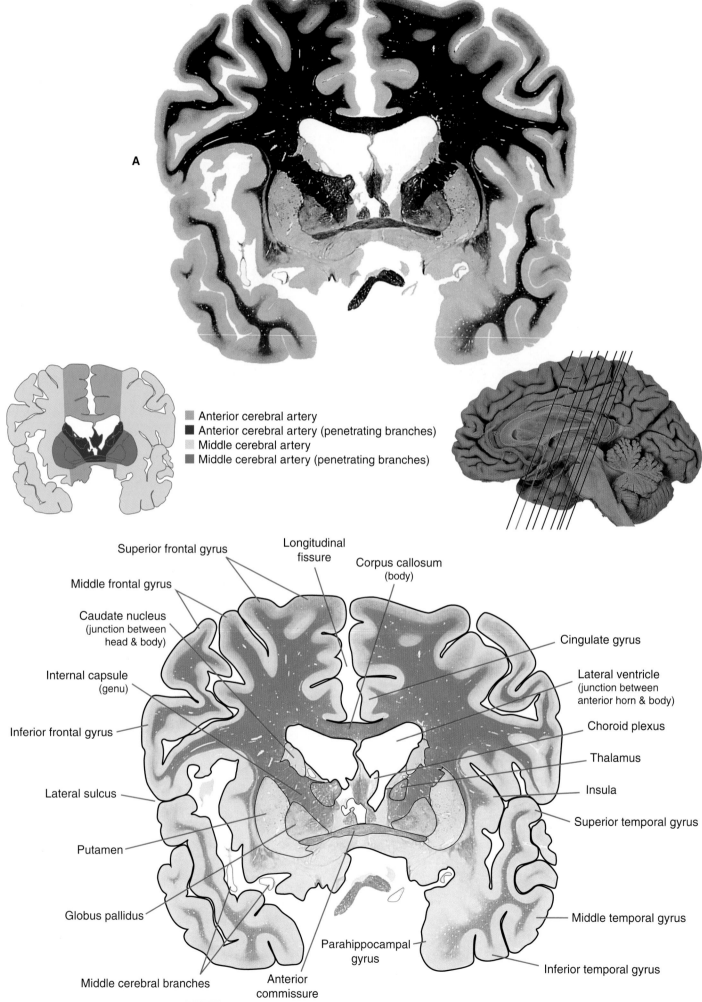

A

Anterior cerebral artery
Anterior cerebral artery (penetrating branches)
Middle cerebral artery
Middle cerebral artery (penetrating branches)

Superior frontal gyrus
Middle frontal gyrus
Caudate nucleus (junction between head & body)
Internal capsule (genu)
Inferior frontal gyrus
Lateral sulcus
Putamen
Globus pallidus
Middle cerebral branches

Longitudinal fissure
Corpus callosum (body)
Cingulate gyrus
Lateral ventricle (junction between anterior horn & body)
Choroid plexus
Thalamus
Insula
Superior temporal gyrus
Middle temporal gyrus
Inferior temporal gyrus
Parahippocampal gyrus
Anterior commissure

Figure 5–5   A, A coronal section at the level of the anterior commissure. Actual size.

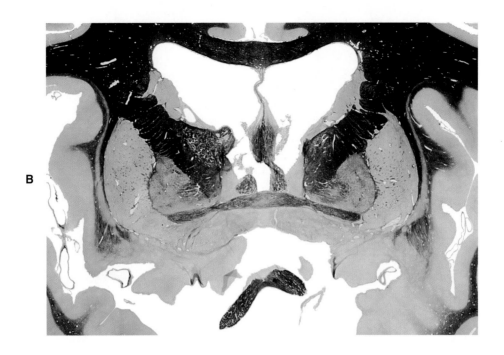

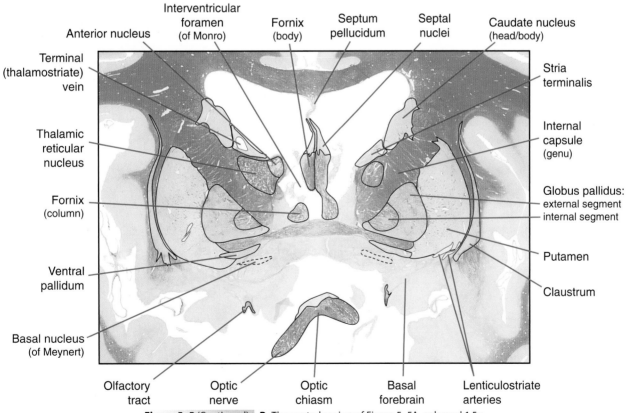

Figure 5–5 (Continued) **B,** The central region of Figure 5–5A, enlarged 1.5×.

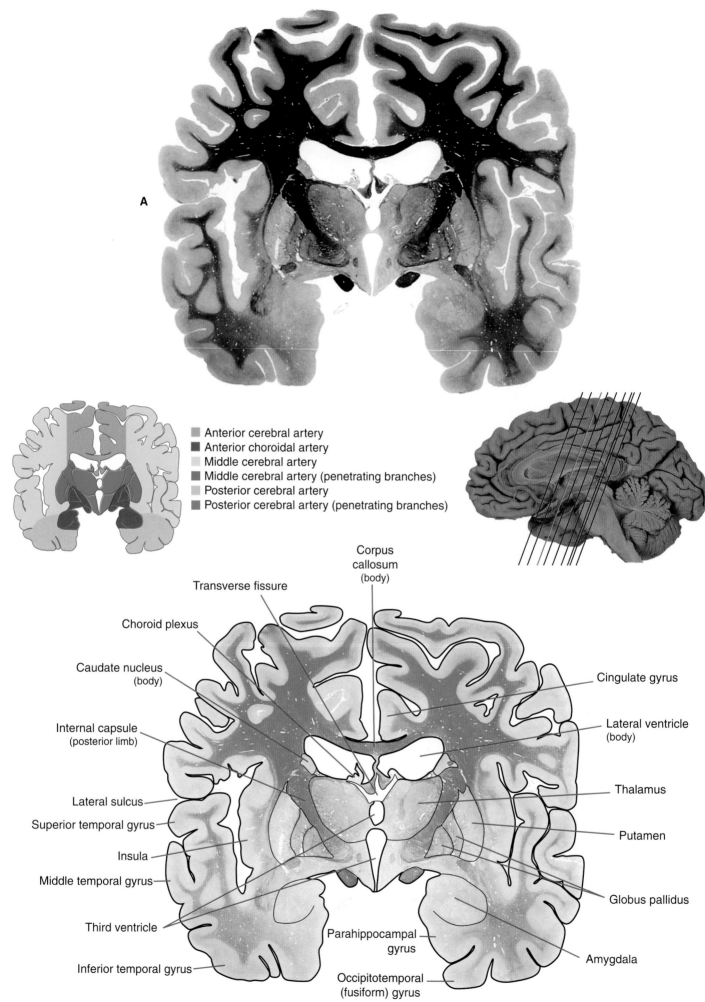

A

Anterior cerebral artery
Anterior choroidal artery
Middle cerebral artery
Middle cerebral artery (penetrating branches)
Posterior cerebral artery
Posterior cerebral artery (penetrating branches)

Corpus callosum (body)

Transverse fissure

Choroid plexus

Caudate nucleus (body)

Internal capsule (posterior limb)

Lateral sulcus

Superior temporal gyrus

Insula

Middle temporal gyrus

Third ventricle

Inferior temporal gyrus

Cingulate gyrus

Lateral ventricle (body)

Thalamus

Putamen

Globus pallidus

Amygdala

Parahippocampal gyrus

Occipitotemporal (fusiform) gyrus

Figure 5–6 **A,** A coronal section at the level of the ansa lenticularis and the anterior thalamus. Actual size.

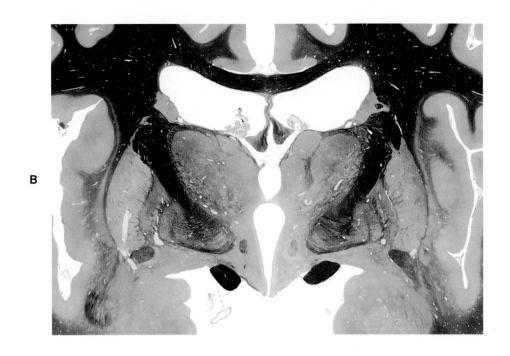

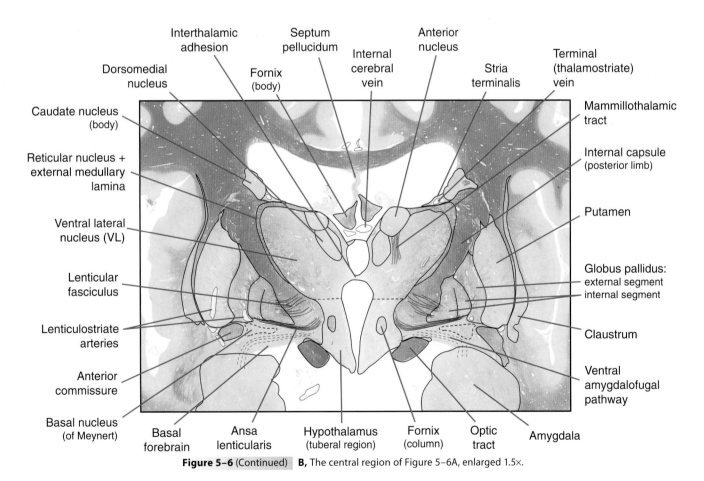

Figure 5–6 (Continued) **B,** The central region of Figure 5–6A, enlarged 1.5×.

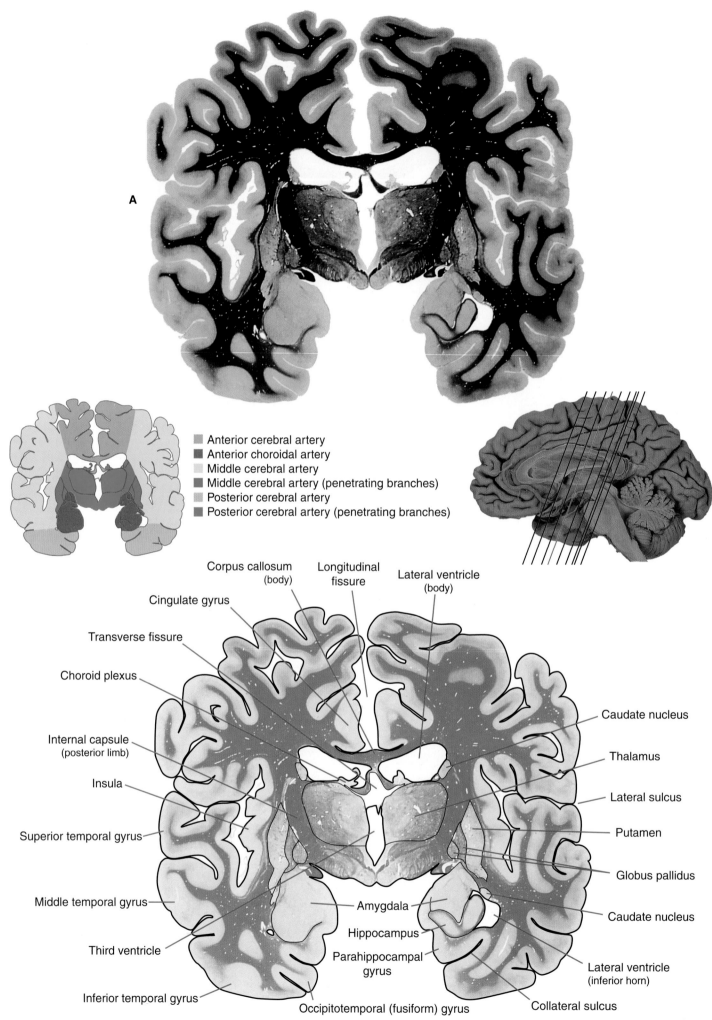

A

Anterior cerebral artery
Anterior choroidal artery
Middle cerebral artery
Middle cerebral artery (penetrating branches)
Posterior cerebral artery
Posterior cerebral artery (penetrating branches)

Corpus callosum (body)
Longitudinal fissure
Lateral ventricle (body)
Cingulate gyrus
Transverse fissure
Choroid plexus
Caudate nucleus
Internal capsule (posterior limb)
Thalamus
Insula
Lateral sulcus
Superior temporal gyrus
Putamen
Globus pallidus
Middle temporal gyrus
Caudate nucleus
Amygdala
Third ventricle
Hippocampus
Parahippocampal gyrus
Lateral ventricle (inferior horn)
Inferior temporal gyrus
Occipitotemporal (fusiform) gyrus
Collateral sulcus

Figure 5–7   **A,** A coronal section at the level of the mammillary bodies. Actual size.

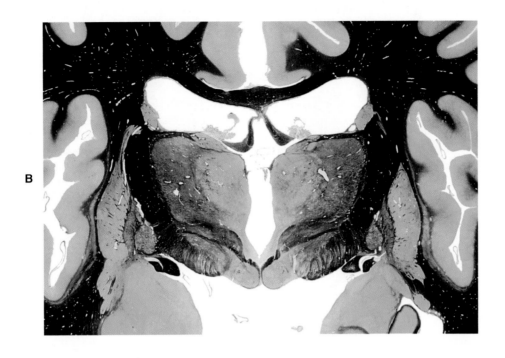

B

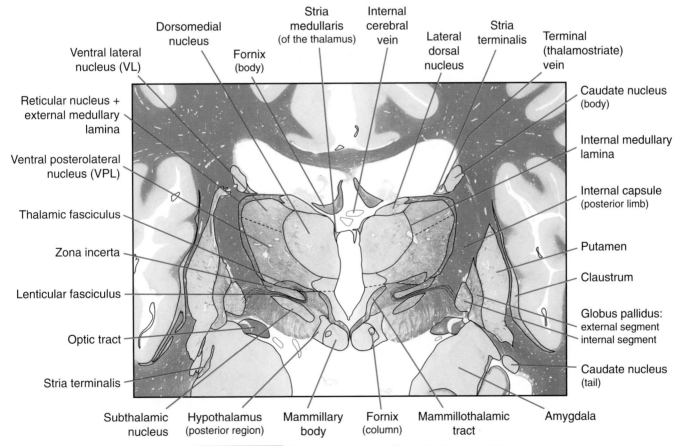

Dorsomedial nucleus

Stria medullaris (of the thalamus)

Internal cerebral vein

Lateral dorsal nucleus

Stria terminalis

Terminal (thalamostriate) vein

Ventral lateral nucleus (VL)

Fornix (body)

Reticular nucleus + external medullary lamina

Ventral posterolateral nucleus (VPL)

Thalamic fasciculus

Zona incerta

Lenticular fasciculus

Optic tract

Stria terminalis

Caudate nucleus (body)

Internal medullary lamina

Internal capsule (posterior limb)

Putamen

Claustrum

Globus pallidus: external segment internal segment

Caudate nucleus (tail)

Subthalamic nucleus

Hypothalamus (posterior region)

Mammillary body

Fornix (column)

Mammillothalamic tract

Amygdala

Figure 5–7 (Continued) **B,** The central region of Figure 5–7A, enlarged 1.5×.

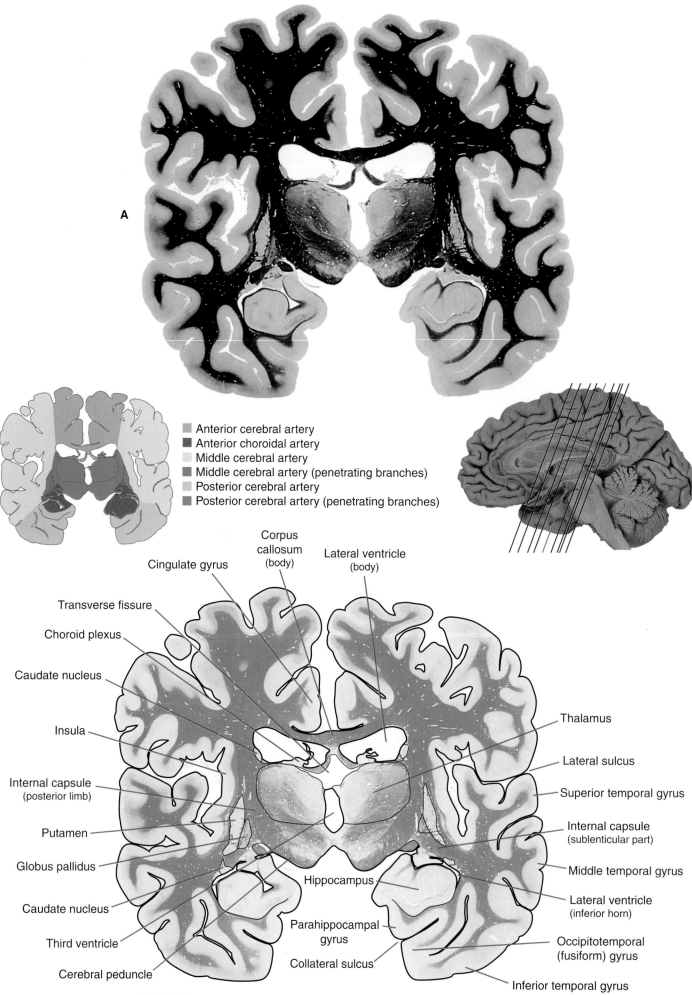

A

Anterior cerebral artery
Anterior choroidal artery
Middle cerebral artery
Middle cerebral artery (penetrating branches)
Posterior cerebral artery
Posterior cerebral artery (penetrating branches)

Corpus callosum (body)

Cingulate gyrus

Lateral ventricle (body)

Transverse fissure

Choroid plexus

Caudate nucleus

Insula

Thalamus

Internal capsule (posterior limb)

Lateral sulcus

Superior temporal gyrus

Putamen

Internal capsule (sublenticular part)

Globus pallidus

Middle temporal gyrus

Hippocampus

Caudate nucleus

Lateral ventricle (inferior horn)

Third ventricle

Parahippocampal gyrus

Occipitotemporal (fusiform) gyrus

Cerebral peduncle

Collateral sulcus

Inferior temporal gyrus

Figure 5–8   A, A coronal section at the level of the anterior end of the hippocampus. Actual size.

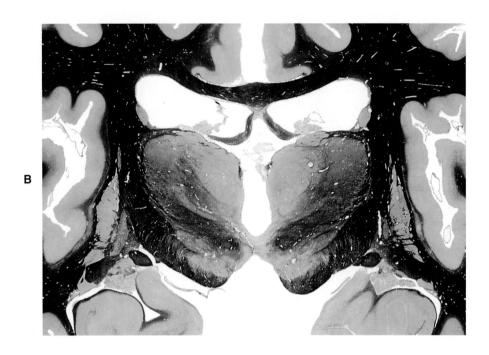

B

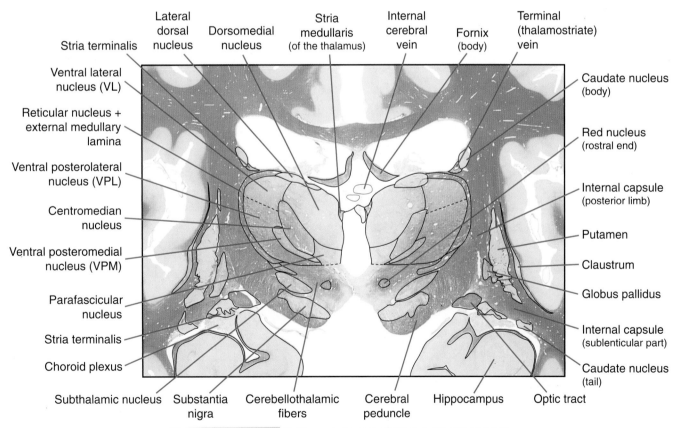

Stria terminalis

Lateral dorsal nucleus

Dorsomedial nucleus

Stria medullaris (of the thalamus)

Internal cerebral vein

Fornix (body)

Terminal (thalamostriate) vein

Ventral lateral nucleus (VL)

Reticular nucleus + external medullary lamina

Ventral posterolateral nucleus (VPL)

Centromedian nucleus

Ventral posteromedial nucleus (VPM)

Parafascicular nucleus

Stria terminalis

Choroid plexus

Caudate nucleus (body)

Red nucleus (rostral end)

Internal capsule (posterior limb)

Putamen

Claustrum

Globus pallidus

Internal capsule (sublenticular part)

Caudate nucleus (tail)

Subthalamic nucleus

Substantia nigra

Cerebellothalamic fibers

Cerebral peduncle

Hippocampus

Optic tract

Figure 5-8 (Continued)   **B,** The central region of Figure 5–8A, enlarged 1.5×.

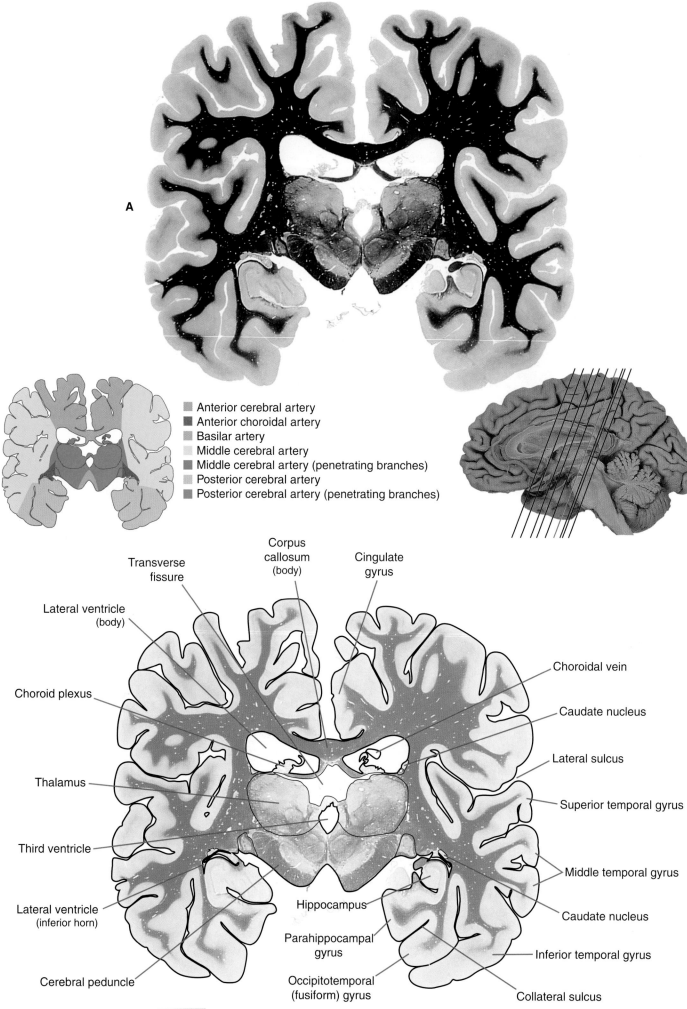

A

Anterior cerebral artery
Anterior choroidal artery
Basilar artery
Middle cerebral artery
Middle cerebral artery (penetrating branches)
Posterior cerebral artery
Posterior cerebral artery (penetrating branches)

Transverse fissure

Corpus callosum (body)

Cingulate gyrus

Lateral ventricle (body)

Choroid plexus

Thalamus

Third ventricle

Lateral ventricle (inferior horn)

Cerebral peduncle

Hippocampus

Parahippocampal gyrus

Occipitotemporal (fusiform) gyrus

Choroidal vein

Caudate nucleus

Lateral sulcus

Superior temporal gyrus

Middle temporal gyrus

Caudate nucleus

Inferior temporal gyrus

Collateral sulcus

Figure 5–9   A, A coronal section through the posterior third of the thalamus. Actual size.

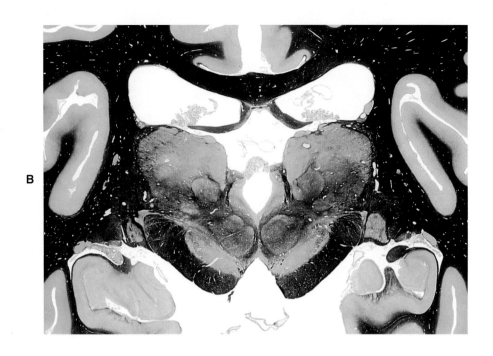

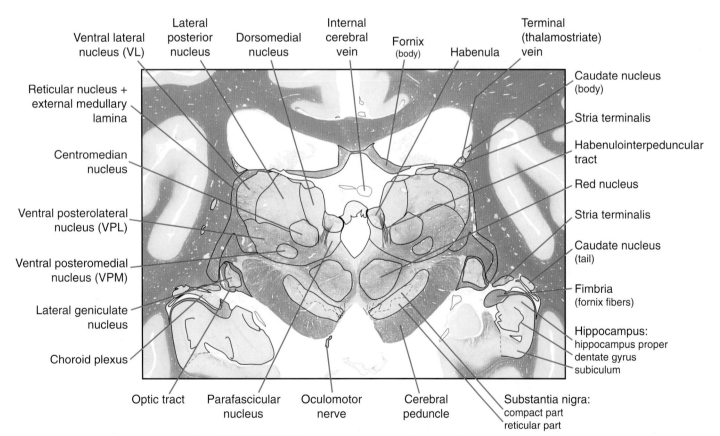

Figure 5–9 (Continued) **B,** The central region of Figure 5–9A, enlarged 1.5×.

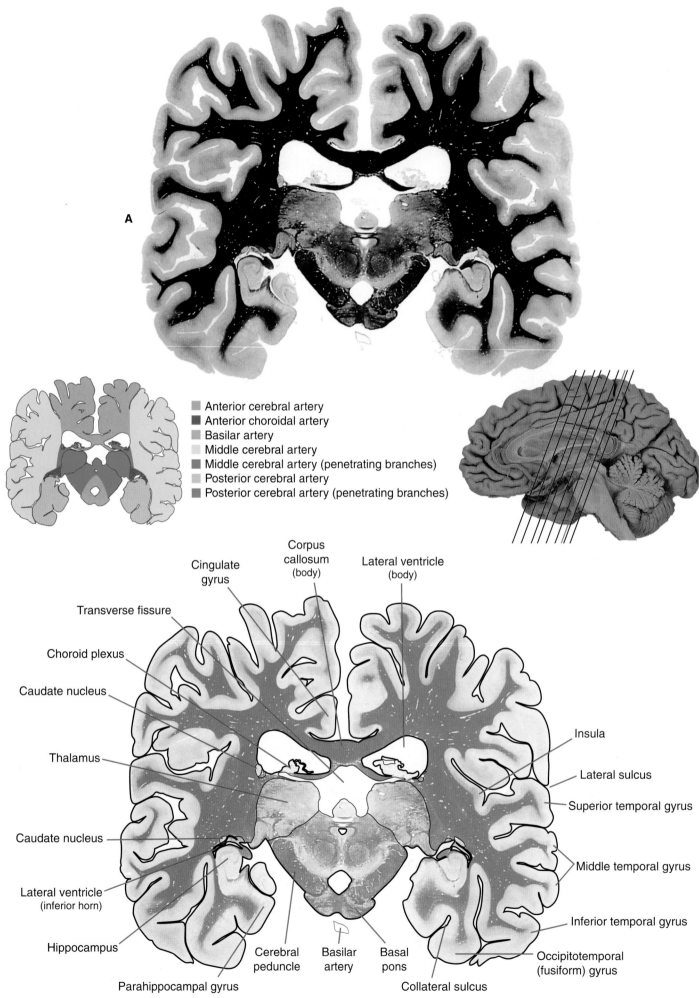

A

Anterior cerebral artery
Anterior choroidal artery
Basilar artery
Middle cerebral artery
Middle cerebral artery (penetrating branches)
Posterior cerebral artery
Posterior cerebral artery (penetrating branches)

Cingulate gyrus

Corpus callosum (body)

Lateral ventricle (body)

Transverse fissure

Choroid plexus

Caudate nucleus

Thalamus

Caudate nucleus

Lateral ventricle (inferior horn)

Hippocampus

Parahippocampal gyrus

Cerebral peduncle

Basilar artery

Basal pons

Collateral sulcus

Insula

Lateral sulcus

Superior temporal gyrus

Middle temporal gyrus

Inferior temporal gyrus

Occipitotemporal (fusiform) gyrus

Figure 5–10   **A,** A coronal section at the level of the posterior commissure. Actual size.

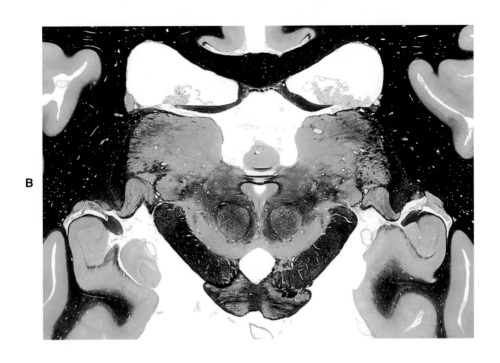

B

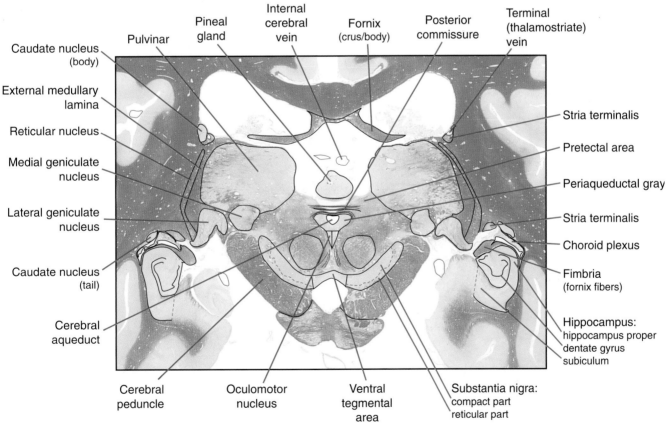

Caudate nucleus
(body)

External medullary
lamina

Reticular nucleus

Medial geniculate
nucleus

Lateral geniculate
nucleus

Caudate nucleus
(tail)

Cerebral
aqueduct

Pulvinar

Pineal
gland

Internal
cerebral
vein

Fornix
(crus/body)

Posterior
commissure

Terminal
(thalamostriate)
vein

Stria terminalis

Pretectal area

Periaqueductal gray

Stria terminalis

Choroid plexus

Fimbria
(fornix fibers)

Hippocampus:
hippocampus proper
dentate gyrus
subiculum

Cerebral
peduncle

Oculomotor
nucleus

Ventral
tegmental
area

Substantia nigra:
compact part
reticular part

Figure 5–10 (Continued)   **B,** The central region of Figure 5–10A, enlarged 1.5×.

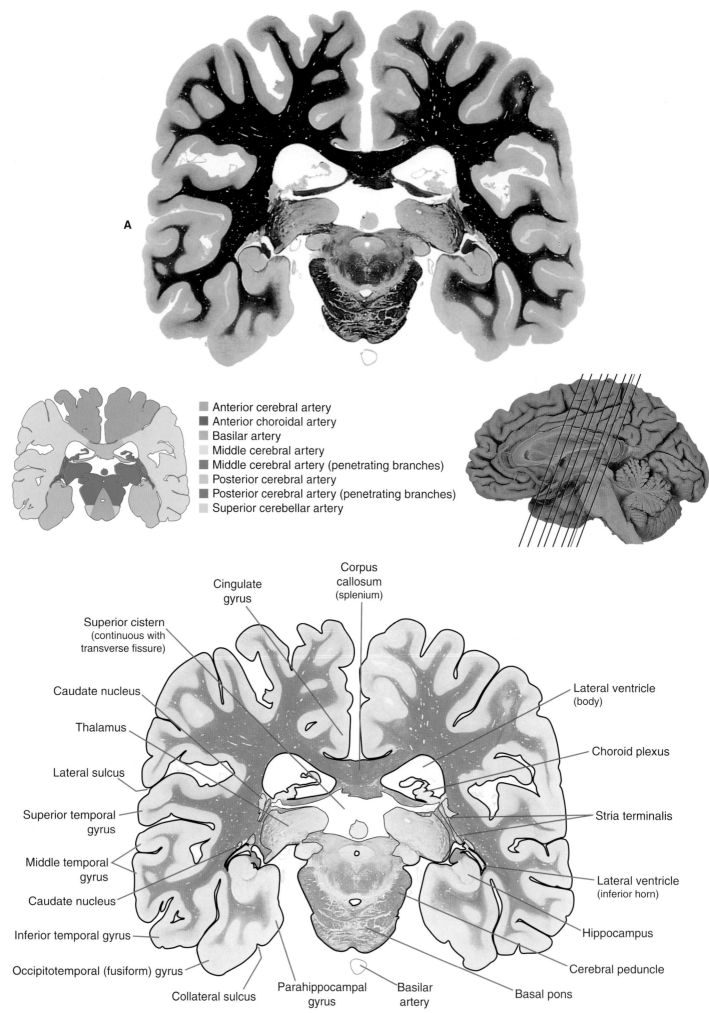

A

Anterior cerebral artery
Anterior choroidal artery
Basilar artery
Middle cerebral artery
Middle cerebral artery (penetrating branches)
Posterior cerebral artery
Posterior cerebral artery (penetrating branches)
Superior cerebellar artery

Cingulate gyrus

Corpus callosum (splenium)

Superior cistern (continuous with transverse fissure)

Caudate nucleus

Thalamus

Lateral sulcus

Superior temporal gyrus

Middle temporal gyrus

Caudate nucleus

Inferior temporal gyrus

Occipitotemporal (fusiform) gyrus

Collateral sulcus

Parahippocampal gyrus

Basilar artery

Lateral ventricle (body)

Choroid plexus

Stria terminalis

Lateral ventricle (inferior horn)

Hippocampus

Cerebral peduncle

Basal pons

Figure 5-11   A, A coronal section that passes tangentially through the stria terminalis. Actual size.

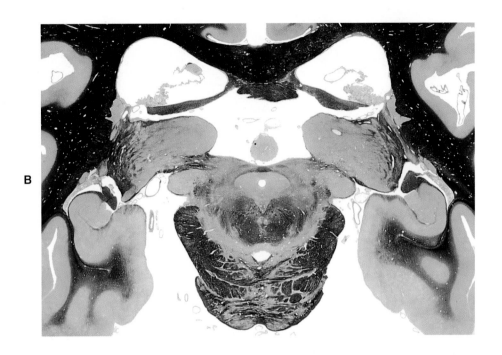

B

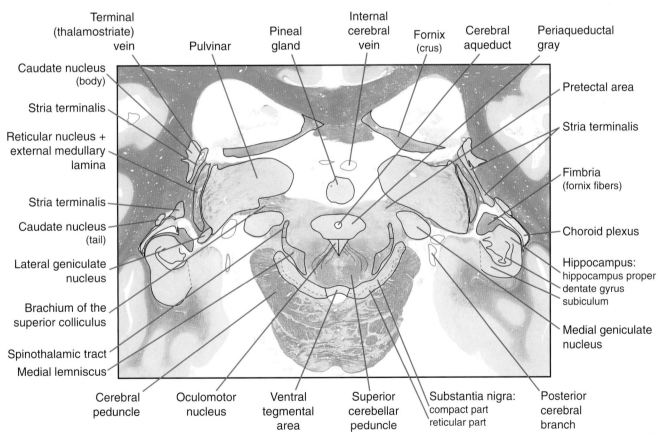

Terminal
(thalamostriate)
vein

Pulvinar

Pineal
gland

Internal
cerebral
vein

Fornix
(crus)

Cerebral
aqueduct

Periaqueductal
gray

Caudate nucleus
(body)

Stria terminalis

Reticular nucleus +
external medullary
lamina

Stria terminalis

Caudate nucleus
(tail)

Lateral geniculate
nucleus

Brachium of the
superior colliculus

Spinothalamic tract

Medial lemniscus

Pretectal area

Stria terminalis

Fimbria
(fornix fibers)

Choroid plexus

Hippocampus:
hippocampus proper
dentate gyrus
subiculum

Medial geniculate
nucleus

Cerebral
peduncle

Oculomotor
nucleus

Ventral
tegmental
area

Superior
cerebellar
peduncle

Substantia nigra:
compact part
reticular part

Posterior
cerebral
branch

Figure 5–11 (Continued)   **B,** The central region of Figure 5–11A, enlarged 1.5×.

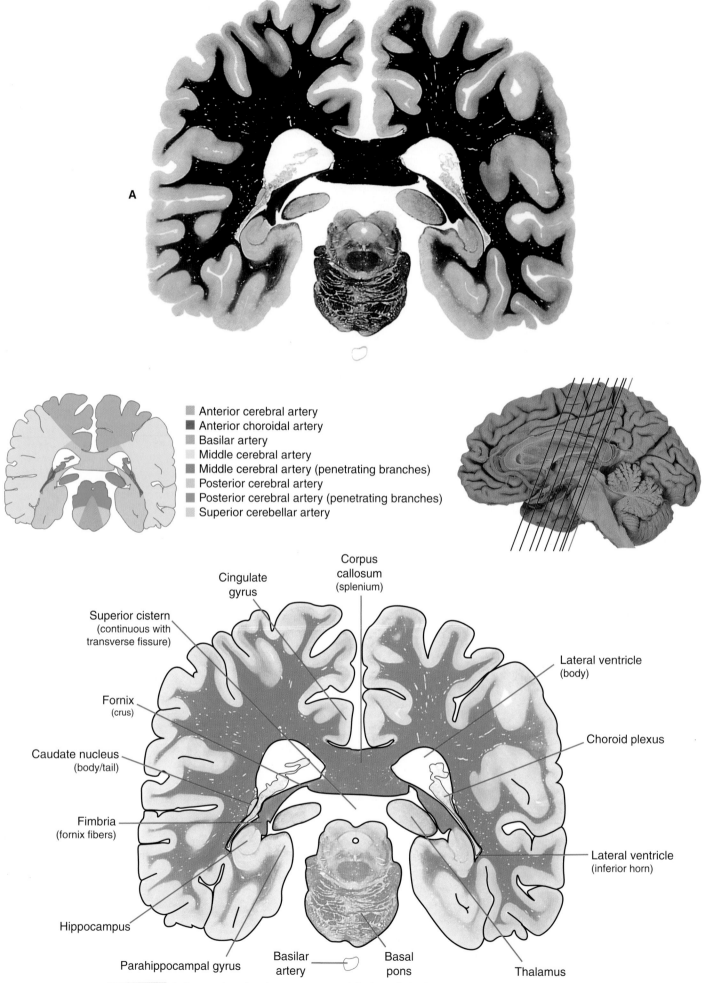

A

Anterior cerebral artery
Anterior choroidal artery
Basilar artery
Middle cerebral artery
Middle cerebral artery (penetrating branches)
Posterior cerebral artery
Posterior cerebral artery (penetrating branches)
Superior cerebellar artery

Cingulate gyrus

Corpus callosum (splenium)

Superior cistern (continuous with transverse fissure)

Lateral ventricle (body)

Fornix (crus)

Caudate nucleus (body/tail)

Choroid plexus

Fimbria (fornix fibers)

Lateral ventricle (inferior horn)

Hippocampus

Parahippocampal gyrus

Basilar artery

Basal pons

Thalamus

Figure 5-12   **A,** A coronal section that passes tangentially through the fornix and caudate nucleus. Actual size.

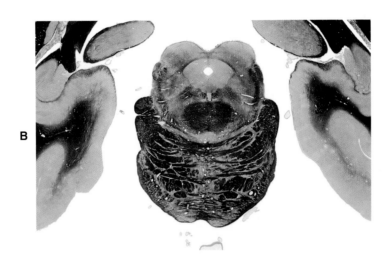

B

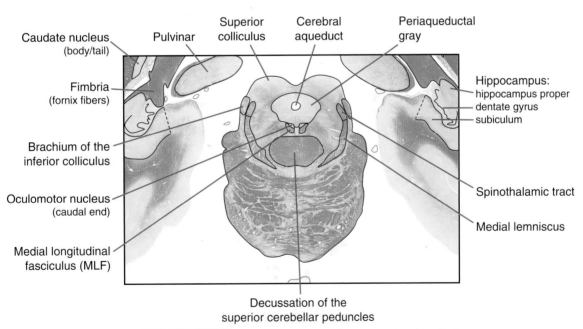

Caudate nucleus
(body/tail)

Pulvinar

Superior
colliculus

Cerebral
aqueduct

Periaqueductal
gray

Fimbria
(fornix fibers)

Brachium of the
inferior colliculus

Oculomotor nucleus
(caudal end)

Medial longitudinal
fasciculus (MLF)

Hippocampus:
hippocampus proper
dentate gyrus
subiculum

Spinothalamic tract

Medial lemniscus

Decussation of the
superior cerebellar peduncles

Figure 5–12 (Continued)   **B,** The central region of Figure 5–12A, enlarged 1.5×.

Horizontal Sections

6

This chapter, the second of three showing sections of entire human brains, illustrates approximately horizontal planes. Forebrain structures continue to be emphasized, but parts of the brainstem and cerebellum are indicated as well. The organization of various functional systems in the forebrain (e.g., thalamus, hippocampus) is presented in Chapter 8.

Drawings showing typical areas of arterial supply in each section are provided in this chapter and Chapters 5 and 7. We have simplified these in two major ways. First, arterial territories are shown as sharply demarcated from each other, when in reality there is significant interdigitation and overlap. Second, penetrating arteries arise from all the vessels of the circle of Willis; however, we have incorporated those from the anterior and posterior communicating arteries with those from the anterior and posterior cerebral arteries.

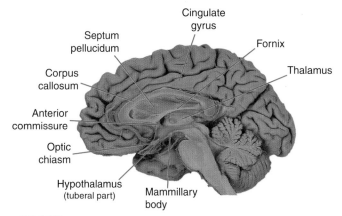

Figure 6–1 The hemisected brain from Figure 1–6, used in much of this chapter to indicate planes of section.

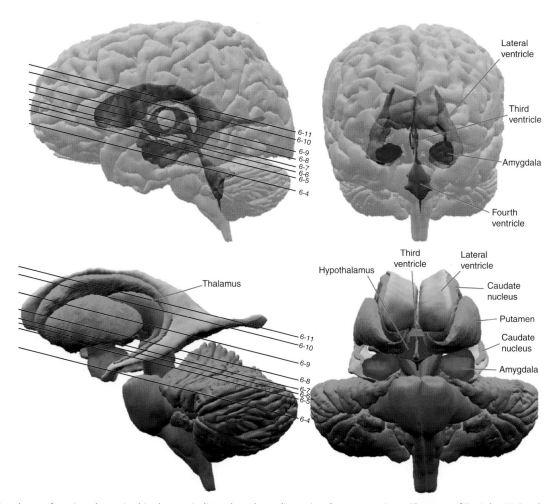

Figure 6–2 The planes of section shown in this chapter, indicated on three-dimensional reconstructions. *(Courtesy of Dr. John W. Sundsten, Department of Biological Structure, University of Washington School of Medicine.)*

Figure 6-3   A–X, Twenty-four horizontal sections of a brain, arranged in an inferior-to-superior sequence extending from the orbital surface of the frontal lobe to just above the corpus callosum. Anterior is toward the top, as in the conventional orientation of computed tomography (CT) and magnetic resonance imaging (MRI).

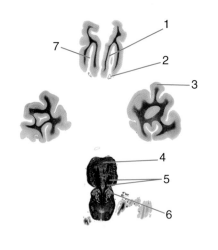

A, The first section just reaches the orbital surface of the frontal lobe, including gyrus rectus (1), and passes through the olfactory sulcus (7) and olfactory tract (2). The temporal pole (3) also can be seen. The brainstem is cut at an odd angle in these sections, with more rostral parts toward the top. This section passes through the basal pons (4) and the inferior olivary nucleus (6) of the medulla. The corticospinal tract (5) can be seen passing from the basal pons into the medullary pyramid.

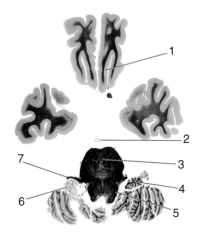

B, Gyrus rectus (1) is still present and is now joined by a little more of the orbital frontal cortex. The section again passes through the basal pons (3) and the basilar artery (2) anterior to it and parts of the rostral medulla. It includes the cerebellar flocculus (4), the inferior cerebellar peduncle (5), the vestibulocochlear (7) nerve, and choroid plexus (6) in the lateral aperture of the fourth ventricle.

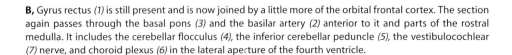

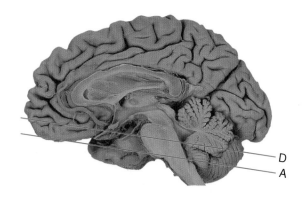

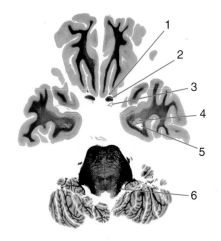

C, The olfactory tract (1) has reached the posterior end of the olfactory sulcus, near where it attaches to the base of the forebrain. The optic nerve (2) moves posteriorly toward the optic chiasm; the internal carotid artery (3) is just lateral to where the optic chiasm will soon be located. The inferior horn of the lateral ventricle (5) and adjacent amygdala (4) begin to appear in the temporal lobe. The inferior cerebellar peduncle (6) turns posteriorly toward the cerebellum.

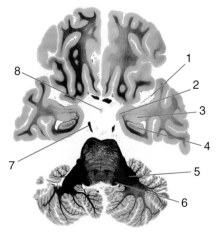

D, The middle cerebral artery (1) moves laterally into the lateral sulcus. The amygdala (3) is larger, and the hippocampus (4) appears; both structures underlie the uncus (2). The plane of section moves closer to the hypothalamus and passes through the infundibulum (8). The middle cerebellar peduncle (5) connects the basal pons to the cerebellum. The inferior cerebellar peduncle (6) has completed its posterior turn and is cut in cross section as it moves into the cerebellum. The abducens nerve (7) moves anteriorly from its point of emergence from the brainstem.

Figure 6–3 (Continued)   Horizontal sections.

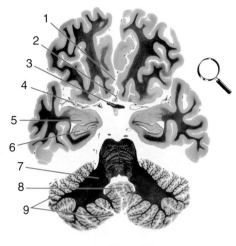

E, The anterior cerebral artery *(2)* moves into the longitudinal fissure *(1)*, and the middle cerebral artery *(4)* continues on its course toward the insula. The optic nerves partially decussate in the optic chiasm *(3)*. The amygdala *(5)* and hippocampus *(6)* continue to increase in size. The cerebellar vermis *(8)* and hemispheres *(9)* can be distinguished, and the middle cerebellar peduncle *(7)* still connects the basal pons to the cerebellum. Shown enlarged in Figure 6–4.

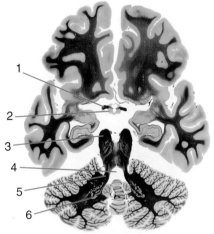

F, The optic tract *(1)* begins to move posteriorly from the optic chiasm, and the plane of section reaches the tuberal zone of the hypothalamus *(2)*. The superior cerebellar peduncle *(5)* leaves the deep cerebellar nuclei, represented here by the dentate nucleus *(6)*, forms part of the wall of the fourth ventricle *(4)*, and enters the pons. The first part of the midbrain to appear in this plane of section is the cerebral peduncle *(3)*.

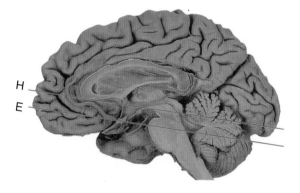

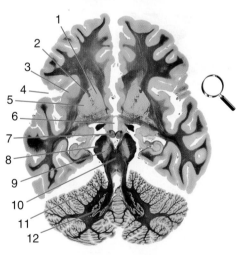

G, The base of the forebrain, beginning to pass through the head of the caudate nucleus *(1)*, the putamen *(5)*, and the anterior limb of the internal capsule *(2)*. The insula *(3)*, buried in the lateral sulcus *(4)*, overlies the putamen. The mammillary bodies *(7)* and other parts of the hypothalamus border the third ventricle *(6)*. The cerebral peduncle *(8)* and substantia nigra *(9)* are apparent in the midbrain. The superior cerebellar peduncle *(11)* leaves the dentate nucleus *(12)*, enters the brainstem, and decussates *(10)*. Shown enlarged in Figure 6–5.

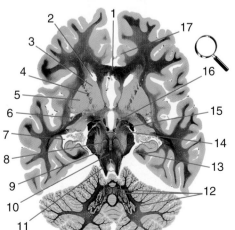

H, The lateral ventricle is cut twice, through the anterior *(2)* and inferior *(7)* horns, and the corpus callosum *(1)* makes its first appearance. The limbic lobe also is cut twice, through the cingulate *(17)* and parahippocampal *(13)* gyri. The head of the caudate nucleus *(3)*, the putamen *(5)*, and the anterior limb of the internal capsule *(4)* all increase in size. Fibers that cross in the anterior commissure *(6)* begin to move toward the midline, and the optic tract *(15)* continues to move posteriorly. The column of the fornix *(16)* and the mammillothalamic tract *(14)* are transected just above each mammillary body. All of the deep cerebellar nuclei *(12)* are now apparent. Most efferents from these nuclei travel through the superior cerebellar peduncle *(11)* and decussate *(10)*, and then most of them *(9)* pass through or around the red nucleus *(8)*. Shown enlarged in Figure 6–6.

Illustration continued on following page

Figure 6–3 (Continued) Horizontal sections.

I, The subcallosal gyrus *(1)*, the last bit of limbic cortex adjacent to the corpus callosum, borders the longitudinal fissure *(12)*. The head of the caudate nucleus *(2)* continues; both parts of the lenticular nucleus—the putamen *(3)* and the globus pallidus *(4)*—are apparent, and the subthalamic nucleus *(5)* can be seen just across the internal capsule from the globus pallidus. Fornix fibers are cut twice, once through the fimbria *(8)* as it leaves the hippocampus *(7)* and again through the column of the fornix *(10)* as it approaches the mammillary body. The mammillothalamic tract *(9)* continues on its course toward the anterior nucleus of the thalamus. Fibers of the anterior commissure *(11)* cross the midline. The dentate nucleus *(6)* is the only deep cerebellar nucleus remaining.

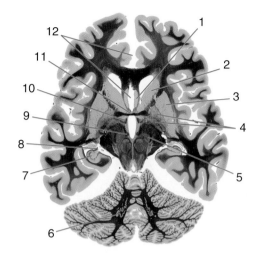

J, The section passes tangentially through the corpus callosum as the genu *(1)* tapers into the rostrum *(2)*. The anterior commissure *(3)*, column of the fornix *(4)*, and subthalamic nucleus *(5)* are still visible, and the inferior colliculus *(6)* appears. Shown enlarged in Figure 6–7.

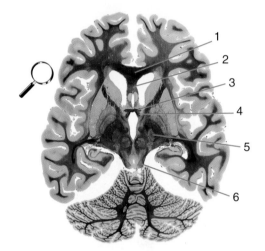

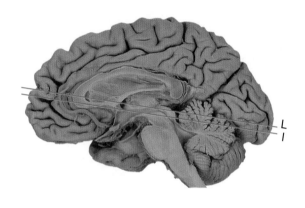

K, The septum pellucidum *(1)*, merging with the septal nuclei *(2)*, succeeds the rostrum of the corpus callosum. The lateral *(3)* and medial *(4)* geniculate nuclei (the most inferior parts of the thalamus) can be seen, and the continuity of the third ventricle *(6)* and the cerebral aqueduct *(5)* is apparent.

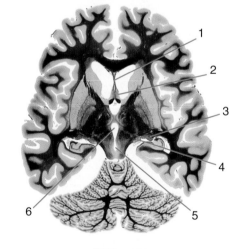

L, Choroid plexus *(1)* passes through each interventricular foramen adjacent to the body of the fornix *(10)*. Four of the five parts of the internal capsule—the anterior limb *(2)*, genu *(3)*, posterior limb *(4)*, and retrolenticular part *(5)*—are present, as is much more of the thalamus *(6)*. The mammillothalamic tract *(9)* continues on its path toward the anterior nucleus of the thalamus. The posterior commissure *(7)* crosses the midline near the periaqueductal gray *(8)*. Shown enlarged in Figure 6–8.

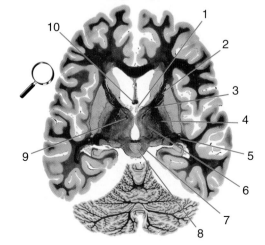

Figure 6–3 (Continued) Horizontal sections.

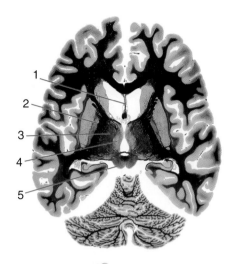

M, The septum pellucidum *(1)* still separates the anterior horns of the two lateral ventricles from each other. The globus pallidus *(2)* gets smaller as the plane of section moves superiorly through the lenticular nucleus. Lateral *(3)* and medial *(4)* divisions of the thalamus can be distinguished because of differences in the numbers of myelinated fibers entering and leaving them. The superior colliculus *(5)* appears in the midbrain.

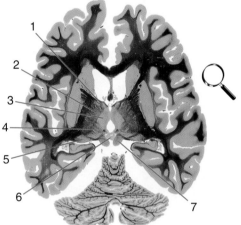

N, More parts of the thalamus can be seen: the lateral *(2)* and medial *(3)* divisions, the anterior *(1)* and centromedian *(4)* nuclei, and the pulvinar *(5)*. (The mammillothalamic tract has terminated in the anterior nucleus and is no longer visible.) The pineal gland *(6)* protrudes posteriorly between the superior colliculi *(7)*. Shown enlarged in Figure 6–9.

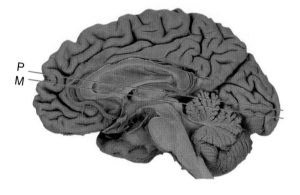

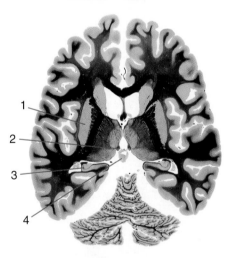

O, The plane of section is above the globus pallidus, and the putamen *(1)* begins to get smaller. The stria medullaris of the thalamus terminates in the habenula *(2)*. The hippocampus *(3)* and pineal gland *(4)* are still apparent.

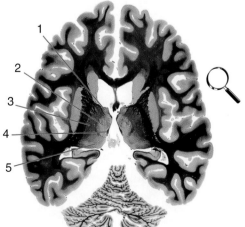

P, In the thalamus, lateral *(3)* and medial *(2)* divisions, the anterior nucleus *(1)*, and the pulvinar *(5)* can still be distinguished. Fibers travel posteriorly in the stria medullaris *(4)* of the thalamus toward the habenula. Shown enlarged in Figure 6–10.

Illustration continued on following page

Figure 6–3 (Continued)   Horizontal sections.

Q, The putamen *(3)* continues to get smaller, as does the overlying insula *(4)*. As the plane of section moves upward through the cerebral hemisphere, the profiles of twice-cut structures, such as the lateral ventricle *(1, 6)* and fornix fibers *(2, 5)*, draw progressively closer to each other until these C-shaped structures are finally cut tangentially (e.g., *T, V*).

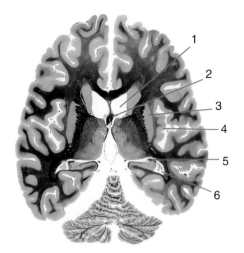

R, Near the top of the putamen *(3)* and internal capsule *(2)*. The fornix *(1)* is now cut obliquely as it begins to curve downward toward the interventricular foramen. Although the thalamus *(4)* begins to get smaller, medial and lateral divisions, the anterior nucleus, and the pulvinar can still be distinguished.

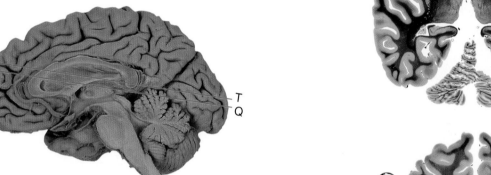

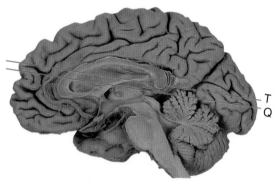

S, Just below the splenium of the corpus callosum and completely above the putamen. The head of the caudate nucleus *(1)* begins to taper into the body of the caudate nucleus, and the posterior part of the hippocampus *(5)* has a distinctive pattern of folding (compare with *R*). The plane of section still passes through the inferior horn *(4)*, but soon enters the atrium and posterior horn of the lateral ventricle. The fornix *(2)* is cut obliquely again. The internal cerebral vein *(3)* travels posteriorly toward the great cerebral vein. Enlarged in Figure 6–11.

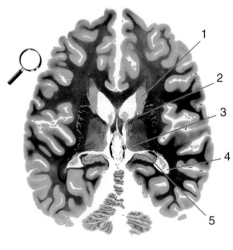

T, The corpus callosum is cut twice, through the body *(9)* and the splenium *(4)*. The thalamus *(3)* continues to dwindle, the distinctive appearance of the hippocampus *(7)* continues, and the two profiles of the lateral ventricle *(1, 6)* draw closer together. On the right side of the section, fornix fibers are still cut twice *(2, 5)*, but on the left side the section cuts tangentially through these fibers *(8)*, showing their entire course as they pass from the fimbria to the fornix.

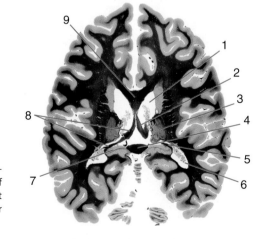

Figure 6–3 (Continued)   Horizontal sections.

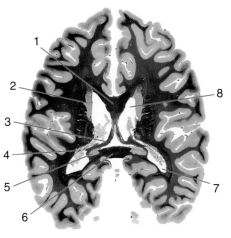

U, The plane of section has nearly reached the top of several C-shaped forebrain structures. It passes tangentially through the fornix *(3)*, but still cuts the corpus callosum *(1, 6)*, caudate nucleus *(2, 4)*, and lateral ventricle *(7, 8)* twice. The last bit of the hippocampus *(5)* can be seen adjacent to the splenium of the corpus callosum *(6)*.

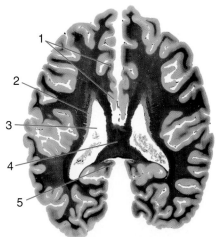

V, A tangential section through the body of the caudate nucleus *(2)*, the lateral ventricle *(3)*, and the body of the corpus callosum *(4)*. The limbic lobe is still cut twice, once (nearly tangentially) through the cingulate gyrus *(1)* and again through the narrow isthmus *(5)* joining the cingulate and parahippocampal gyri.

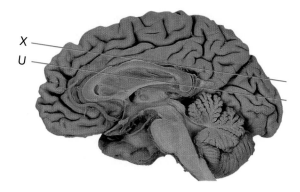

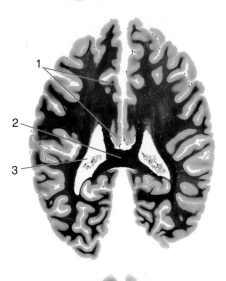

W, A tangential cut through the corpus callosum *(2)*, lateral ventricle *(3)*, and a larger expanse of the cingulate gyrus *(1)*.

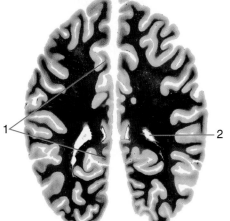

X, Finally, a tangential cut through the cingulate gyrus *(1)* just above the corpus callosum and near the roof of the lateral ventricle *(2)*.

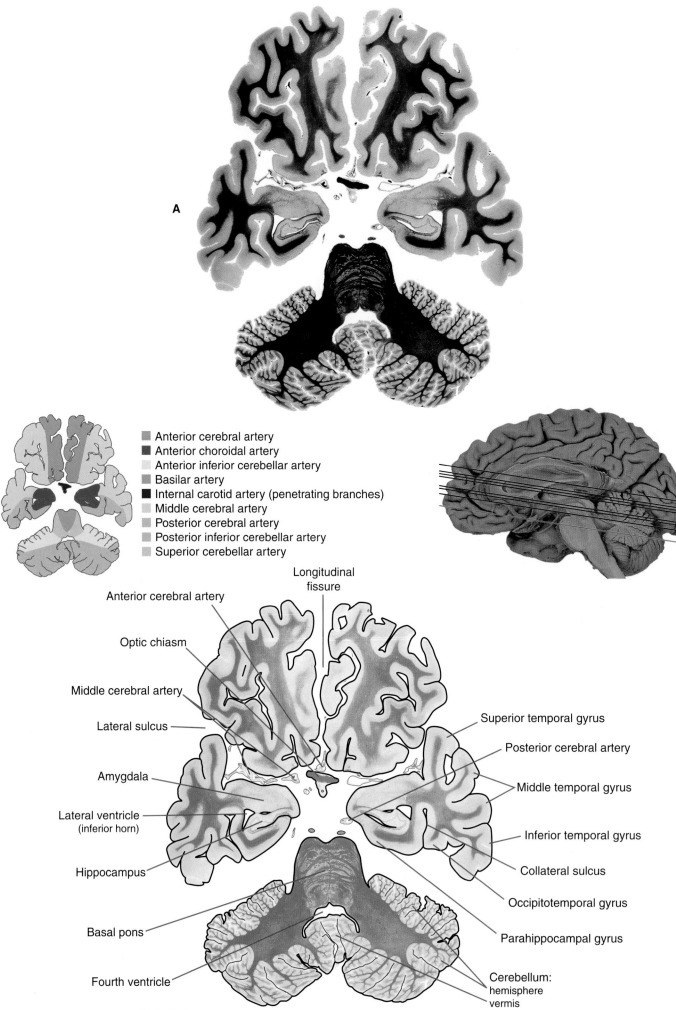

A

Anterior cerebral artery
Anterior choroidal artery
Anterior inferior cerebellar artery
Basilar artery
Internal carotid artery (penetrating branches)
Middle cerebral artery
Posterior cerebral artery
Posterior inferior cerebellar artery
Superior cerebellar artery

Longitudinal fissure

Anterior cerebral artery

Optic chiasm

Middle cerebral artery

Lateral sulcus

Amygdala

Lateral ventricle (inferior horn)

Hippocampus

Basal pons

Fourth ventricle

Superior temporal gyrus

Posterior cerebral artery

Middle temporal gyrus

Inferior temporal gyrus

Collateral sulcus

Occipitotemporal gyrus

Parahippocampal gyrus

Cerebellum:
hemisphere
vermis

Figure 6–4 **A,** A horizontal section through the uncus and optic chiasm. Three fourths actual size.

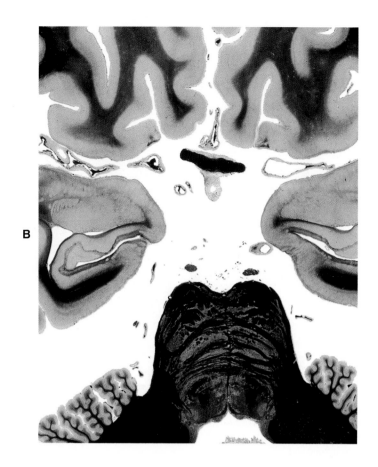

B

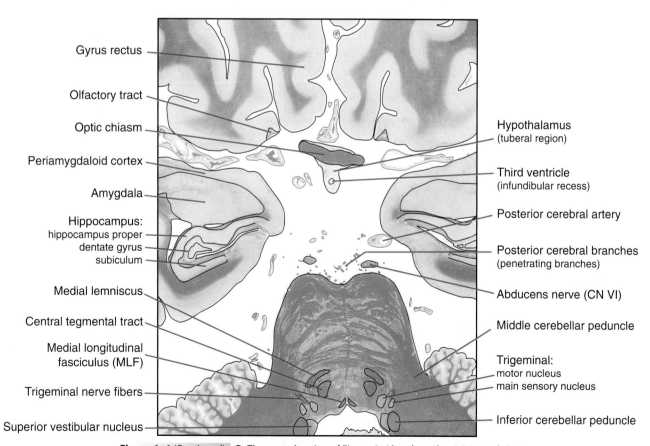

Gyrus rectus

Olfactory tract

Optic chiasm

Periamygdaloid cortex

Amygdala

Hippocampus:
hippocampus proper
dentate gyrus
subiculum

Medial lemniscus

Central tegmental tract

Medial longitudinal
fasciculus (MLF)

Trigeminal nerve fibers

Superior vestibular nucleus

Hypothalamus
(tuberal region)

Third ventricle
(infundibular recess)

Posterior cerebral artery

Posterior cerebral branches
(penetrating branches)

Abducens nerve (CN VI)

Middle cerebellar peduncle

Trigeminal:
motor nucleus
main sensory nucleus

Inferior cerebellar peduncle

Figure 6–4 (Continued)   **B,** The central region of Figure 6–4A, enlarged to 1.5× actual size.

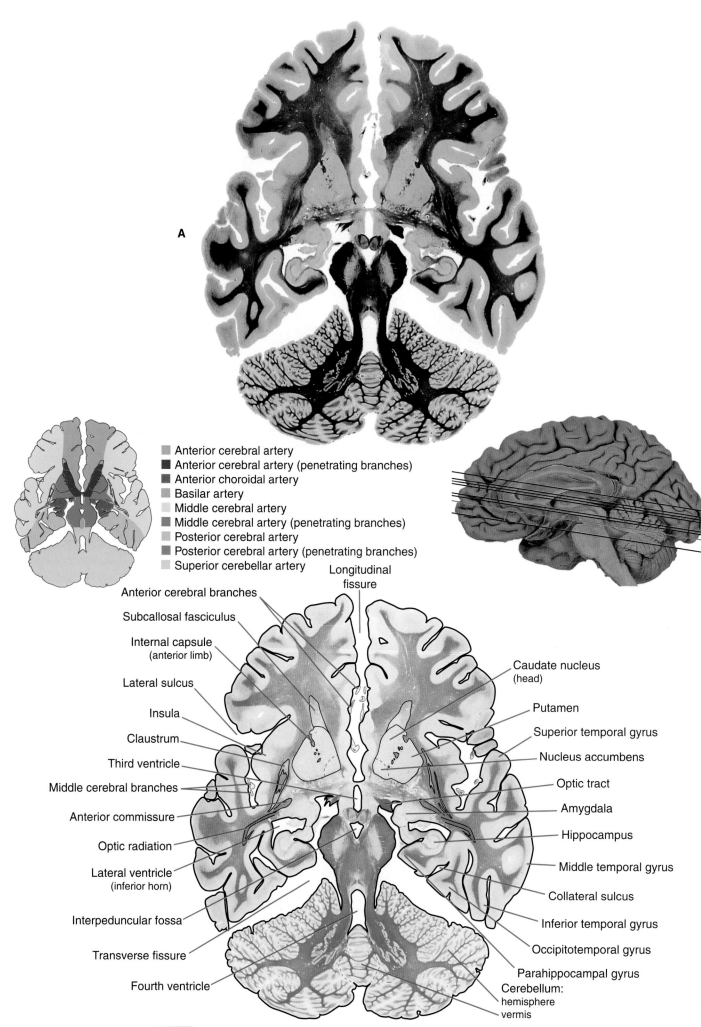

A

Anterior cerebral artery
Anterior cerebral artery (penetrating branches)
Anterior choroidal artery
Basilar artery
Middle cerebral artery
Middle cerebral artery (penetrating branches)
Posterior cerebral artery
Posterior cerebral artery (penetrating branches)
Superior cerebellar artery

Longitudinal fissure

Anterior cerebral branches

Subcallosal fasciculus

Internal capsule
(anterior limb)

Lateral sulcus

Insula

Claustrum

Third ventricle

Middle cerebral branches

Anterior commissure

Optic radiation

Lateral ventricle
(inferior horn)

Interpeduncular fossa

Transverse fissure

Fourth ventricle

Caudate nucleus
(head)

Putamen

Superior temporal gyrus

Nucleus accumbens

Optic tract

Amygdala

Hippocampus

Middle temporal gyrus

Collateral sulcus

Inferior temporal gyrus

Occipitotemporal gyrus

Parahippocampal gyrus

Cerebellum:
hemisphere
vermis

Figure 6–5   A, A horizontal section through the base of the diencephalon. Three fourths actual size.

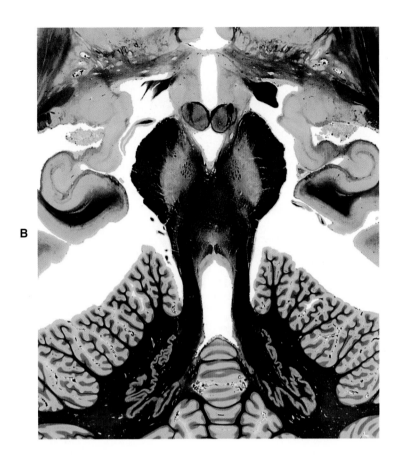

B

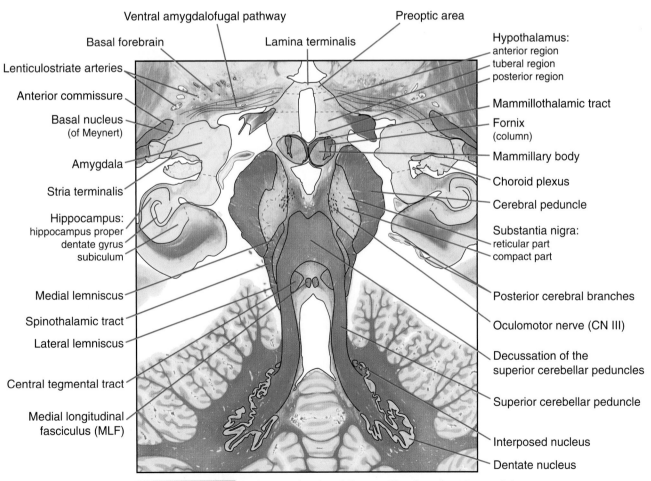

Ventral amygdalofugal pathway

Preoptic area

Basal forebrain

Lamina terminalis

Hypothalamus:
anterior region
tuberal region
posterior region

Lenticulostriate arteries

Anterior commissure

Mammillothalamic tract

Basal nucleus
(of Meynert)

Fornix
(column)

Amygdala

Mammillary body

Stria terminalis

Choroid plexus

Cerebral peduncle

Hippocampus:
hippocampus proper
dentate gyrus
subiculum

Substantia nigra:
reticular part
compact part

Medial lemniscus

Posterior cerebral branches

Spinothalamic tract

Oculomotor nerve (CN III)

Lateral lemniscus

Decussation of the
superior cerebellar peduncles

Central tegmental tract

Superior cerebellar peduncle

Medial longitudinal
fasciculus (MLF)

Interposed nucleus

Dentate nucleus

Figure 6–5 (Continued) **B,** The central region of Figure 6–5A, enlarged to 1.5× actual size.

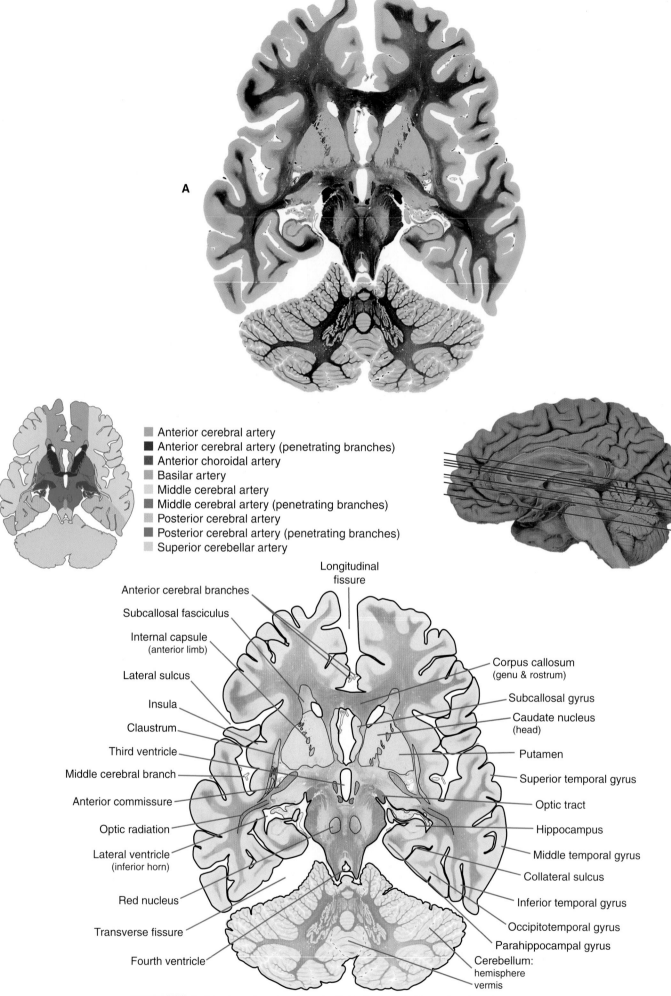

A

Anterior cerebral artery
Anterior cerebral artery (penetrating branches)
Anterior choroidal artery
Basilar artery
Middle cerebral artery
Middle cerebral artery (penetrating branches)
Posterior cerebral artery
Posterior cerebral artery (penetrating branches)
Superior cerebellar artery

Longitudinal fissure

Anterior cerebral branches

Subcallosal fasciculus

Internal capsule (anterior limb)

Lateral sulcus

Insula

Claustrum

Third ventricle

Middle cerebral branch

Anterior commissure

Optic radiation

Lateral ventricle (inferior horn)

Red nucleus

Transverse fissure

Fourth ventricle

Corpus callosum (genu & rostrum)

Subcallosal gyrus

Caudate nucleus (head)

Putamen

Superior temporal gyrus

Optic tract

Hippocampus

Middle temporal gyrus

Collateral sulcus

Inferior temporal gyrus

Occipitotemporal gyrus

Parahippocampal gyrus

Cerebellum: hemisphere vermis

Figure 6–6   A, A horizontal section through all the deep cerebellar nuclei. Three fourths actual size.

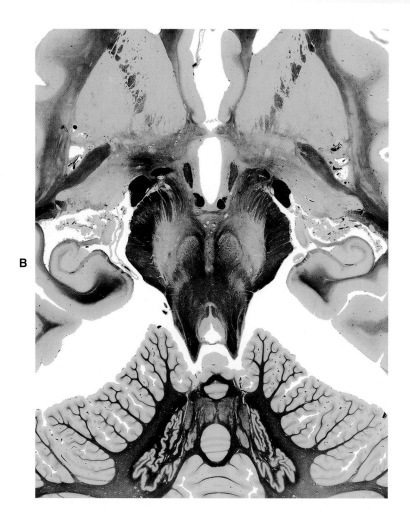

B

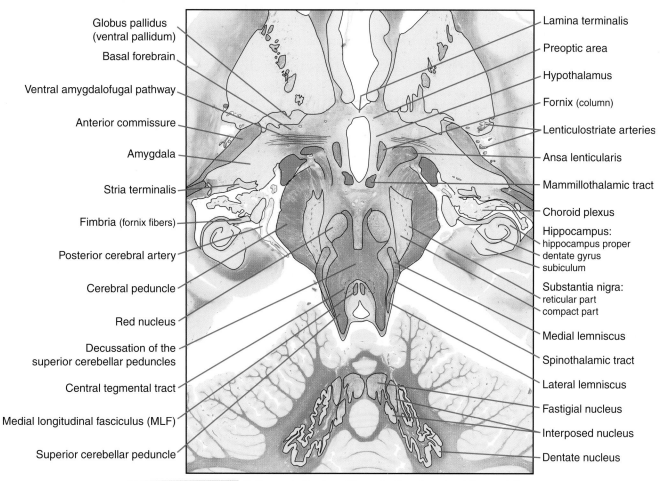

Globus pallidus
(ventral pallidum)

Basal forebrain

Ventral amygdalofugal pathway

Anterior commissure

Amygdala

Stria terminalis

Fimbria (fornix fibers)

Posterior cerebral artery

Cerebral peduncle

Red nucleus

Decussation of the
superior cerebellar peduncles

Central tegmental tract

Medial longitudinal fasciculus (MLF)

Superior cerebellar peduncle

Lamina terminalis

Preoptic area

Hypothalamus

Fornix (column)

Lenticulostriate arteries

Ansa lenticularis

Mammillothalamic tract

Choroid plexus

Hippocampus:
hippocampus proper
dentate gyrus
subiculum

Substantia nigra:
reticular part
compact part

Medial lemniscus

Spinothalamic tract

Lateral lemniscus

Fastigial nucleus

Interposed nucleus

Dentate nucleus

Figure 6–6 (Continued)   **B,** The central region of Figure 6–6A, enlarged to 1.5× actual size.

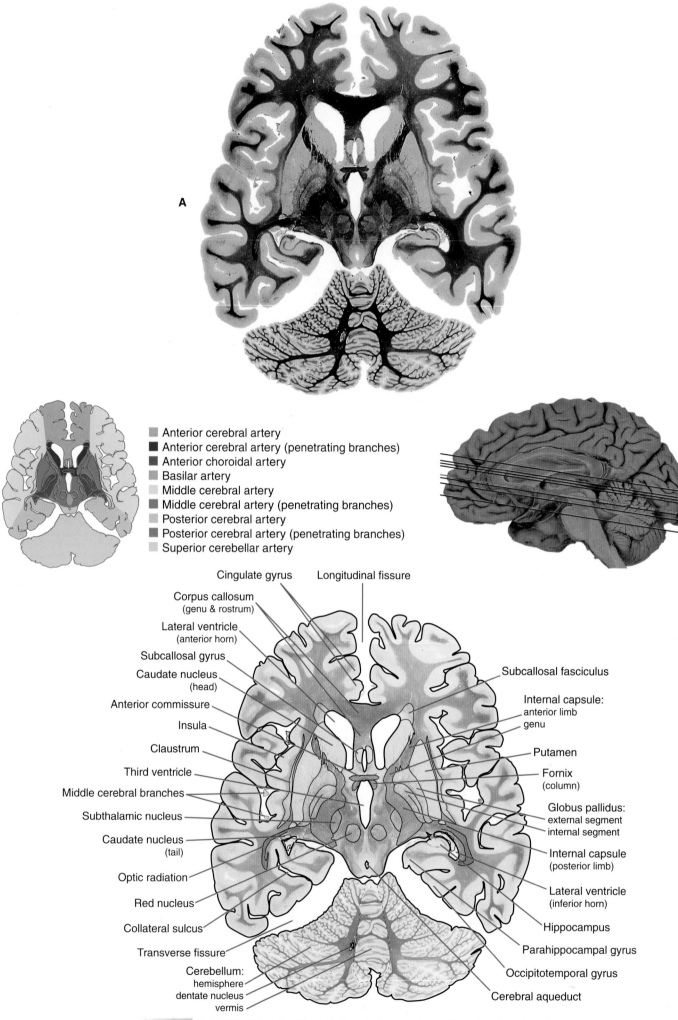

A

■ Anterior cerebral artery
■ Anterior cerebral artery (penetrating branches)
■ Anterior choroidal artery
■ Basilar artery
■ Middle cerebral artery
■ Middle cerebral artery (penetrating branches)
■ Posterior cerebral artery
■ Posterior cerebral artery (penetrating branches)
■ Superior cerebellar artery

Cingulate gyrus   Longitudinal fissure

Corpus callosum
(genu & rostrum)

Lateral ventricle
(anterior horn)

Subcallosal gyrus

Caudate nucleus
(head)

Anterior commissure

Insula

Claustrum

Third ventricle

Middle cerebral branches

Subthalamic nucleus

Caudate nucleus
(tail)

Optic radiation

Red nucleus

Collateral sulcus

Transverse fissure

Cerebellum:
hemisphere
dentate nucleus
vermis

Subcallosal fasciculus

Internal capsule:
anterior limb
genu

Putamen

Fornix
(column)

Globus pallidus:
external segment
internal segment

Internal capsule
(posterior limb)

Lateral ventricle
(inferior horn)

Hippocampus

Parahippocampal gyrus

Occipitotemporal gyrus

Cerebral aqueduct

Figure 6–7   A, A horizontal section through the anterior commissure. Three fourths actual size.

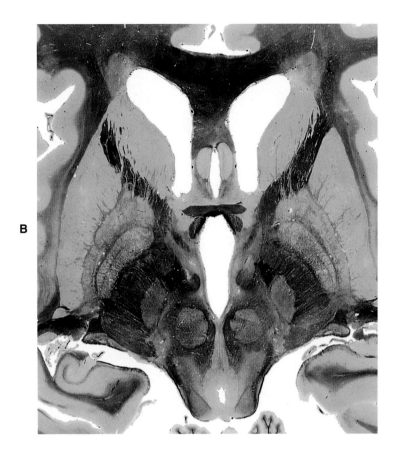

B

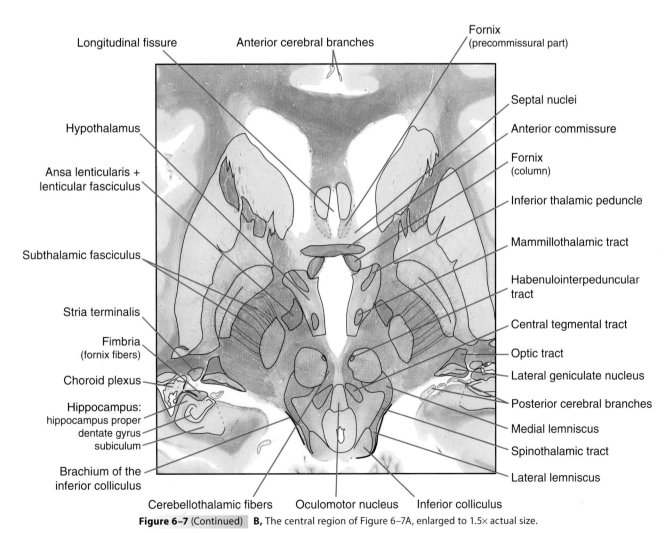

Longitudinal fissure

Anterior cerebral branches

Fornix
(precommissural part)

Hypothalamus

Ansa lenticularis +
lenticular fasciculus

Subthalamic fasciculus

Stria terminalis

Fimbria
(fornix fibers)

Choroid plexus

Hippocampus:
hippocampus proper
dentate gyrus
subiculum

Brachium of the
inferior colliculus

Septal nuclei

Anterior commissure

Fornix
(column)

Inferior thalamic peduncle

Mammillothalamic tract

Habenulointerpeduncular
tract

Central tegmental tract

Optic tract

Lateral geniculate nucleus

Posterior cerebral branches

Medial lemniscus

Spinothalamic tract

Lateral lemniscus

Cerebellothalamic fibers   Oculomotor nucleus   Inferior colliculus

Figure 6–7 (Continued)   **B,** The central region of Figure 6–7A, enlarged to 1.5× actual size.

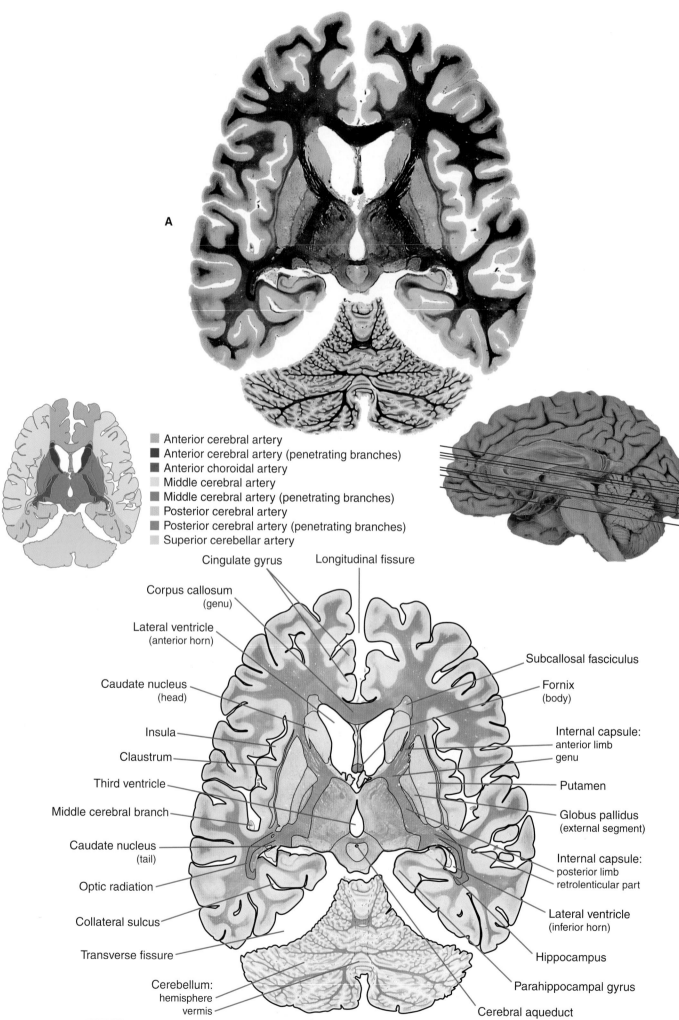

A

- Anterior cerebral artery
- Anterior cerebral artery (penetrating branches)
- Anterior choroidal artery
- Middle cerebral artery
- Middle cerebral artery (penetrating branches)
- Posterior cerebral artery
- Posterior cerebral artery (penetrating branches)
- Superior cerebellar artery

Cingulate gyrus

Longitudinal fissure

Corpus callosum (genu)

Lateral ventricle (anterior horn)

Caudate nucleus (head)

Insula

Claustrum

Third ventricle

Middle cerebral branch

Caudate nucleus (tail)

Optic radiation

Collateral sulcus

Transverse fissure

Cerebellum: hemisphere vermis

Subcallosal fasciculus

Fornix (body)

Internal capsule: anterior limb genu

Putamen

Globus pallidus (external segment)

Internal capsule: posterior limb retrolenticular part

Lateral ventricle (inferior horn)

Hippocampus

Parahippocampal gyrus

Cerebral aqueduct

Figure 6–8   A, A horizontal section through the interventricular foramen and posterior commissure. Three fourths actual size.

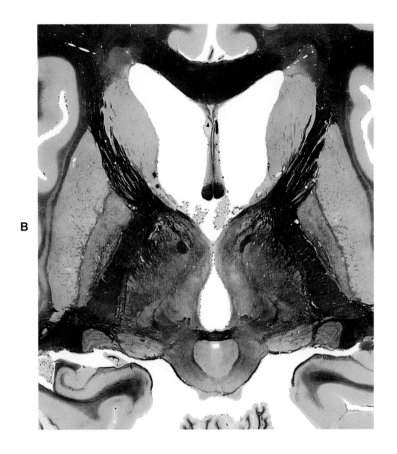

B

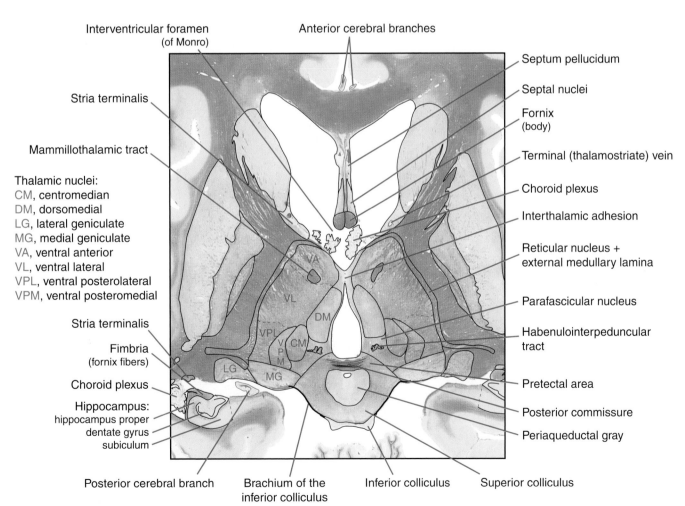

Interventricular foramen
(of Monro)

Anterior cerebral branches

Septum pellucidum

Stria terminalis

Septal nuclei

Fornix
(body)

Mammillothalamic tract

Terminal (thalamostriate) vein

Thalamic nuclei:
CM, centromedian
DM, dorsomedial
LG, lateral geniculate
MG, medial geniculate
VA, ventral anterior
VL, ventral lateral
VPL, ventral posterolateral
VPM, ventral posteromedial

Choroid plexus

Interthalamic adhesion

Reticular nucleus +
external medullary lamina

Parafascicular nucleus

Stria terminalis

Habenulointerpeduncular
tract

Fimbria
(fornix fibers)

Choroid plexus

Pretectal area

Hippocampus:
hippocampus proper
dentate gyrus
subiculum

Posterior commissure

Periaqueductal gray

Posterior cerebral branch

Brachium of the
inferior colliculus

Inferior colliculus

Superior colliculus

Figure 6–8 (Continued)   **B,** The central region of Figure 6–8A, enlarged to 1.5× actual size.

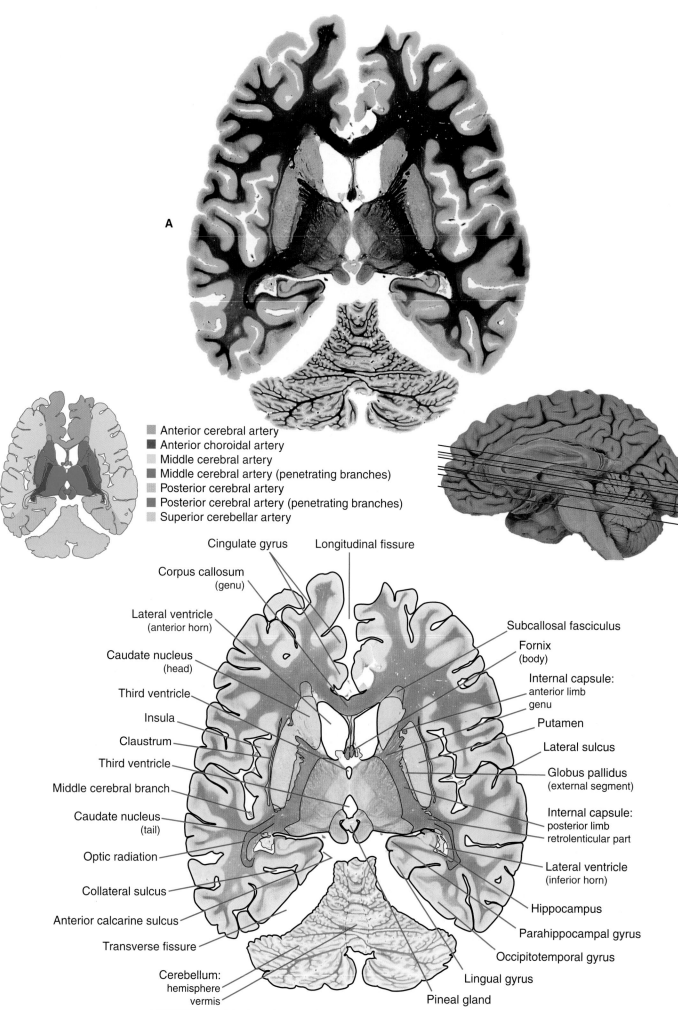

A

■ Anterior cerebral artery
■ Anterior choroidal artery
■ Middle cerebral artery
■ Middle cerebral artery (penetrating branches)
▒ Posterior cerebral artery
■ Posterior cerebral artery (penetrating branches)
■ Superior cerebellar artery

Cingulate gyrus   Longitudinal fissure

Corpus callosum
(genu)

Lateral ventricle
(anterior horn)

Caudate nucleus
(head)

Third ventricle

Insula

Claustrum

Third ventricle

Middle cerebral branch

Caudate nucleus
(tail)

Optic radiation

Collateral sulcus

Anterior calcarine sulcus

Transverse fissure

Cerebellum:
hemisphere
vermis

Subcallosal fasciculus

Fornix
(body)

Internal capsule:
anterior limb
genu

Putamen

Lateral sulcus

Globus pallidus
(external segment)

Internal capsule:
posterior limb
retrolenticular part

Lateral ventricle
(inferior horn)

Hippocampus

Parahippocampal gyrus

Occipitotemporal gyrus

Lingual gyrus

Pineal gland

Figure 6–9   A, A horizontal section through the midthalamus. Three fourths actual size.

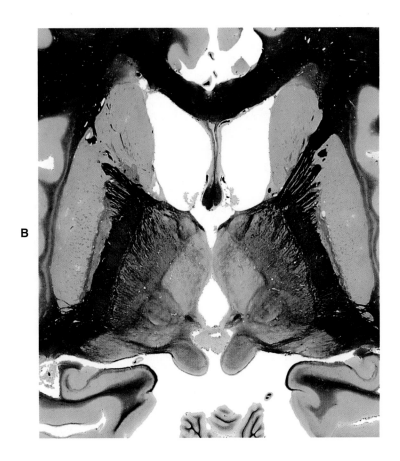

B

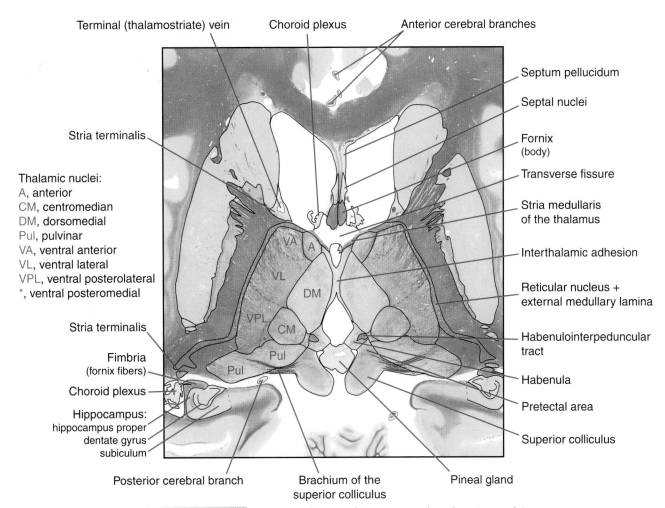

Terminal (thalamostriate) vein   Choroid plexus   Anterior cerebral branches

Stria terminalis

Thalamic nuclei:
A, anterior
CM, centromedian
DM, dorsomedial
Pul, pulvinar
VA, ventral anterior
VL, ventral lateral
VPL, ventral posterolateral
*, ventral posteromedial

Stria terminalis

Fimbria
(fornix fibers)

Choroid plexus

Hippocampus:
hippocampus proper
dentate gyrus
subiculum

Septum pellucidum

Septal nuclei

Fornix
(body)

Transverse fissure

Stria medullaris
of the thalamus

Interthalamic adhesion

Reticular nucleus +
external medullary lamina

Habenulointerpeduncular
tract

Habenula

Pretectal area

Superior colliculus

Posterior cerebral branch   Brachium of the   Pineal gland
                            superior colliculus

VA A
VL
DM
VPL
CM
Pul
Pul

Figure 6–9 (Continued)   **B,** The central region of Figure 6–9A, enlarged to 1.5× actual size.

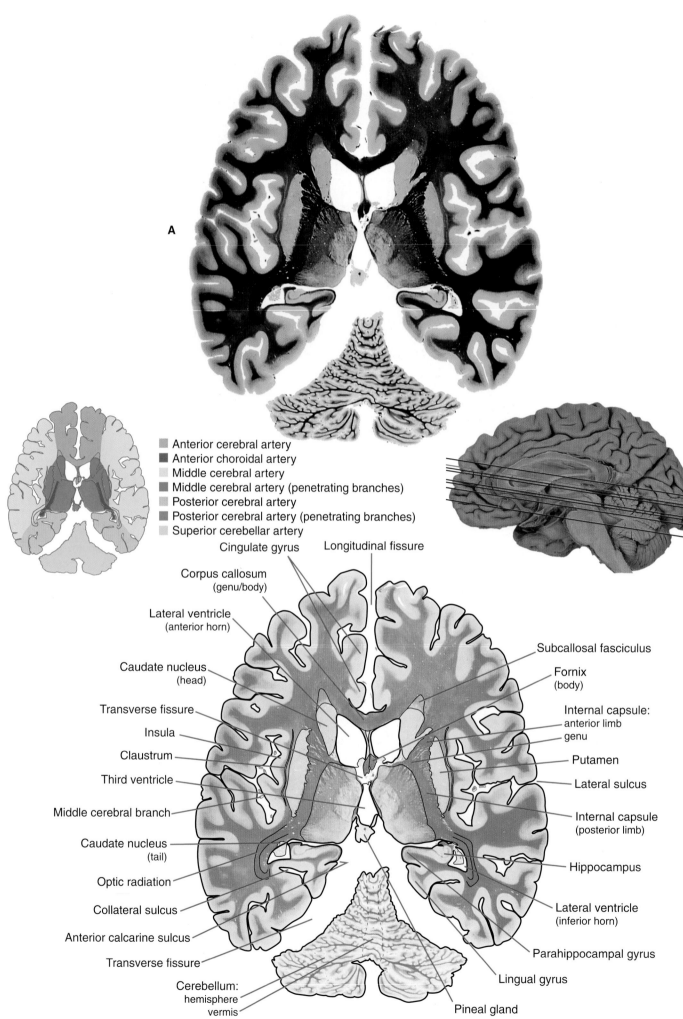

A,

Anterior cerebral artery
Anterior choroidal artery
Middle cerebral artery
Middle cerebral artery (penetrating branches)
Posterior cerebral artery
Posterior cerebral artery (penetrating branches)
Superior cerebellar artery

Cingulate gyrus   Longitudinal fissure

Corpus callosum (genu/body)

Lateral ventricle (anterior horn)

Caudate nucleus (head)

Transverse fissure

Insula

Claustrum

Third ventricle

Middle cerebral branch

Caudate nucleus (tail)

Optic radiation

Collateral sulcus

Anterior calcarine sulcus

Transverse fissure

Cerebellum: hemisphere vermis

Subcallosal fasciculus

Fornix (body)

Internal capsule: anterior limb genu

Putamen

Lateral sulcus

Internal capsule (posterior limb)

Hippocampus

Lateral ventricle (inferior horn)

Parahippocampal gyrus

Lingual gyrus

Pineal gland

Figure 6–10   A, A horizontal section at the level of the roof of the third ventricle. Three fourths actual size.

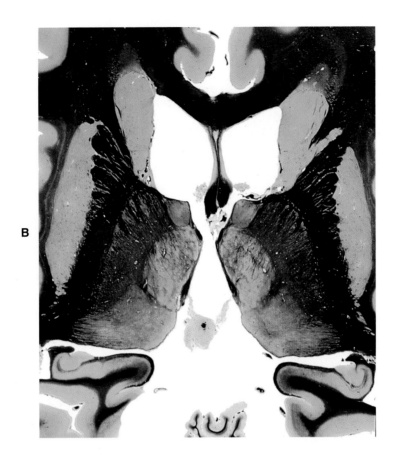

B

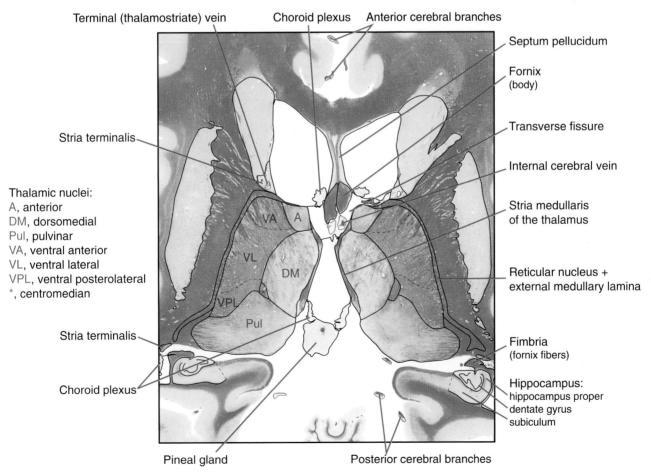

Terminal (thalamostriate) vein   Choroid plexus   Anterior cerebral branches

Septum pellucidum

Fornix
(body)

Transverse fissure

Internal cerebral vein

Stria medullaris
of the thalamus

Stria terminalis

Thalamic nuclei:
A, anterior
DM, dorsomedial
Pul, pulvinar
VA, ventral anterior
VL, ventral lateral
VPL, ventral posterolateral
*, centromedian

VA   A

VL

DM

VPL

Pul

Reticular nucleus +
external medullary lamina

Stria terminalis

Fimbria
(fornix fibers)

Choroid plexus

Hippocampus:
hippocampus proper
dentate gyrus
subiculum

Pineal gland   Posterior cerebral branches

Figure 6–10 (Continued)   **B,** The central region of Figure 6–10A, enlarged to 1.5× actual size.

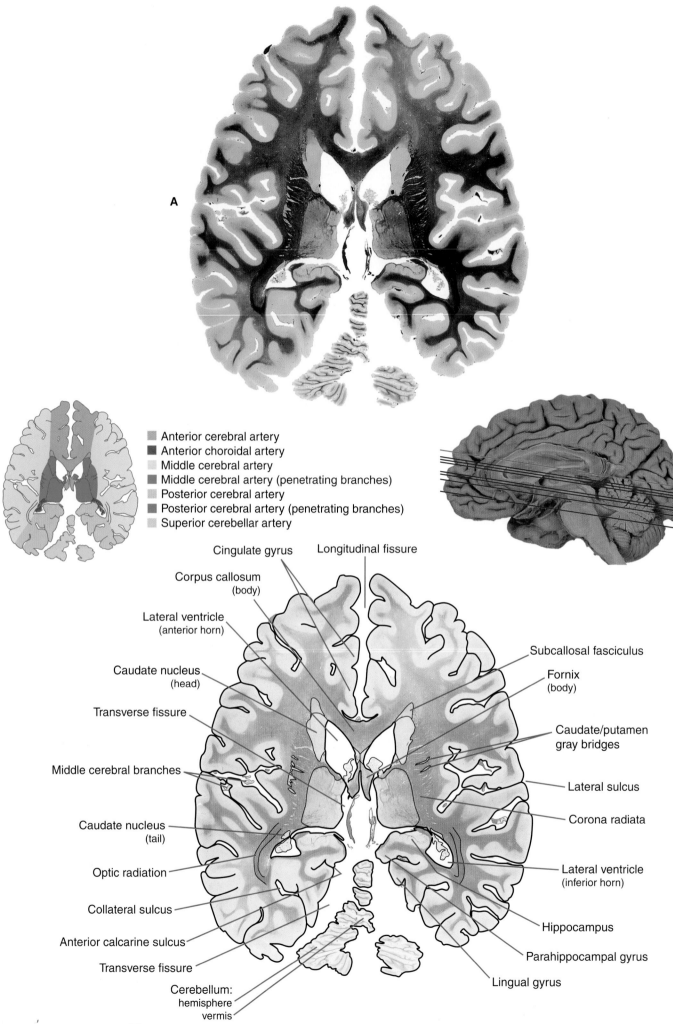

A

Anterior cerebral artery
Anterior choroidal artery
Middle cerebral artery
Middle cerebral artery (penetrating branches)
Posterior cerebral artery
Posterior cerebral artery (penetrating branches)
Superior cerebellar artery

Cingulate gyrus
Longitudinal fissure
Corpus callosum (body)
Lateral ventricle (anterior horn)
Caudate nucleus (head)
Transverse fissure
Middle cerebral branches
Caudate nucleus (tail)
Optic radiation
Collateral sulcus
Anterior calcarine sulcus
Transverse fissure
Cerebellum: hemisphere vermis

Subcallosal fasciculus
Fornix (body)
Caudate/putamen gray bridges
Lateral sulcus
Corona radiata
Lateral ventricle (inferior horn)
Hippocampus
Parahippocampal gyrus
Lingual gyrus

Figure 6–11   A, A horizontal section through the transverse fissure and internal cerebral veins. Three fourths actual size.

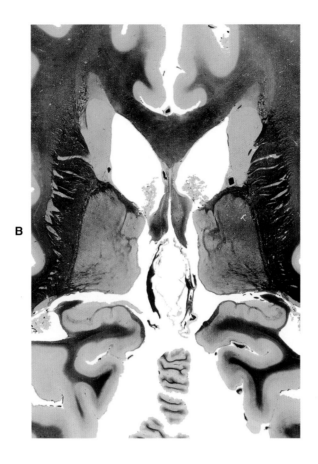

B

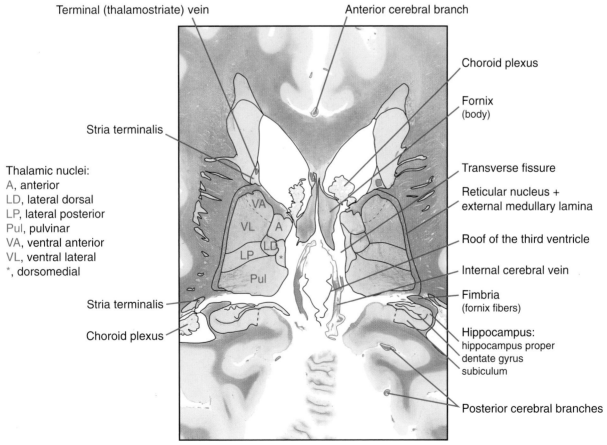

Terminal (thalamostriate) vein

Anterior cerebral branch

Choroid plexus

Fornix
(body)

Stria terminalis

Thalamic nuclei:
A, anterior
LD, lateral dorsal
LP, lateral posterior
Pul, pulvinar
VA, ventral anterior
VL, ventral lateral
*, dorsomedial

VA

VL   A

LD

LP   *

Pul

Transverse fissure

Reticular nucleus +
external medullary lamina

Roof of the third ventricle

Internal cerebral vein

Stria terminalis

Choroid plexus

Fimbria
(fornix fibers)

Hippocampus:
hippocampus proper
dentate gyrus
subiculum

Posterior cerebral branches

Figure 6–11 (Continued)   **B,** The central region of Figure 6–11A, enlarged to 1.5× actual size.

7

Sagittal Sections

This chapter, the last of three showing sections of entire human brains, illustrates parasagittal planes. Forebrain structures continue to be emphasized, but parts of the brainstem and cerebellum are indicated as well. The organization of various functional systems in the forebrain (e.g., thalamus, hippocampus) is presented in Chapter 8.

Drawings showing typical areas of arterial supply in each section are provided in this chapter and the preceding two chapters. We have simplified these in two major ways. First, arterial territories are shown as sharply demarcated from each other, when in reality there is significant interdigitation and overlap. Second, penetrating arteries arise from all the vessels of the circle of Willis; however, we have incorporated those from the anterior and posterior communicating arteries with those from the anterior and posterior cerebral arteries.

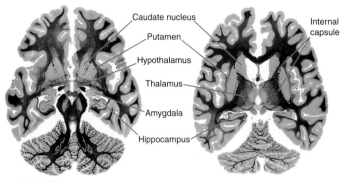

Figure 7–1 The horizontal sections from Figures 6–3G and N, used in much of this chapter to indicate planes of section.

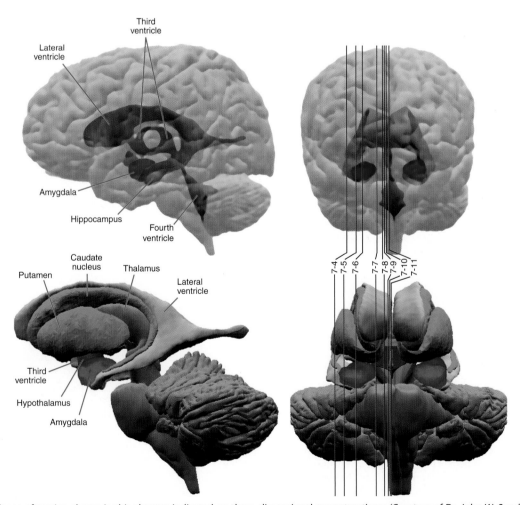

Figure 7–2 The planes of section shown in this chapter, indicated on three-dimensional reconstructions. *(Courtesy of Dr. John W. Sundsten, Department of Biological Structure, University of Washington School of Medicine.)*

Figure 7–3   A–P, Sixteen sagittal sections of the right hemisphere of a brain. The sections are arranged in a lateral-to-medial sequence extending from the insula to the midline. Anterior is toward the left, so the view is as though you were backing through the brain, always looking from inside the brain out toward the lateral sulcus.

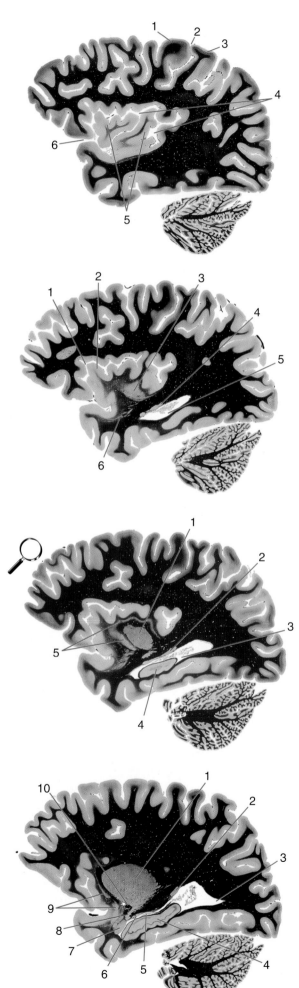

A, The first section passes tangentially through the insula (5) and shows nicely how the lateral sulcus (6) leads to it, and the circular sulcus (4) outlines it. The precentral (1) and postcentral (3) gyri also can be seen, separated from each other by the central sulcus (2), which, cut obliquely, seems deeper than it really is.

B, The circular sulcus (1) is still present, partially surrounding the insula (2), but now the plane of section begins to reveal structures just deep to insular cortex—in this case, the claustrum (3, 6). The most lateral part of the lateral ventricle, the inferior horn (5), also appears, with the tail of the caudate nucleus (4) cut tangentially in its wall.

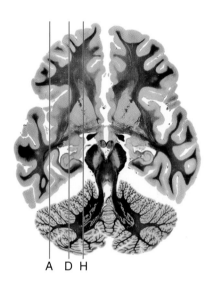

C, The putamen (1) appears, and the claustrum (5), a sheet of gray matter that covers the curved lateral aspect of the putamen, appears to surround it partially in this two-dimensional view. The tail of the caudate nucleus (2) is cut tangentially in the wall of the inferior horn of the lateral ventricle (3). Across the ventricle, the hippocampus (4) makes its appearance. Shown enlarged in Figure 7–4.

D, The putamen (1) continues to increase in size, still partially surrounded by the claustrum (9). The tail of the caudate nucleus (2, 6) is cut in two places as it curves into the temporal lobe with the inferior horn of the lateral ventricle (5). The posterior horn of the lateral ventricle (3) extends back toward the occipital lobe. The hippocampus (4) increases in size, and the amygdala (7) appears at its anterior end. A downward extension (8) of the putamen merges with the amygdala, much as the tail of the caudate nucleus merges with both in a nearby plane (see Fig. 7–3E). Fibers that have collected from the temporal lobe and will cross in the anterior commissure (10) mass underneath the putamen.

Figure 7–3 (Continued)   Sagittal sections.

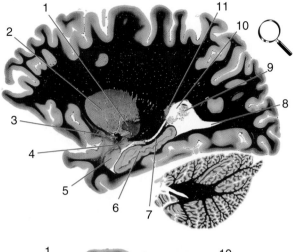

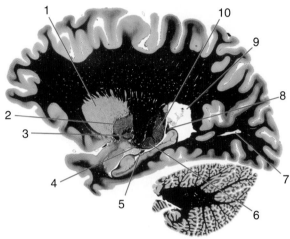

E, The globus pallidus (*1*, part of its external segment) appears adjacent to the putamen (*2*), with fibers of the anterior commissure (*3*) traveling beneath them. The caudate nucleus is again cut twice, once (*11*) as it curves around from the body to the inferior horn of the lateral ventricle and a second time (*4*) as it merges with the amygdala (*5*). Fibers of the fimbria (*7*) are cut tangentially as they emerge from the hippocampus (*6*). An enlarged mass of choroid plexus (*9*, the glomus) protrudes into the atrium of the lateral ventricle (*10*), and the posterior horn of the ventricle (*8*) extends back into the occipital lobe. Shown enlarged in Figure 7–5.

F, The internal (*3*) and external (*2*) segments of the globus pallidus can be seen adjacent to the putamen (*1*). The plane of section has reached the thalamus—the pulvinar (*10*) appears, as well as the lateral geniculate nucleus (*6*) with the optic tract (*4*) ending in it. The fimbria, cut tangentially in Figure 7–3E, is now cut in two places (*5, 8*). The posterior horn of the lateral ventricle (*7*) appears in this plane to be a detached cavity in the occipital lobe, but is in fact continuous with the atrium (*9*).

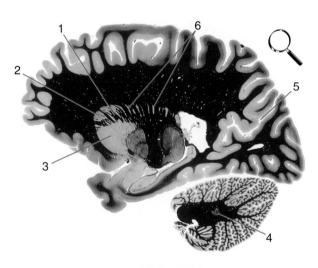

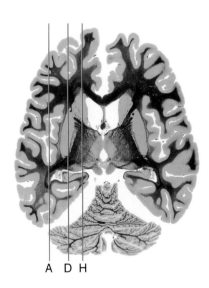

A D H

G, The head of the caudate nucleus (*2*) appears, with fibers of the anterior limb of the internal capsule (*1*) emerging from the cleft between it and the putamen (*3*). Strands of gray matter (*6*) extend between the caudate nucleus and putamen, emphasizing the common embryological origin and similar pattern of connections of these two parts of the striatum. The most lateral of the deep cerebellar nuclei, the dentate nucleus (*4*), can be seen, and the parietooccipital sulcus (*5*) is now distinct. Shown enlarged in Figure 7–6.

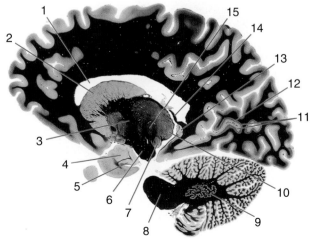

H, The head of the caudate nucleus (*2*) is cut tangentially in the wall of the anterior horn of the lateral ventricle (*1*). The continuity between the internal capsule (*3*, here the genu) and cerebral peduncle (*6*) is apparent. In the temporal lobe, the amygdala (*4*) and the anterior end of the hippocampus (*5*) underlie the uncus, and the fimbria is in the process of separating from the most caudal bit of hippocampus (*13*) and continuing as the crus of the fornix (*14*). The plane of section has moved deeper into the thalamus, and the medial geniculate nucleus (*7*), pulvinar (*10*), and nuclei of the lateral division (*15*, here VPL) can be seen. The dentate nucleus (*9*) is more fully formed, and visual cortex (*11*) occupies the banks of the calcarine sulcus (*12*). The middle cerebellar peduncle (*8*) leaves the basal pons and enters the cerebellum.

Illustration continued on following page

Figure 7–3 (Continued) Sagittal sections.

I, As the plane of section moves medially, progressively more of the prominent sulci of the medial surface of the brain become apparent—in this case, the cingulate sulcus (1) and its marginal branch (2). The subthalamic nucleus (4) and substantia nigra (5) appear beneath the thalamus, and the continuous white matter path from the internal capsule (3) through the cerebral peduncle (6) and into the basal pons (7) is shown nicely. The optic tract (8) proceeds posteriorly toward the lateral geniculate nucleus, and fibers of the anterior commissure (9) proceed toward (or away from) the midline.

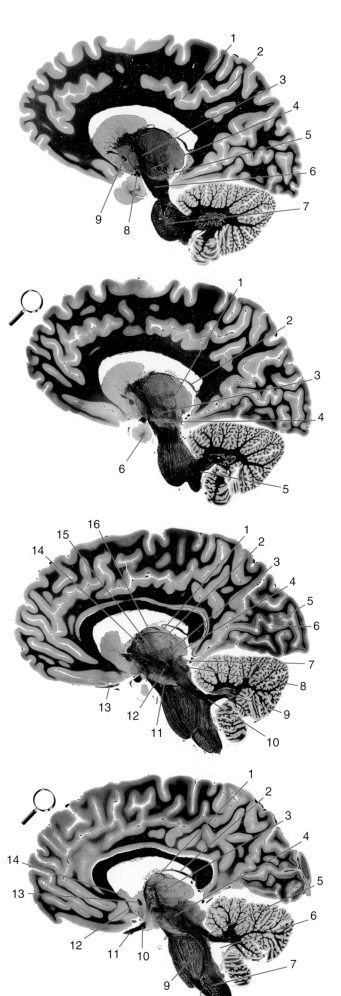

J, The subthalamic nucleus (3) and substantia nigra (4) are still apparent, and the centromedian nucleus (1) can be seen in the thalamus. Fibers that formed the fimbria in previous sections of this series are now separated from the hippocampus and proceeding anteriorly as the crus of the fornix (2). The inferior cerebellar peduncle (5) turns dorsally and enters the cerebellum. The uncus (6) appears for the last time. Shown enlarged in Figure 7–7.

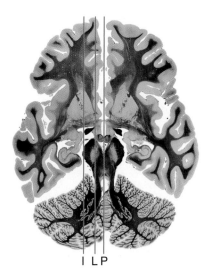

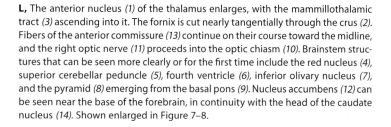

K, Many thalamic nuclei are now distinct, including the lateral dorsal (1), dorsomedial (2), centromedian (3), pulvinar (4), ventral anterior (14), ventral lateral (15), and anterior (16) nuclei. The olfactory tract (13) moves posteriorly across the orbital surface of the frontal lobe. As the plane of section approaches the midline, more brainstem components begin to become apparent, including the superior (7) and inferior (8) colliculi and the red nucleus (12), adjacent to the substantia nigra (11). The superior cerebellar peduncle (10) emerges from the cerebellum, and the interposed nucleus (9) largely replaces the dentate nucleus. Visual cortex (5) lines the calcarine sulcus (6).

L, The anterior nucleus (1) of the thalamus enlarges, with the mammillothalamic tract (3) ascending into it. The fornix is cut nearly tangentially through the crus (2). Fibers of the anterior commissure (13) continue on their course toward the midline, and the right optic nerve (11) proceeds into the optic chiasm (10). Brainstem structures that can be seen more clearly or for the first time include the red nucleus (4), superior cerebellar peduncle (5), fourth ventricle (6), inferior olivary nucleus (7), and the pyramid (8) emerging from the basal pons (9). Nucleus accumbens (12) can be seen near the base of the forebrain, in continuity with the head of the caudate nucleus (14). Shown enlarged in Figure 7–8.

Figure 7–3 (Continued) Sagittal sections.

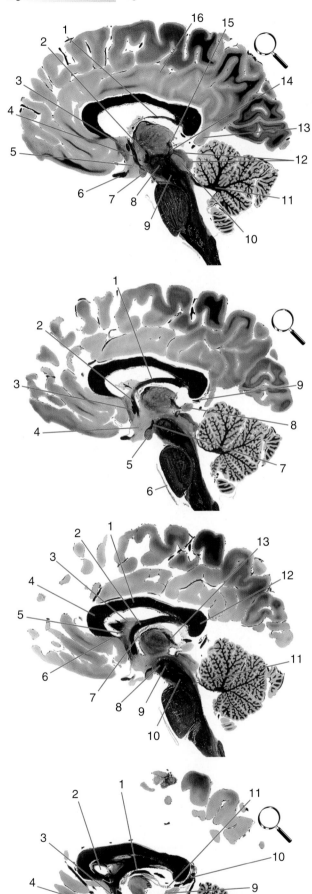

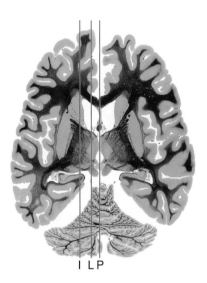

I L P

M, The fornix is cut twice (although nearly tangentially in each instance)—through the crus and body (1) and as the column (4) ends in the mammillary body (7), from which the mammillothalamic tract (2) emanates. The physical continuity between the septal nuclei (3) and the hypothalamus (5) is apparent. The cingulate gyrus (16) narrows into an isthmus (13), through which it is continuous with the parahippocampal gyrus. Half the fibers from each optic nerve cross the midline in the optic chiasm (6), and the habenulointerpeduncular tract leaves the habenula (15). Brainstem and cerebellar structures include posterior commissure fibers (14), the superior and inferior colliculi (12), periaqueductal gray (10), fastigial nucleus (11), and fibers of the superior cerebellar peduncle that emerge from their decussation (9) and pass through or around the red nucleus (8). Shown enlarged in Figure 7–9.

N, The plane of section, now very near the midline, passes through the body (1) and column (2) of the fornix as the latter travels just behind the anterior commissure (3). The hypothalamus (4), including the mammillary body (5) and emerging mammillothalamic fibers (7), forms the wall and floor of the third ventricle. Other near-midline structures include the basilar artery (6), pineal gland (8), and great cerebral vein of Galen (9). Shown enlarged in Figure 7–10.

O, All the parts of the corpus callosum—the body (1), genu (4), rostrum (6), and splenium (12)—are now apparent. The septum pellucidum (3) merges with the septal nuclei (5), the fornix (2) is again cut tangentially, and choroid plexus (7) passes through the interventricular foramen. The stria medullaris of the thalamus (13) proceeds posteriorly toward the habenula. Brainstem structures include the medial longitudinal fasciculus (11), the decussating superior cerebellar peduncles (10), and their continuation as cerebellothalamic fibers (8) surrounding the red nucleus (9).

P, Almost exactly in the midline, the internal cerebral vein (1) travels posteriorly to join the great cerebral vein of Galen (10). Much of the ventricular system also can be seen, including the cerebral aqueduct (7) and the fourth ventricle (8). The section did not quite follow the entire septum pellucidum, and part of the anterior horn of the lateral ventricle (2) is visible through the resulting hole. The third ventricle (3) and its parts and boundaries are shown nicely: the lamina terminalis (4) at the rostral end of the ventricle and the optic (5), infundibular (6), pineal (9), and suprapineal (11) recesses. Shown enlarged in Figure 7–11.

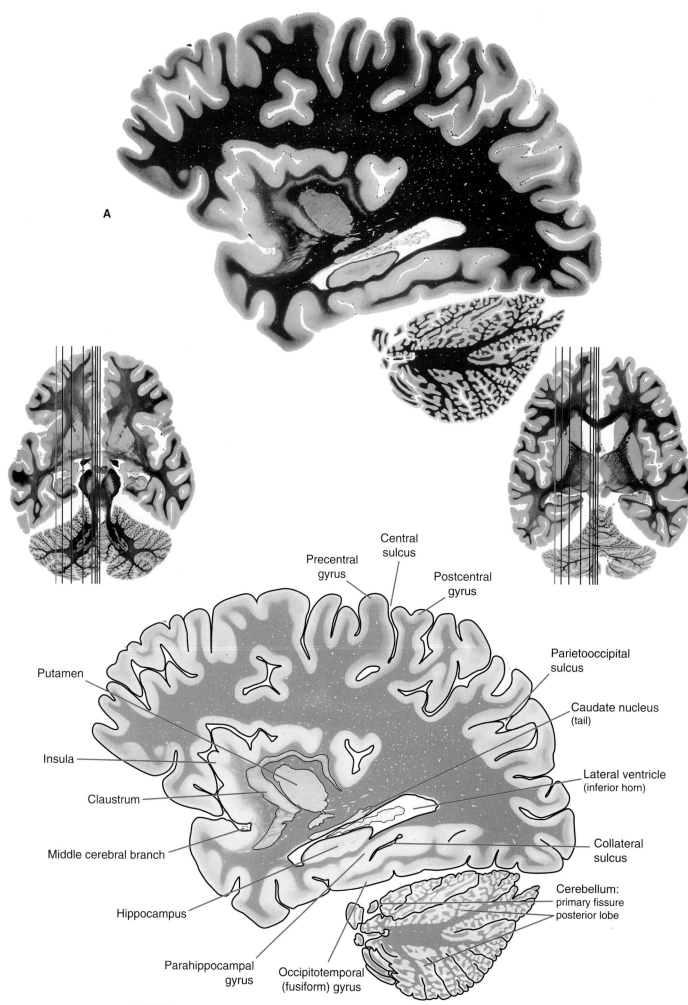

A

Central
sulcus
Precentral   Postcentral
gyrus   gyrus

Parietooccipital
sulcus

Putamen   Caudate nucleus
                                                                          (tail)

Insula   Lateral ventricle
                                                                          (inferior horn)
Claustrum

Middle cerebral branch   Collateral
                                                                          sulcus

                                                                      Cerebellum:
                                                                      primary fissure
                                                                      posterior lobe
Hippocampus

Parahippocampal   Occipitotemporal
gyrus   (fusiform) gyrus

Figure 7–4   A, A parasagittal section through lateral parts of the putamen and hippocampus. Actual size.

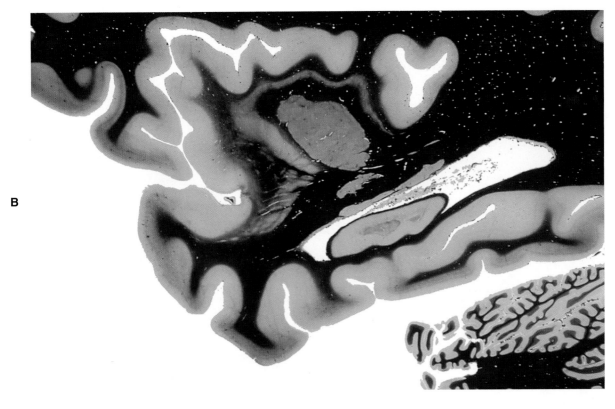

B

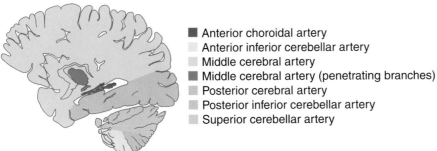

■ Anterior choroidal artery
  Anterior inferior cerebellar artery
  Middle cerebral artery
■ Middle cerebral artery (penetrating branches)
  Posterior cerebral artery
  Posterior inferior cerebellar artery
  Superior cerebellar artery

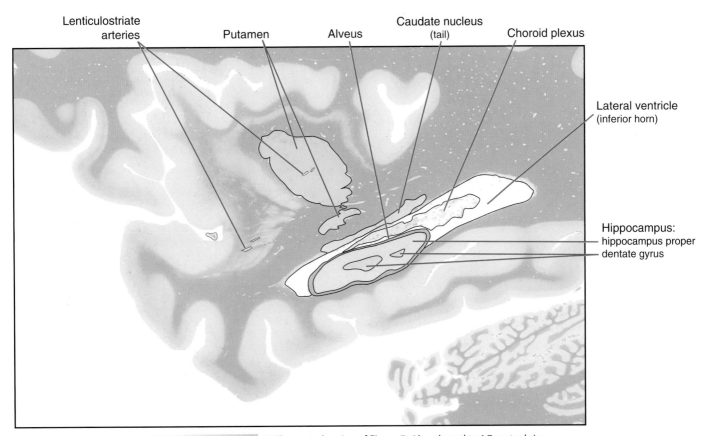

Lenticulostriate
arteries   Putamen   Alveus   Caudate nucleus
                                     (tail)   Choroid plexus

                                                   Lateral ventricle
                                                   (inferior horn)

                                                   Hippocampus:
                                                   hippocampus proper
                                                   dentate gyrus

Figure 7–4 (Continued) **B,** The central region of Figure 7–4A, enlarged to 1.7× actual size.

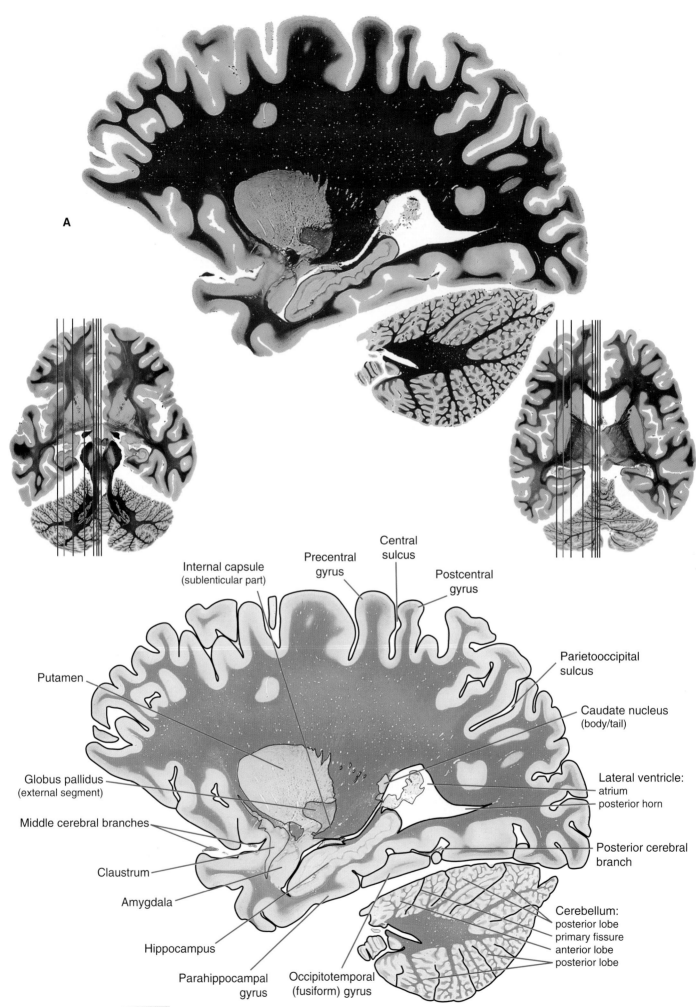

A

Internal capsule
(sublenticular part)

Precentral
gyrus

Central
sulcus

Postcentral
gyrus

Parietooccipital
sulcus

Putamen

Caudate nucleus
(body/tail)

Globus pallidus
(external segment)

Lateral ventricle:
atrium
posterior horn

Middle cerebral branches

Posterior cerebral
branch

Claustrum

Amygdala

Cerebellum:
posterior lobe
primary fissure
anterior lobe
posterior lobe

Hippocampus

Parahippocampal
gyrus

Occipitotemporal
(fusiform) gyrus

Figure 7–5 **A,** A parasagittal section passing longitudinally through much of the hippocampus. Actual size.

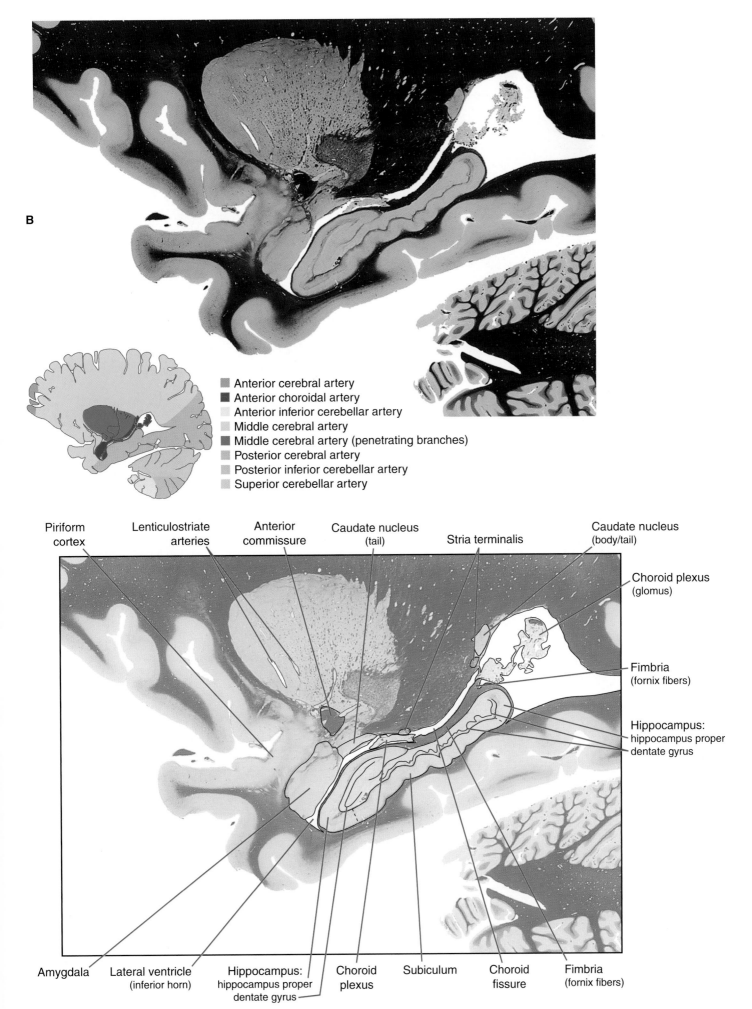

Anterior cerebral artery
Anterior choroidal artery
Anterior inferior cerebellar artery
Middle cerebral artery
Middle cerebral artery (penetrating branches)
Posterior cerebral artery
Posterior inferior cerebellar artery
Superior cerebellar artery

Piriform cortex
Lenticulostriate arteries
Anterior commissure
Caudate nucleus (tail)
Stria terminalis
Caudate nucleus (body/tail)
Choroid plexus (glomus)
Fimbria (fornix fibers)
Hippocampus: hippocampus proper dentate gyrus

Amygdala
Lateral ventricle (inferior horn)
Hippocampus: hippocampus proper dentate gyrus
Choroid plexus
Subiculum
Choroid fissure
Fimbria (fornix fibers)

Figure 7–5 (Continued) **B,** The central region of Figure 7–5A, enlarged to 1.7× actual size.

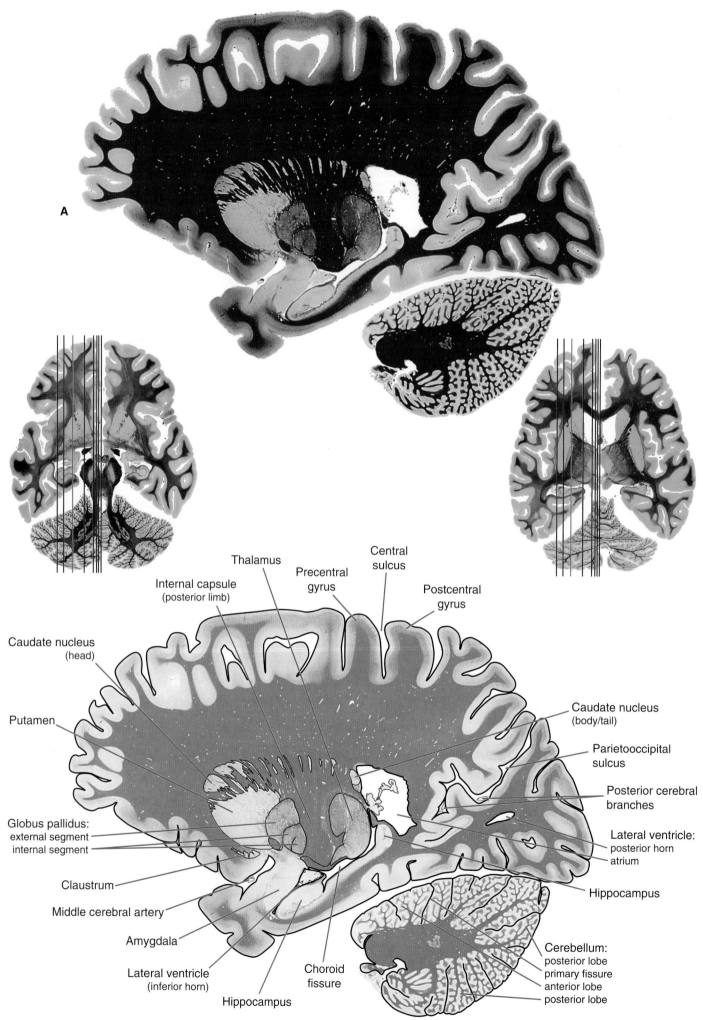

A

Thalamus

Central sulcus

Precentral gyrus

Postcentral gyrus

Internal capsule (posterior limb)

Caudate nucleus (head)

Caudate nucleus (body/tail)

Putamen

Parietooccipital sulcus

Posterior cerebral branches

Globus pallidus: external segment internal segment

Lateral ventricle: posterior horn atrium

Claustrum

Hippocampus

Middle cerebral artery

Amygdala

Lateral ventricle (inferior horn)

Choroid fissure

Hippocampus

Cerebellum: posterior lobe primary fissure anterior lobe posterior lobe

Figure 7–6 **A,** A parasagittal section through the amygdala and hippocampus. Actual size.

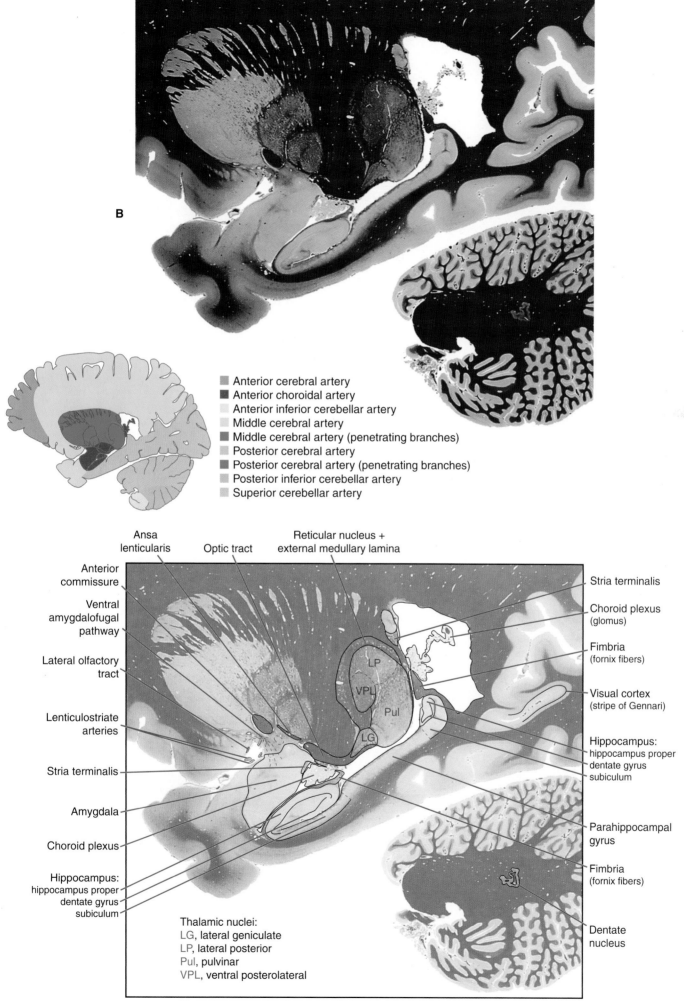

B

Anterior cerebral artery
Anterior choroidal artery
Anterior inferior cerebellar artery
Middle cerebral artery
Middle cerebral artery (penetrating branches)
Posterior cerebral artery
Posterior cerebral artery (penetrating branches)
Posterior inferior cerebellar artery
Superior cerebellar artery

Ansa
lenticularis

Optic tract

Reticular nucleus +
external medullary lamina

Anterior
commissure

Ventral
amygdalofugal
pathway

Lateral olfactory
tract

Lenticulostriate
arteries

Stria terminalis

Amygdala

Choroid plexus

Hippocampus:
hippocampus proper
dentate gyrus
subiculum

Stria terminalis

Choroid plexus
(glomus)

Fimbria
(fornix fibers)

Visual cortex
(stripe of Gennari)

Hippocampus:
hippocampus proper
dentate gyrus
subiculum

Parahippocampal
gyrus

Fimbria
(fornix fibers)

Dentate
nucleus

LP
VPL
Pul
LG

Thalamic nuclei:
LG, lateral geniculate
LP, lateral posterior
Pul, pulvinar
VPL, ventral posterolateral

Figure 7–6 (Continued)   **B,** The central region of Figure 7–6A, enlarged to 1.7× actual size.

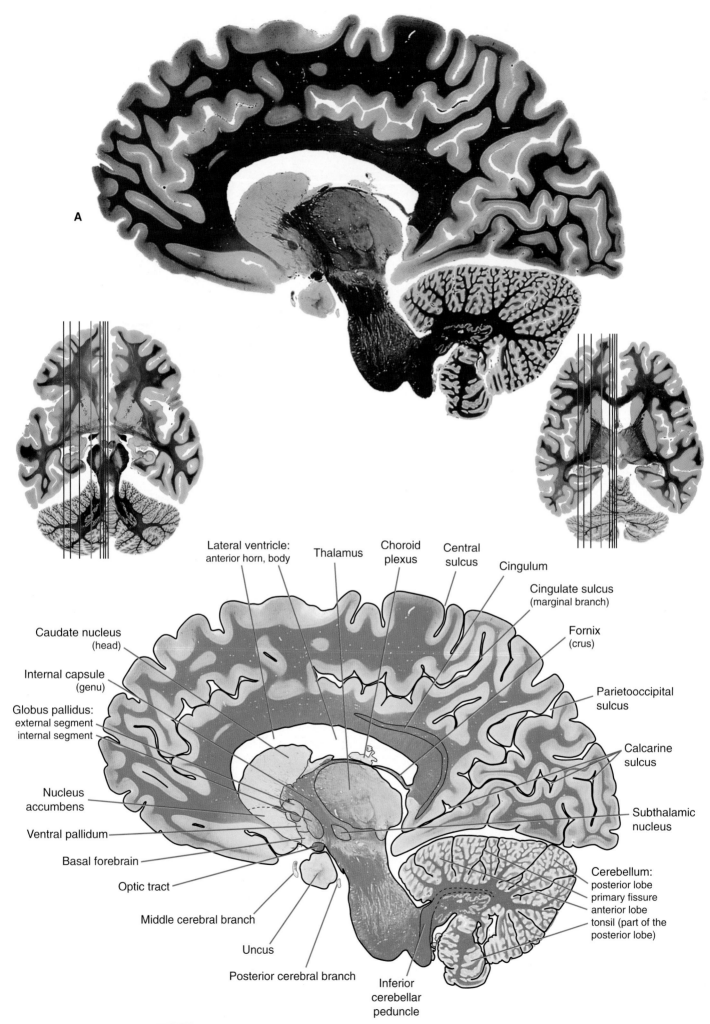

A

Lateral ventricle: anterior horn, body

Thalamus

Choroid plexus

Central sulcus

Cingulum

Cingulate sulcus (marginal branch)

Caudate nucleus (head)

Internal capsule (genu)

Globus pallidus: external segment internal segment

Nucleus accumbens

Ventral pallidum

Basal forebrain

Optic tract

Middle cerebral branch

Uncus

Posterior cerebral branch

Inferior cerebellar peduncle

Fornix (crus)

Parietooccipital sulcus

Calcarine sulcus

Subthalamic nucleus

Cerebellum: posterior lobe primary fissure anterior lobe tonsil (part of the posterior lobe)

Figure 7–7   A, A parasagittal section through the uncus and the middle of the thalamus. Actual size.

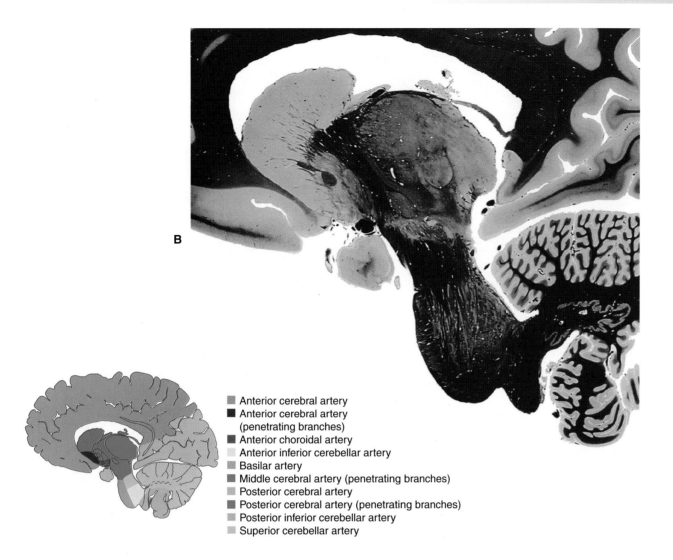

B

Anterior cerebral artery
Anterior cerebral artery
(penetrating branches)
Anterior choroidal artery
Anterior inferior cerebellar artery
Basilar artery
Middle cerebral artery (penetrating branches)
Posterior cerebral artery
Posterior cerebral artery (penetrating branches)
Posterior inferior cerebellar artery
Superior cerebellar artery

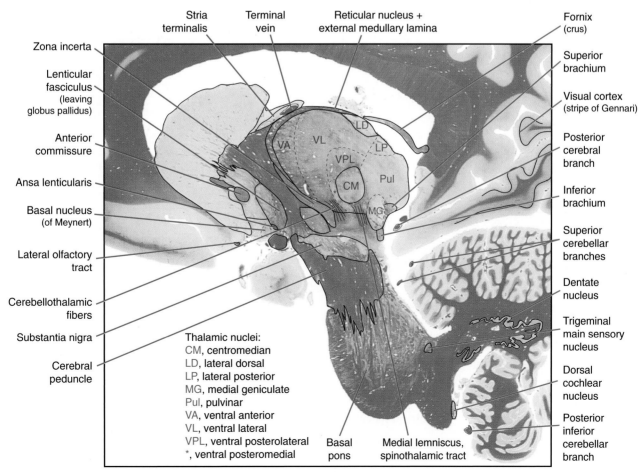

Stria terminalis
Terminal vein
Reticular nucleus + external medullary lamina
Fornix (crus)
Zona incerta
Superior brachium
Lenticular fasciculus (leaving globus pallidus)
Visual cortex (stripe of Gennari)
Anterior commissure
Posterior cerebral branch
Ansa lenticularis
Inferior brachium
Basal nucleus (of Meynert)
Superior cerebellar branches
Lateral olfactory tract
Dentate nucleus
Cerebellothalamic fibers
Trigeminal main sensory nucleus
Substantia nigra
Dorsal cochlear nucleus
Cerebral peduncle
Posterior inferior cerebellar branch

LD
VA
VL
LP
VPL
Pul
CM
MG

Thalamic nuclei:
CM, centromedian
LD, lateral dorsal
LP, lateral posterior
MG, medial geniculate
Pul, pulvinar
VA, ventral anterior
VL, ventral lateral
VPL, ventral posterolateral
*, ventral posteromedial

Basal pons
Medial lemniscus, spinothalamic tract

Figure 7–7 (Continued) **B,** The central region of Figure 7–7A, enlarged to 1.7× actual size.

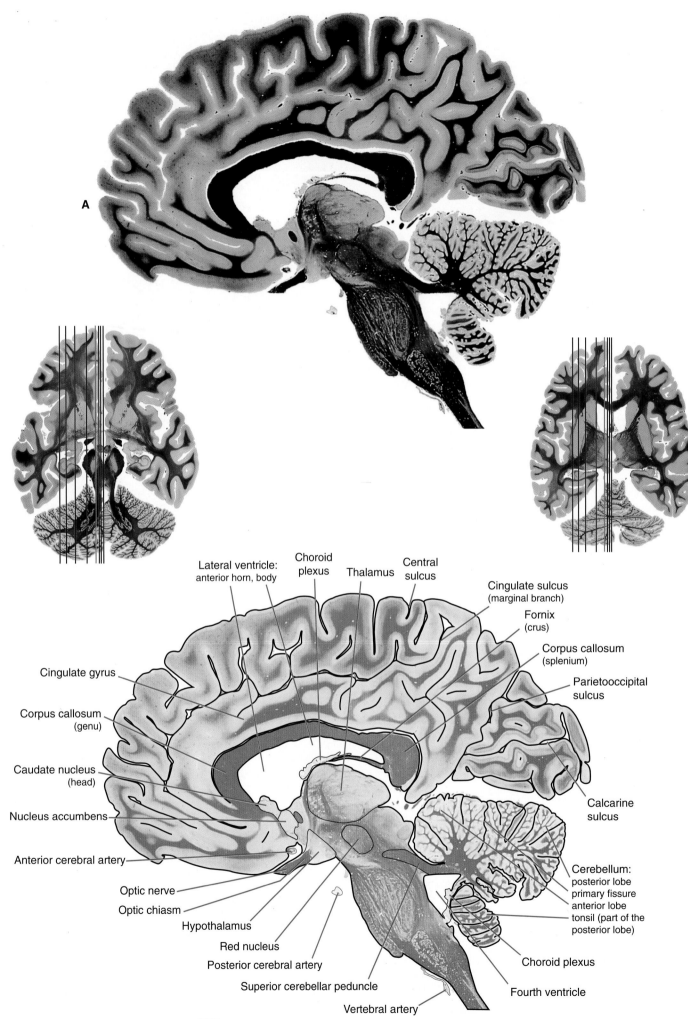

Figure 7–8   A, A parasagittal section through the mammillothalamic tract. Actual size.

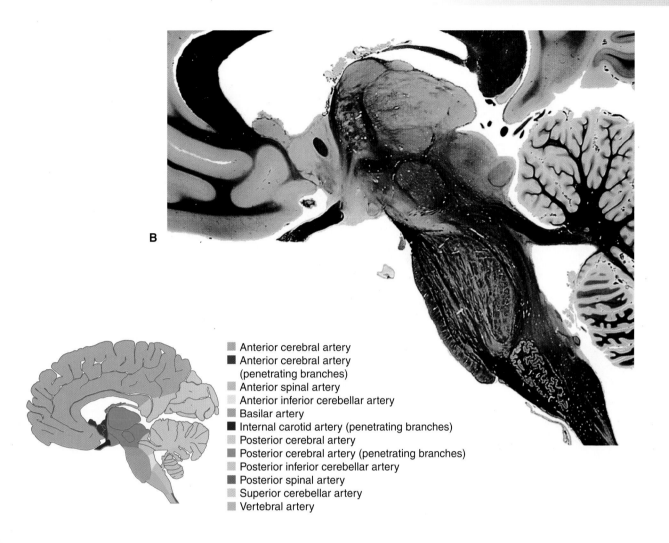

Anterior cerebral artery
Anterior cerebral artery (penetrating branches)
Anterior spinal artery
Anterior inferior cerebellar artery
Basilar artery
Internal carotid artery (penetrating branches)
Posterior cerebral artery
Posterior cerebral artery (penetrating branches)
Posterior inferior cerebellar artery
Posterior spinal artery
Superior cerebellar artery
Vertebral artery

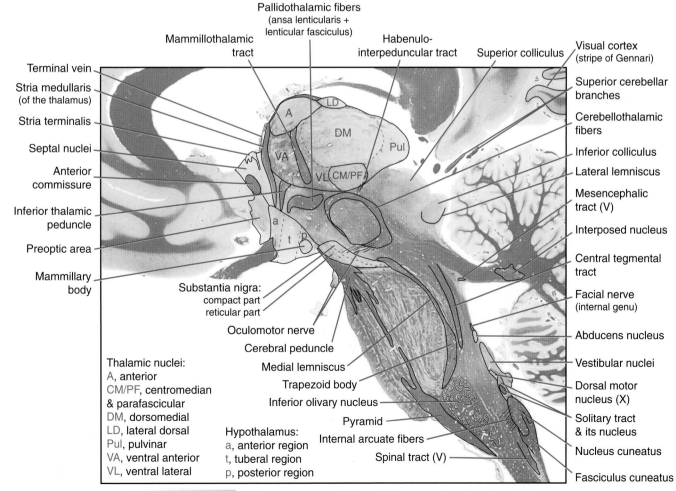

Figure 7–8 (Continued)   **B,** The central region of Figure 7–8A, enlarged to 1.7× actual size.

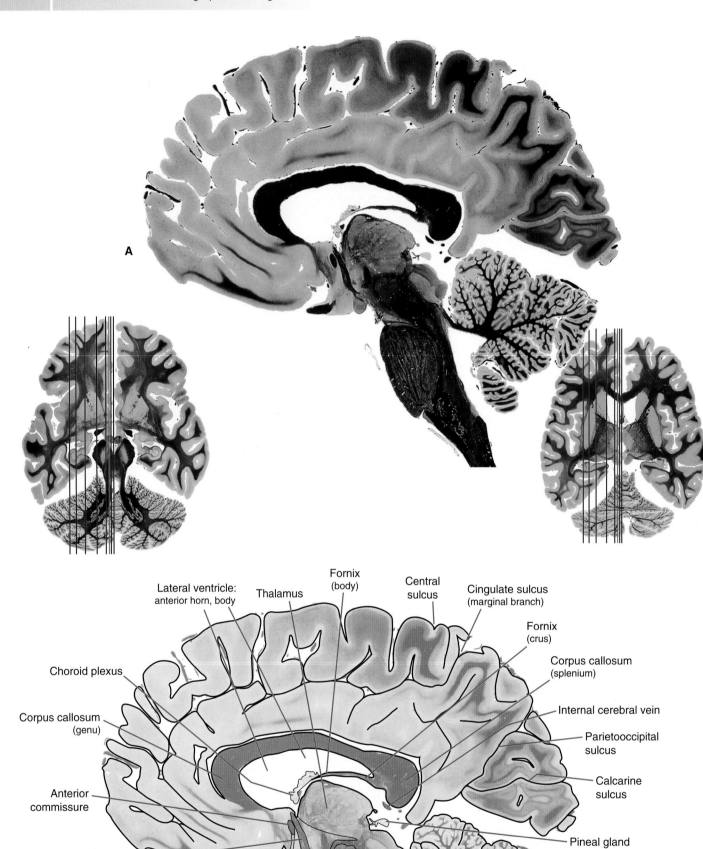

Figure 7–9   A, A parasagittal section through the column of the fornix as it enters the mammillary body. Actual size.

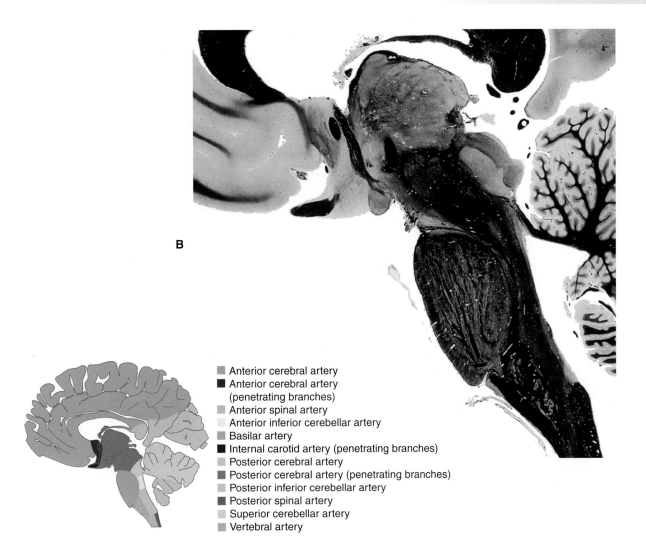

B

Anterior cerebral artery
Anterior cerebral artery (penetrating branches)
Anterior spinal artery
Anterior inferior cerebellar artery
Basilar artery
Internal carotid artery (penetrating branches)
Posterior cerebral artery
Posterior cerebral artery (penetrating branches)
Posterior inferior cerebellar artery
Posterior spinal artery
Superior cerebellar artery
Vertebral artery

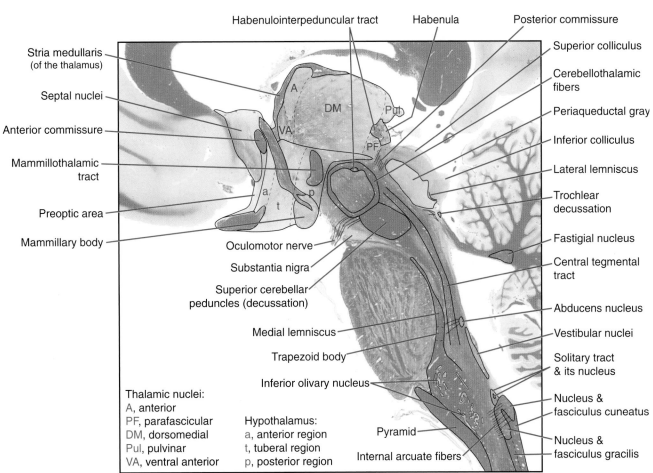

Habenulointerpeduncular tract   Habenula   Posterior commissure

Stria medullaris (of the thalamus)

Septal nuclei

Anterior commissure

Mammillothalamic tract

Preoptic area

Mammillary body

Superior colliculus

Cerebellothalamic fibers

Periaqueductal gray

Inferior colliculus

Lateral lemniscus

Trochlear decussation

Fastigial nucleus

Central tegmental tract

Abducens nucleus

Vestibular nuclei

Solitary tract & its nucleus

Nucleus & fasciculus cuneatus

Nucleus & fasciculus gracilis

Oculomotor nerve

Substantia nigra

Superior cerebellar peduncles (decussation)

Medial lemniscus

Trapezoid body

Inferior olivary nucleus

Pyramid

Internal arcuate fibers

Thalamic nuclei:
A, anterior
PF, parafascicular
DM, dorsomedial
Pul, pulvinar
VA, ventral anterior

Hypothalamus:
a, anterior region
t, tuberal region
p, posterior region

Figure 7–9 (Continued)   **B,** The central region of Figure 7–9A, enlarged to 1.7× actual size.

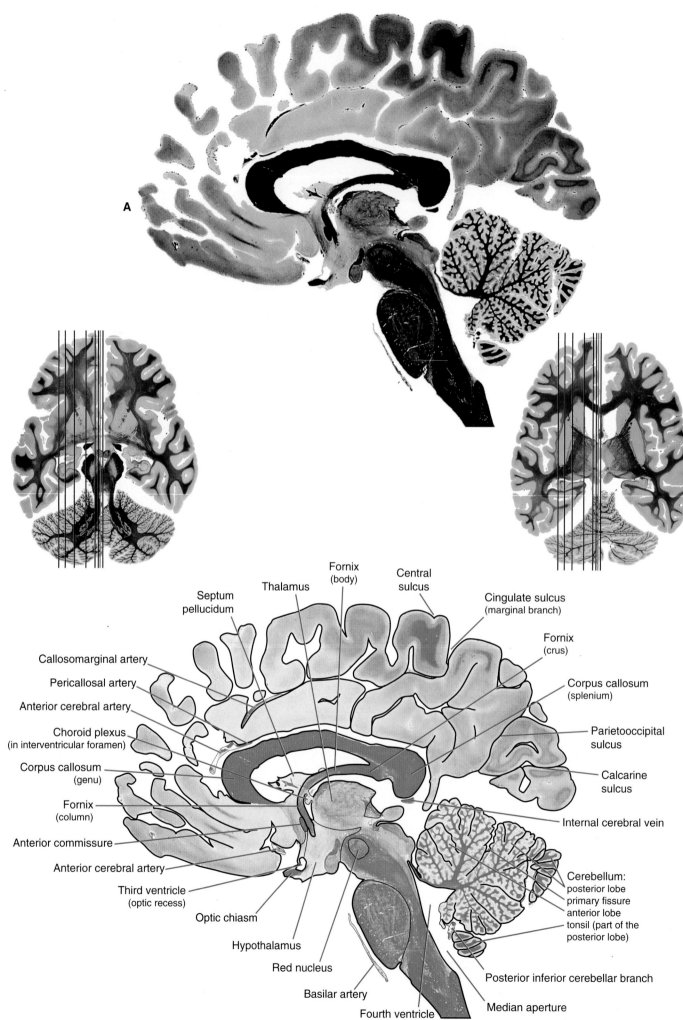

Figure 7–10   A, A parasagittal section near the midline. Actual size.

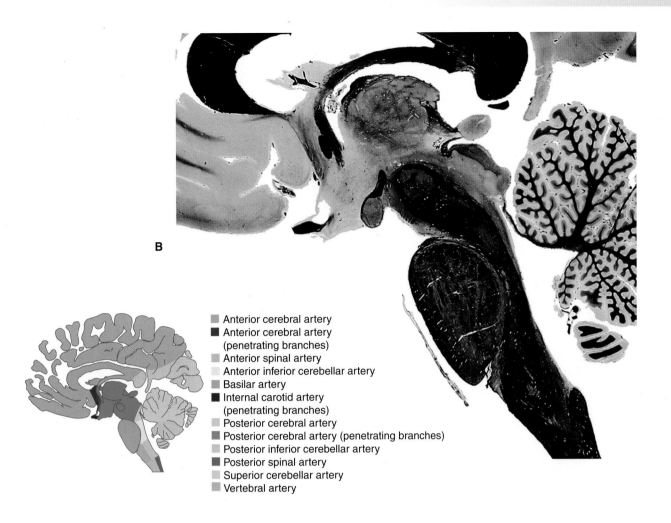

B

- Anterior cerebral artery
- Anterior cerebral artery (penetrating branches)
- Anterior spinal artery
- Anterior inferior cerebellar artery
- Basilar artery
- Internal carotid artery (penetrating branches)
- Posterior cerebral artery
- Posterior cerebral artery (penetrating branches)
- Posterior inferior cerebellar artery
- Posterior spinal artery
- Superior cerebellar artery
- Vertebral artery

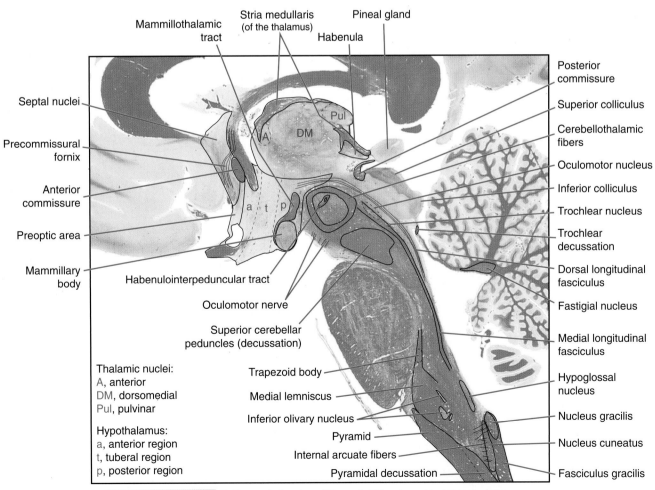

Stria medullaris (of the thalamus)

Mammillothalamic tract

Pineal gland

Habenula

Posterior commissure

Septal nuclei

Precommissural fornix

Anterior commissure

Preoptic area

Mammillary body

Habenulointerpeduncular tract

Oculomotor nerve

Superior cerebellar peduncles (decussation)

Pul

A

DM

a t p

Superior colliculus

Cerebellothalamic fibers

Oculomotor nucleus

Inferior colliculus

Trochlear nucleus

Trochlear decussation

Dorsal longitudinal fasciculus

Fastigial nucleus

Medial longitudinal fasciculus

Hypoglossal nucleus

Nucleus gracilis

Nucleus cuneatus

Fasciculus gracilis

Thalamic nuclei:
A, anterior
DM, dorsomedial
Pul, pulvinar

Hypothalamus:
a, anterior region
t, tuberal region
p, posterior region

Trapezoid body

Medial lemniscus

Inferior olivary nucleus

Pyramid

Internal arcuate fibers

Pyramidal decussation

Figure 7–10 (Continued) **B,** The central region of Figure 7–10A, enlarged to 1.7× actual size.

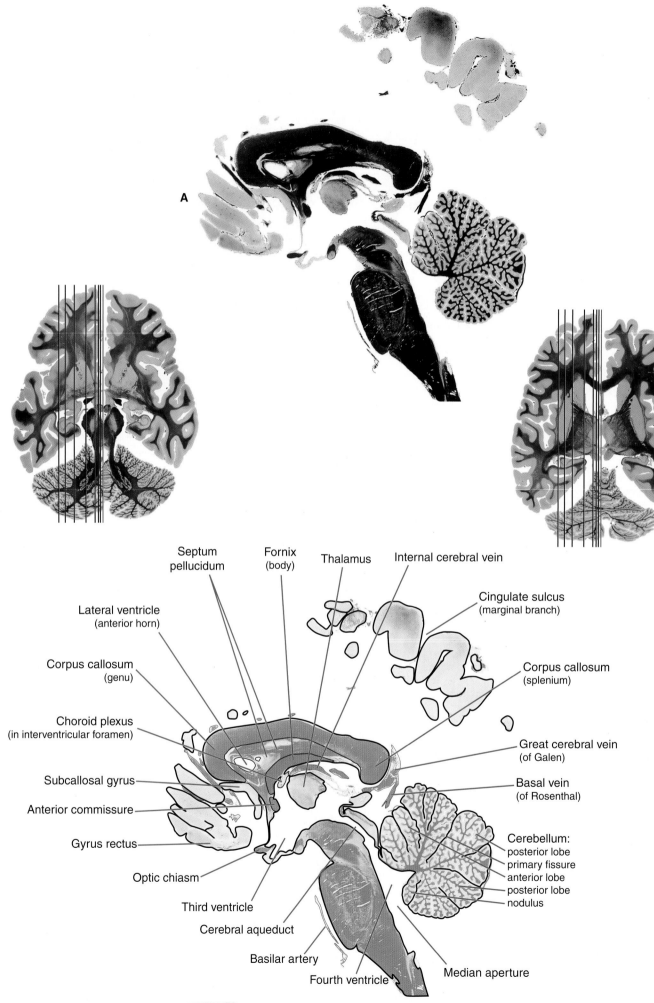

A

Septum
pellucidum

Fornix
(body)

Thalamus

Internal cerebral vein

Cingulate sulcus
(marginal branch)

Lateral ventricle
(anterior horn)

Corpus callosum
(genu)

Corpus callosum
(splenium)

Choroid plexus
(in interventricular foramen)

Great cerebral vein
(of Galen)

Subcallosal gyrus

Basal vein
(of Rosenthal)

Anterior commissure

Gyrus rectus

Cerebellum:
posterior lobe
primary fissure
anterior lobe
posterior lobe
nodulus

Optic chiasm

Third ventricle

Cerebral aqueduct

Basilar artery

Fourth ventricle

Median aperture

Figure 7–11 **A,** A parasagittal section almost exactly in the midline. Actual size.

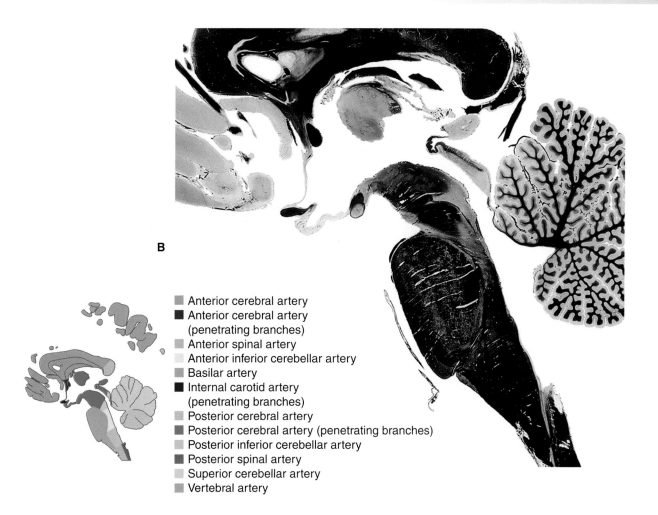

B

- Anterior cerebral artery
- Anterior cerebral artery (penetrating branches)
- Anterior spinal artery
- Anterior inferior cerebellar artery
- Basilar artery
- Internal carotid artery (penetrating branches)
- Posterior cerebral artery
- Posterior cerebral artery (penetrating branches)
- Posterior inferior cerebellar artery
- Posterior spinal artery
- Superior cerebellar artery
- Vertebral artery

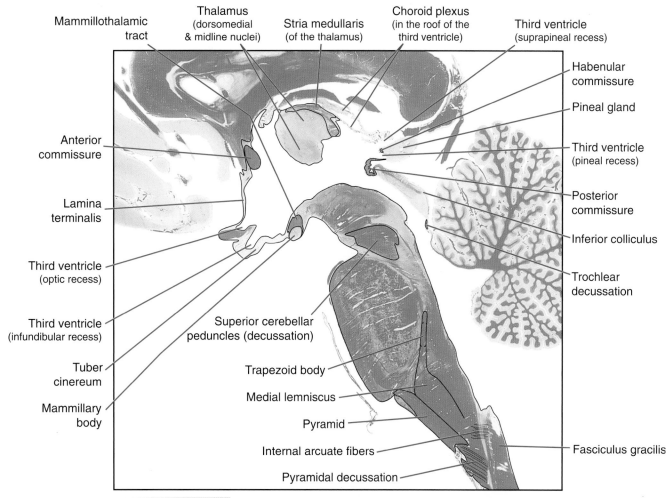

Figure 7–11 (Continued) **B,** The central region of Figure 7–11A, enlarged to 1.7× actual size.

8

Functional Systems

The preceding chapters presented the major structures seen at individual levels of the CNS or in particular views of the brain. This chapter is complementary, using many of the same sections and views to indicate the structures and connections involved in particular neurological functions.

We have taken a "bare bones" approach to this task and indicated only major pathways and connections. Much of the circuitry discussed in standard textbooks has been omitted in the interest of simplicity. The locations of neuronal cell bodies, the trajectories of their axons in tracts, and the locations of their synaptic endings usually are indicated by cartoon neurons such as this one:

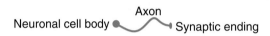

Long tracts of the spinal cord and brainstem

In addition, some anatomical liberties were taken to keep the diagrams relatively simple. The number of lines was minimized by indicating axons as diverging or converging, as follows:

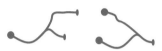

(Axons frequently branch to innervate multiple targets, but this is not what we mean to indicate in any of these figures; moreover, axons from multiple neurons never converge to form a single axon.)

Finally, colors were used to make it easier to follow particular pathways in each figure. Their use is consistent within a given figure, but not across figures: We were unable to devise a meaningful color scheme that would accommodate all the different functional systems. Hence, a given color seldom has a functional implication.

Figure 8–1   A, The posterior column–medial lemniscus system.

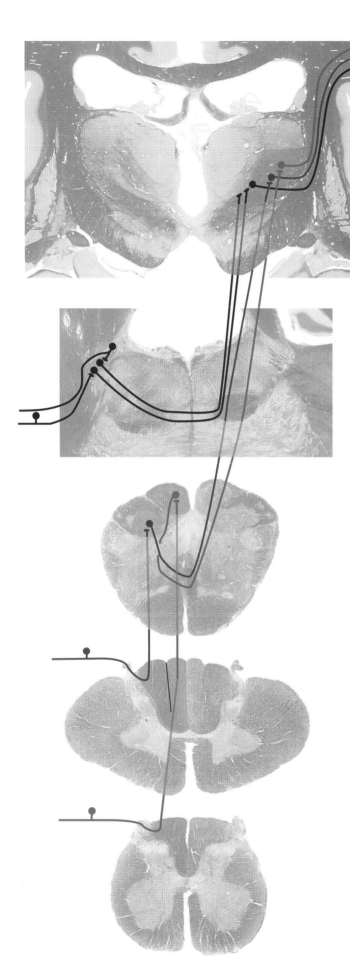

Large-diameter primary afferent fibers, conveying information about limb position and movement and the details of tactile stimuli, enter the spinal cord in the medial division of each dorsal rootlet (Figure 8–1B [inset 1]). The principal route through which this information reaches consciousness is the posterior column–medial lemniscus pathway. Branches of the primary afferents ascend through the ipsilateral posterior funiculus. Entering fibers add onto the lateral aspect of fibers already present in the posterior funiculus (Figure 8–1B [inset 2]), so by the time they reach the medulla, fibers conveying information from the leg are located in the more medial fasciculus gracilis and those conveying information from the arm in the more lateral fasciculus cuneatus. This is the beginning of a somatotopic arrangement that is maintained (with some twists and turns) throughout the remainder of this pathway.

Each posterior column terminates in the ipsilateral posterior column nuclei (nuclei gracilis and cuneatus), whose axons cross the midline and ascend to the ventral posterolateral (VPL) nucleus of the thalamus. VPL in turn projects to primary somatosensory cortex in the postcentral gyrus.

An analogous pathway conveying similar information from the face involves primary afferents with cell bodies in the trigeminal ganglion and the mesencephalic nucleus of the trigeminal nerve (see Fig. 8–4). Central processes of these afferents terminate in the main sensory nucleus of the trigeminal nerve. Their axons cross the midline, join the somatotopically appropriate region of the medial lemniscus, and ascend to the ventral posteromedial (VPM) nucleus of the thalamus. VPM in turn projects to the face area of the postcentral gyrus.

Tactile and proprioceptive information also can reach consciousness via postsynaptic fibers arising from spinal cord neurons. Some of these projections travel in the posterior columns, but others travel in pathways outside the posterior funiculus (e.g., tactile information in the anterolateral system described in Figure 8–2), so posterior column damage does not cause total loss of touch and position sensation.

Figure 8–1 (Continued)   **B,** The posterior column–medial lemniscus system, continued. *(Inset 2 redrawn from Mettler FA: Neuroanatomy, ed 2, St. Louis, 1948, Mosby.)*

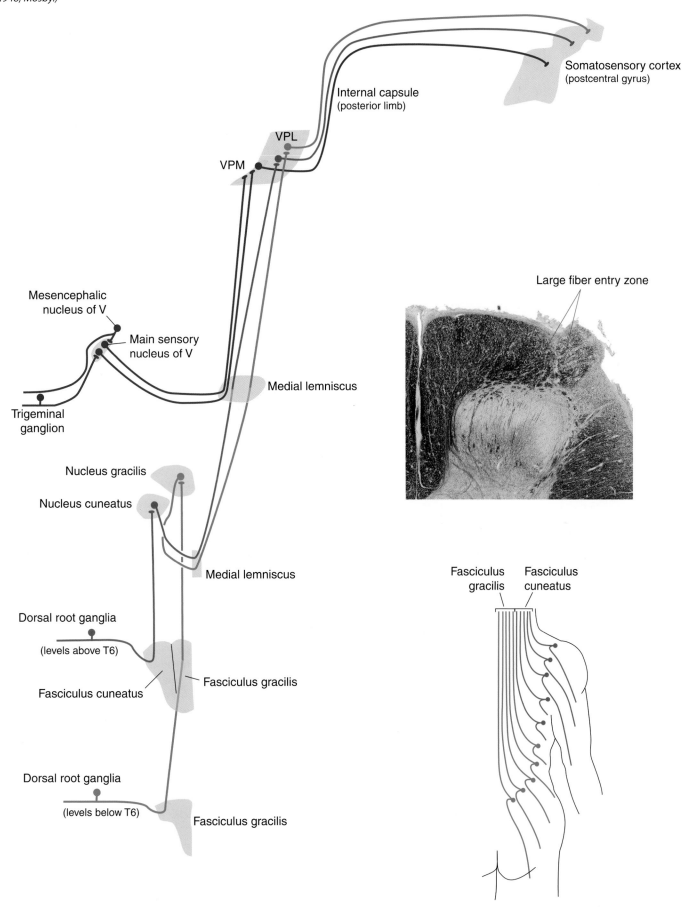

Figure 8–2   A, The anterolateral system.

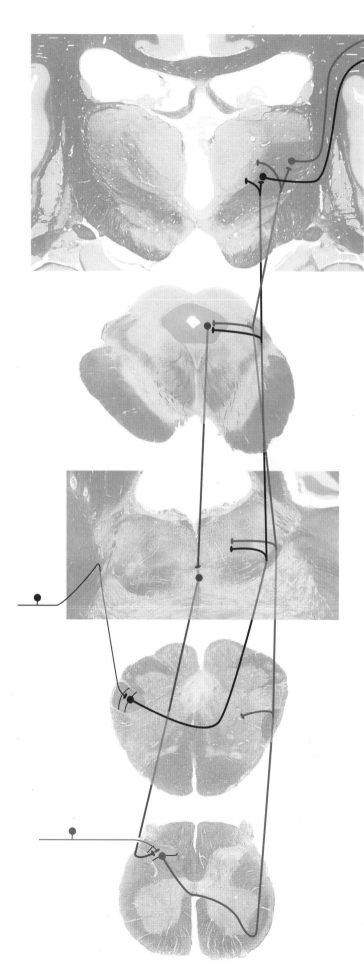

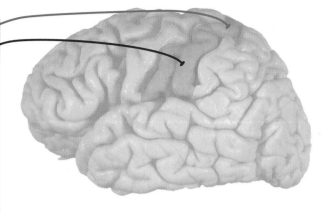

Small-diameter afferent fibers conveying pain and temperature (and a limited amount of tactile) information enter the spinal cord in the lateral division of each dorsal rootlet. The principal route through which this information reaches consciousness is the spinothalamic tract. Primary afferents terminate on tract cells in the posterior horn, whose axons cross and join the spinothalamic tract, adding onto the ventromedial aspect of fibers already present. This initiates a somatotopic arrangement that is maintained (relatively unchanged) throughout the pathway. Spinothalamic fibers then ascend to VPL of the thalamus, which projects to primary somatosensory cortex in the postcentral gyrus.

The analogous trigeminal pathway involves trigeminal ganglion cells whose central processes descend through the spinal trigeminal tract to caudal parts of the spinal trigeminal nucleus (see Fig. 8–4). Axons of these second-order neurons cross the midline, join the somatotopically appropriate region of the spinothalamic tract, and ascend to VPM of the thalamus. VPM in turn projects to the face area of the postcentral gyrus.

Pain and temperature information is in fact more widely distributed than this simplified account would indicate and reaches the reticular formation, additional thalamic nuclei, and multiple cortical areas. Several additional pain pathways travel with or near the spinothalamic tract, and all are commonly referred to collectively as the *anterolateral system.*

Access to the spinothalamic tract is modulated by small neurons of the substantia gelatinosa (and at several other sites). One important pain-control pathway originates in the periaqueductal gray matter of the midbrain and involves a relay in the raphe nuclei (see Fig. 8–38) and nearby reticular formation of the medulla and caudal pons.

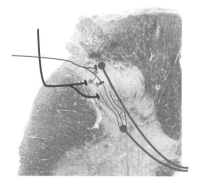

Figure 8–2 (Continued)   **B,** The anterolateral system, continued.

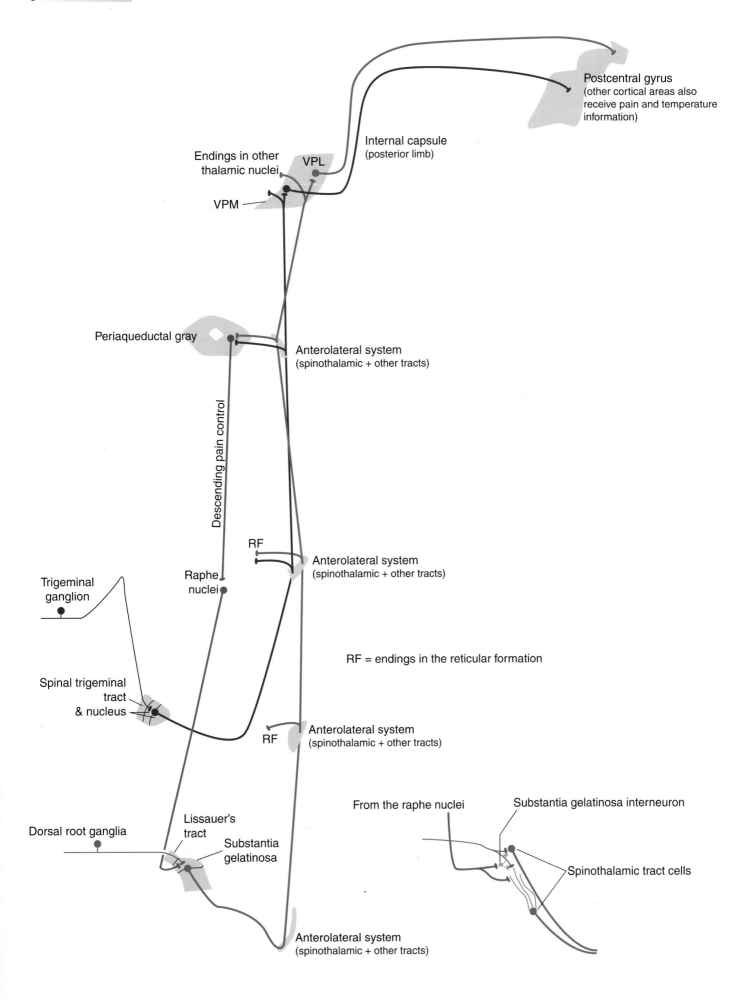

Postcentral gyrus
(other cortical areas also
receive pain and temperature
information)

Internal capsule
(posterior limb)

Endings in other
thalamic nuclei

VPL

VPM

Periaqueductal gray

Anterolateral system
(spinothalamic + other tracts)

Descending pain control

RF

Anterolateral system
(spinothalamic + other tracts)

Raphe
nuclei

Trigeminal
ganglion

RF = endings in the reticular formation

Spinal trigeminal
tract
& nucleus

RF

Anterolateral system
(spinothalamic + other tracts)

From the raphe nuclei

Substantia gelatinosa interneuron

Dorsal root ganglia

Lissauer's
tract

Substantia
gelatinosa

Spinothalamic tract cells

Anterolateral system
(spinothalamic + other tracts)

Figure 8-3   A, The corticospinal tract.

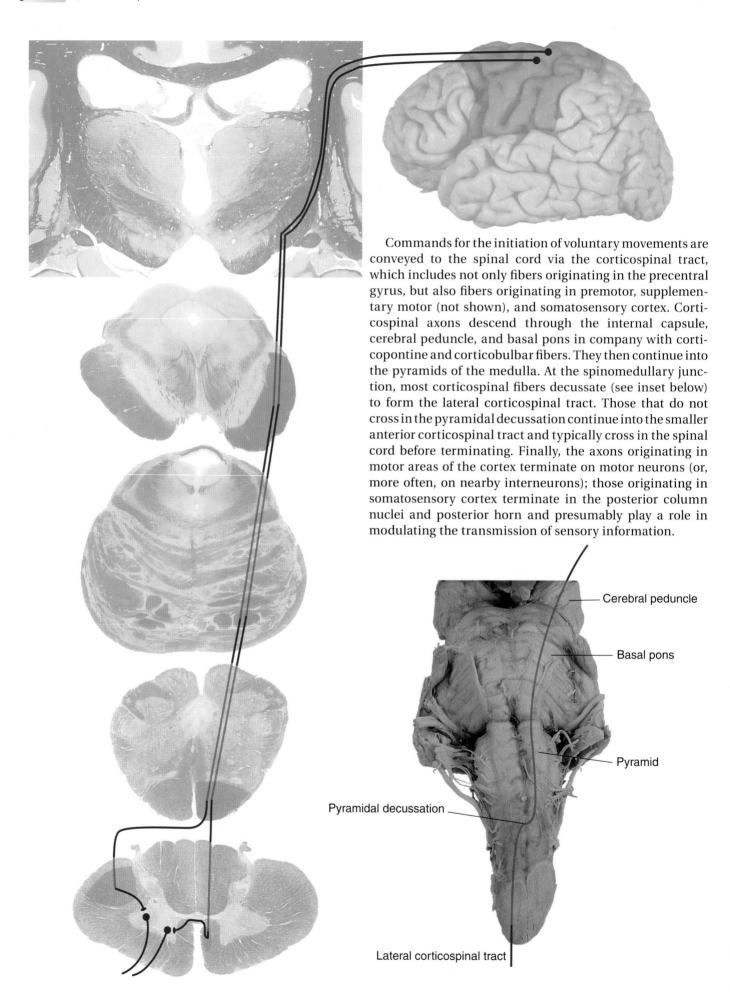

Commands for the initiation of voluntary movements are conveyed to the spinal cord via the corticospinal tract, which includes not only fibers originating in the precentral gyrus, but also fibers originating in premotor, supplementary motor (not shown), and somatosensory cortex. Corticospinal axons descend through the internal capsule, cerebral peduncle, and basal pons in company with corticopontine and corticobulbar fibers. They then continue into the pyramids of the medulla. At the spinomedullary junction, most corticospinal fibers decussate (see inset below) to form the lateral corticospinal tract. Those that do not cross in the pyramidal decussation continue into the smaller anterior corticospinal tract and typically cross in the spinal cord before terminating. Finally, the axons originating in motor areas of the cortex terminate on motor neurons (or, more often, on nearby interneurons); those originating in somatosensory cortex terminate in the posterior column nuclei and posterior horn and presumably play a role in modulating the transmission of sensory information.

Cerebral peduncle

Basal pons

Pyramid

Pyramidal decussation

Lateral corticospinal tract

Figure 8–3 (Continued) **B,** The corticospinal tract, continued.

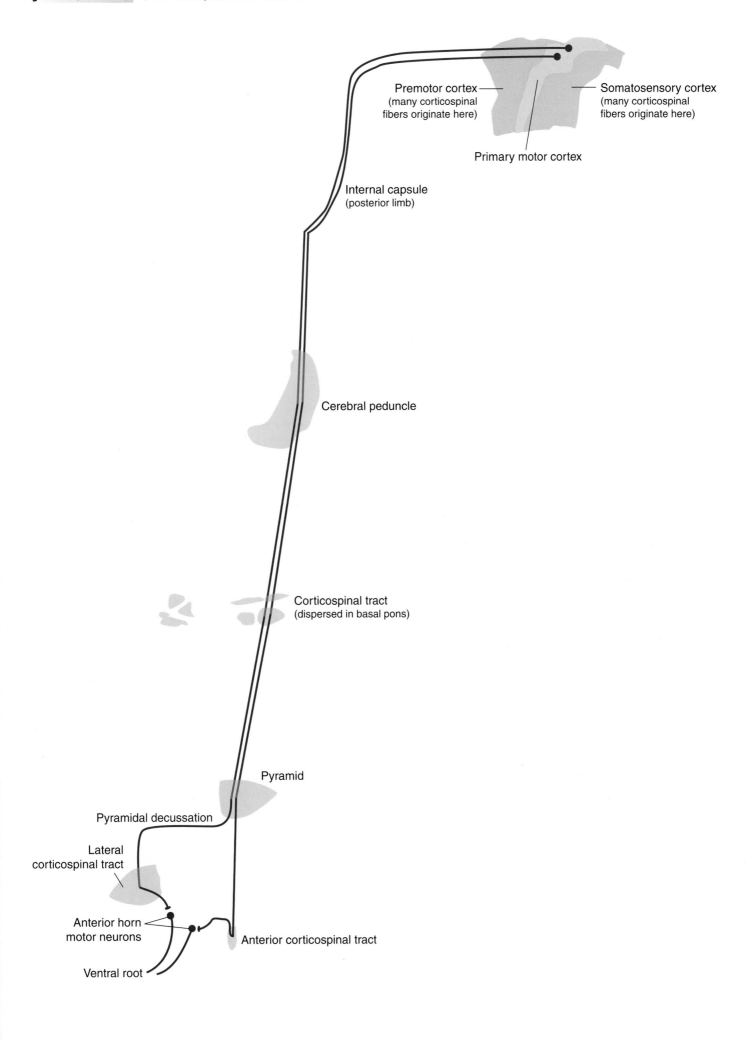

Figure 8-4   A, Central connections of the trigeminal nerve.

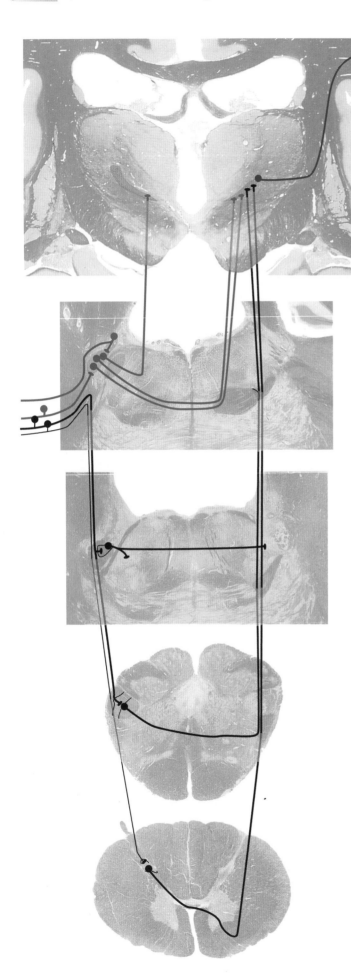

The trigeminal nerve conveys somatic sensory information from most of the head, and it is the motor nerve for most muscles of mastication. Connections of the trigeminal motor nucleus are noted in Figure 8-11, and sensory connections are reviewed here. The connections of somatosensory components bear many similarities to those of spinal nerves (see Figs. 8-1 and 8-2), but there are important differences as well.

Large-diameter trigeminal afferents have cell bodies in the trigeminal ganglion or in the mesencephalic nucleus of the trigeminal (in effect, a bit of the trigeminal ganglion located within the CNS instead of in the periphery). Many central processes terminate in the main sensory nucleus of the trigeminal, which in turn projects through the contralateral medial lemniscus to VPM of the thalamus. (Part of the main sensory nucleus, where the mouth is represented, sends an uncrossed projection, the dorsal trigeminal tract, to the ipsilateral VPM; the functional significance of this uncrossed projection is unclear.) Other central processes project to the trigeminal motor nucleus as part of the masseter stretch reflex arc or to trigeminocerebellar neurons in rostral parts of the spinal trigeminal nucleus.

Small-diameter trigeminal afferents, all with cell bodies in the trigeminal ganglion, travel through the spinal trigeminal tract to termination sites at various levels of the spinal trigeminal nucleus. The most caudal levels of the spinal trigeminal tract and nucleus are essentially rostral extensions of Lissauer's tract and the posterior horn of the upper cervical spinal cord, respectively, and have an analogous function. That is, they convey information about facial pain and temperature to VPM. This seemingly odd location of the second-order neurons for facial pain and temperature ensures that, moving from the spinal cord into the brainstem, there is a smooth continuation of the somatotopic pain/temperature map. More rostral levels participate in trigeminocerebellar projections and in other reflexes, notably the bilateral blink reflex in response to an object touching either cornea.

Figure 8–4 (Continued)   **B,** Central connections of the trigeminal nerve, continued.

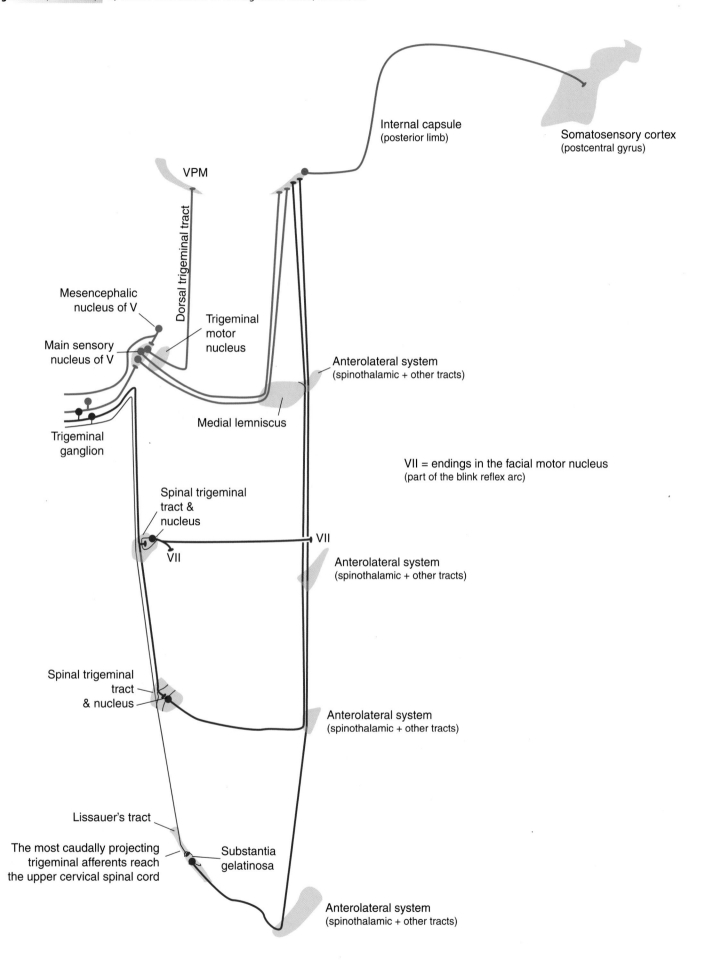

Internal capsule
(posterior limb)

Somatosensory cortex
(postcentral gyrus)

VPM

Dorsal trigeminal tract

Mesencephalic
nucleus of V

Trigeminal
motor
nucleus

Main sensory
nucleus of V

Anterolateral system
(spinothalamic + other tracts)

Medial lemniscus

Trigeminal
ganglion

VII = endings in the facial motor nucleus
(part of the blink reflex arc)

Spinal trigeminal
tract &
nucleus

VII

VII

Anterolateral system
(spinothalamic + other tracts)

Spinal trigeminal
tract
& nucleus

Anterolateral system
(spinothalamic + other tracts)

Lissauer's tract

The most caudally projecting
trigeminal afferents reach
the upper cervical spinal cord

Substantia
gelatinosa

Anterolateral system
(spinothalamic + other tracts)

Figure 8–5   A, Central gustatory connections.

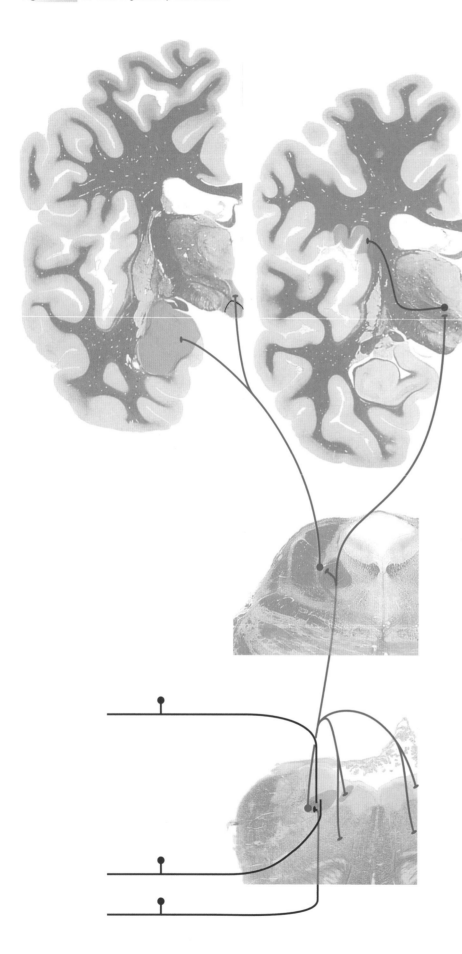

What we commonly refer to as "taste" is actually a complex sensation. Sensory information from taste buds is an important contributor, but this is combined with information from olfactory receptors (aroma) and trigeminal endings (texture, spiciness, temperature). To avoid ambiguity, the sensations initiated in taste buds are referred to as *gustatory* sensations.

The receptor cells in taste buds synapse on peripheral processes of fibers in the facial (CN VII), glossopharyngeal (CN IX), and vagus (CN X) nerves. Facial endings innervate taste buds on the anterior two thirds of the tongue, glossopharyngeal endings innervate those on the posterior third, and vagal endings innervate scattered taste buds of the epiglottis and esophagus. Central processes of these gustatory primary afferents travel through the solitary tract to reach second-order neurons in the nucleus of the solitary tract.

Second-order gustatory neurons influence feeding-related behavior and autonomic functions by projecting to the dorsal motor nucleus of the vagus, to the nearby reticular formation, and even to preganglionic sympathetic neurons in the spinal cord (not indicated in the accompanying figures). Conscious perception of taste is mediated by a largely uncrossed projection from the nucleus of the solitary tract to the thalamus (VPM) and from there to gustatory cortex in the insula and adjacent frontal operculum.

Gustatory information also reaches the hypothalamus and amygdala, where it influences metabolic regulation and feelings of hunger, satiety, and pleasantness or unpleasantness accompanying various tastes. The route used involves, at least partially, a projection from gustatory cortex to the amygdala. In many animals, gustatory information also is transmitted to the hypothalamus and amygdala more directly, through a projection from the parabrachial nuclei of the pontine reticular formation. Whether this pathway is important in humans is uncertain, as implied by question marks in Figure 8–5B.

Figure 8–5 (Continued)   **B,** Central gustatory connections, continued. *(Tongue inset modified from Nolte J: The human brain, ed 5, St. Louis, 2002, Mosby.)*

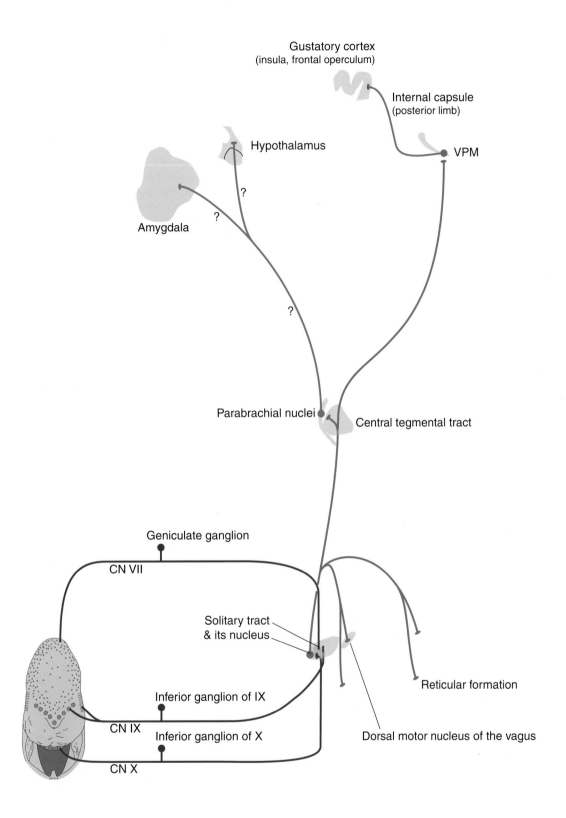

Figure 8–6   A, Central olfactory connections. *(Prosection from Nolte J: The human brain, ed 5, St. Louis, 2002, Mosby.)*

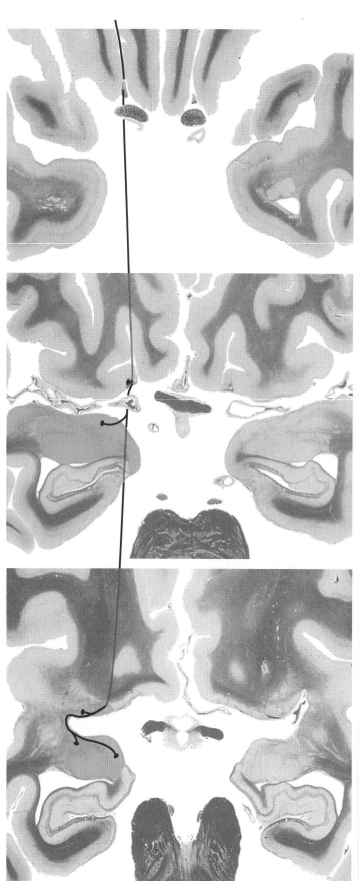

The olfactory bulb develops as an outgrowth of the cerebral hemisphere, leading to a unique arrangement of connections in the olfactory system. The axons of olfactory receptor neurons, collectively composing CN I, pass through the cribriform plate of the ethmoid bone and terminate in the olfactory bulb. Second-order olfactory neurons then project through the olfactory tract to a variety of nearby sites, all part of the cerebral hemisphere. Some olfactory tract fibers terminate in the anterior olfactory nucleus (which in turn projects through the anterior commissure to the contralateral olfactory bulb) or the olfactory tubercle (an inconspicuous part of the anterior perforated substance at the base of the forebrain). The remaining fibers curve toward the temporal lobe as the lateral olfactory tract to reach olfactory cortical areas (piriform cortex adjacent to the lateral olfactory tract, periamygdaloid cortex overlying part of the amygdala, and entorhinal cortex at the anterior end of the parahippocampal gyrus) and a restricted part of the amygdala. This is the only known example of sensory information reaching the cerebral cortex directly, without a stop in the thalamus.

Olfactory information subsequently is distributed more widely, both by projections from these primary olfactory receiving areas and by relays in the thalamus. Some of these olfactory projections converge with gustatory and somatosensory information in an area of orbital cortex important for integrated judgments of flavor.

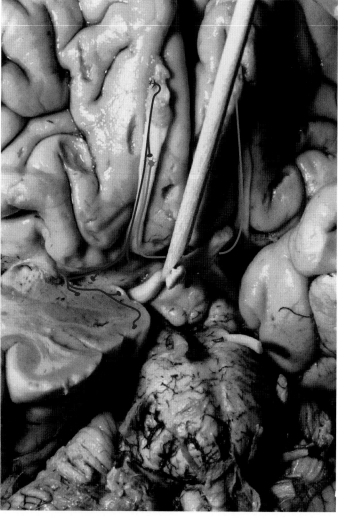

Figure 8–6 (Continued)   **B,** Central olfactory connections, continued.

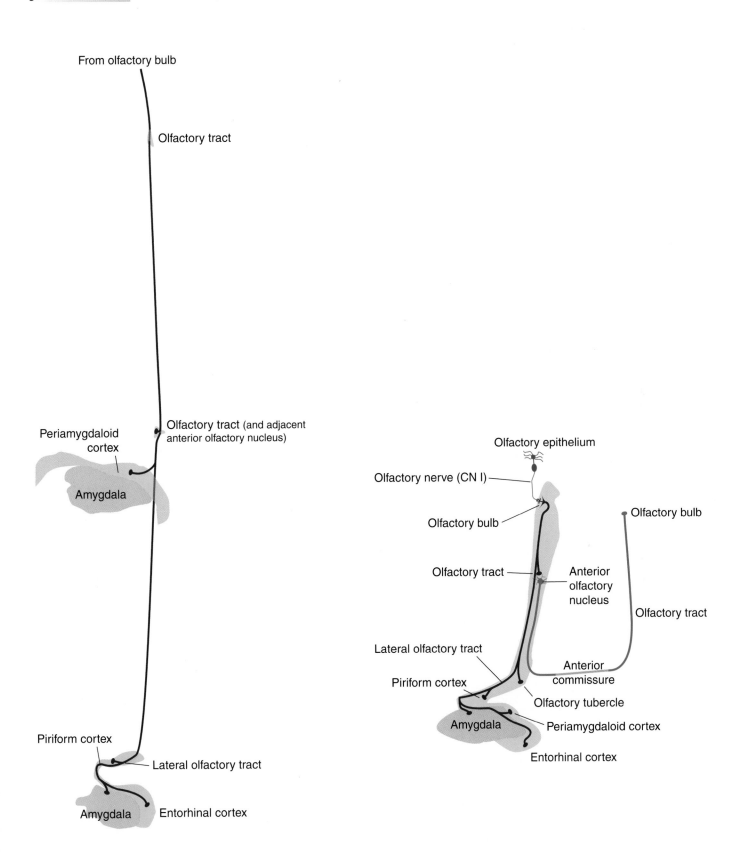

Figure 8–7   A, The auditory system.

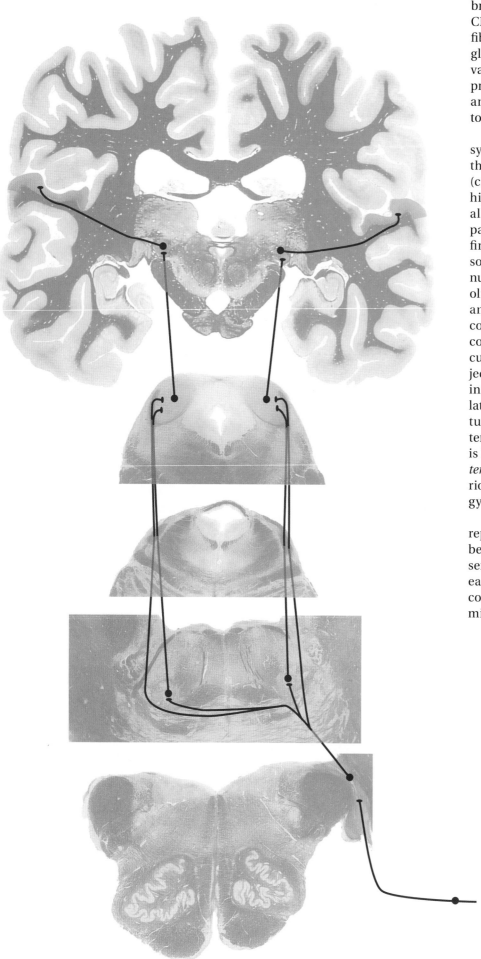

Auditory information reaches the brainstem via the cochlear division of CN VIII, a collection of primary afferent fibers with cell bodies in the spiral ganglion, peripheral processes that innervate cochlear hair cells, and central processes that terminate in the dorsal and ventral cochlear nuclei at the pontomedullary junction.

In contrast to the somatosensory system, the second-order neurons of the cochlear nuclei project bilaterally (crossing in the trapezoid body) to higher levels of the auditory system, allowing for sound localization by comparing inputs from the two ears. The first site where such binaural comparisons occur is the superior olivary nucleus. Efferents from each superior olivary nucleus, together with crossed and uncrossed projections from the cochlear nuclei, ascend to the inferior colliculus through the lateral lemniscus. The inferior colliculus then projects through the brachium of the inferior colliculus to the medial geniculate nucleus of the thalamus, which in turn projects to auditory cortex in the temporal lobe. Primary auditory cortex is located in the aptly named *transverse temporal gyri* (of Heschl) on the superior surface of the superior temporal gyrus.

One consequence of this bilateral representation of each ear at all levels beyond the cochlear nuclei is that serious hearing loss restricted to one ear implies damage at the level of the cochlear nuclei or (more likely) the middle or inner ear.

Figure 8–7 (Continued) **B,** The auditory system, continued. *(Prosection in B from Nolte J: The human brain, ed 5, St. Louis, 2002, Mosby.)*

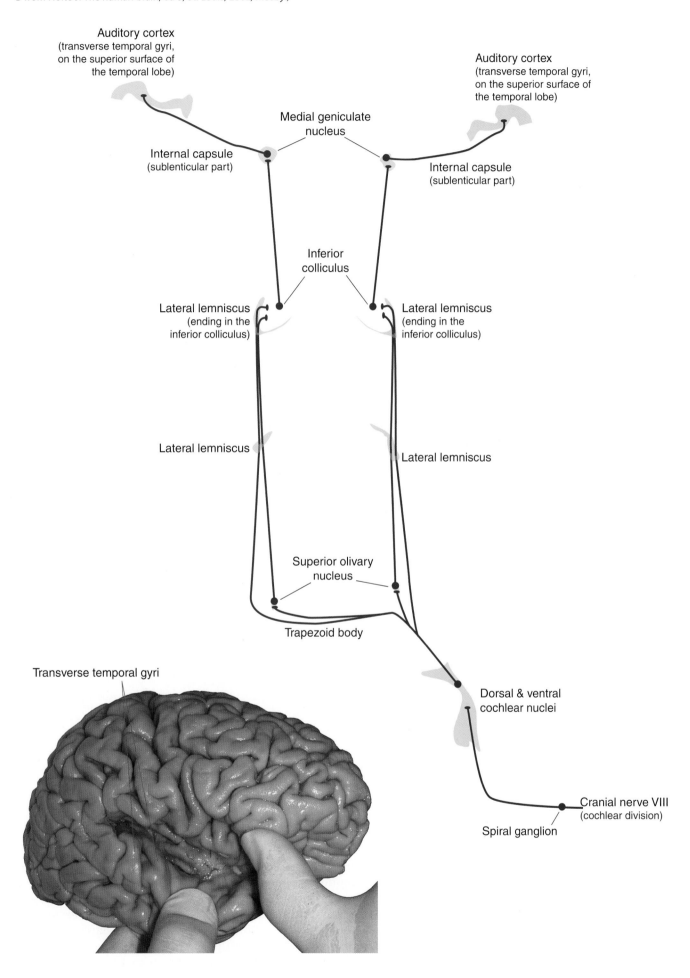

Figure 8–8   A, The vestibular system.

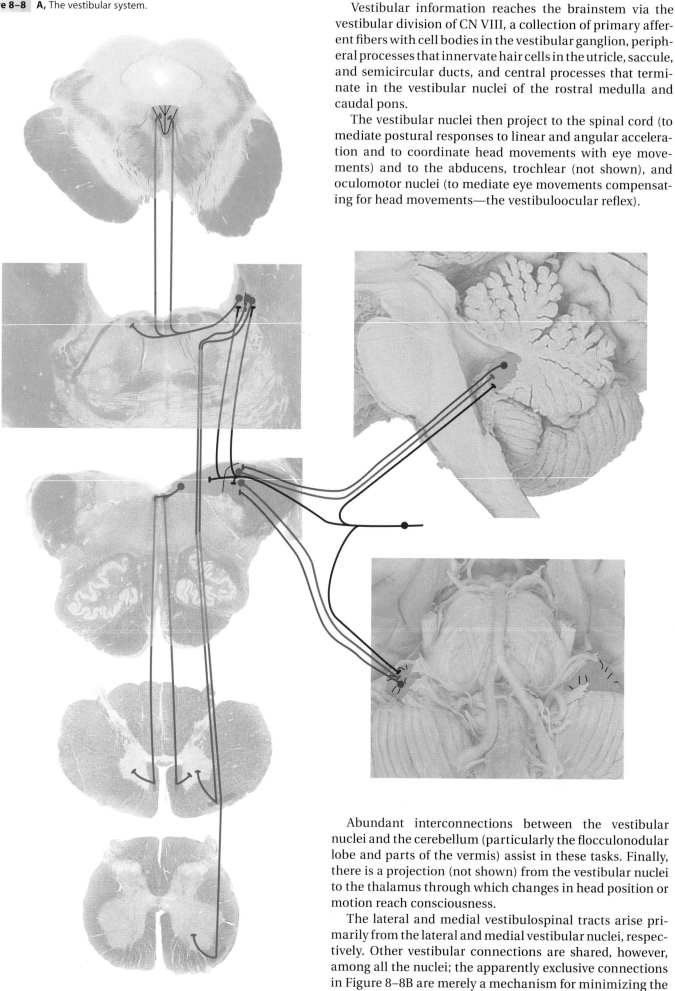

Vestibular information reaches the brainstem via the vestibular division of CN VIII, a collection of primary afferent fibers with cell bodies in the vestibular ganglion, peripheral processes that innervate hair cells in the utricle, saccule, and semicircular ducts, and central processes that terminate in the vestibular nuclei of the rostral medulla and caudal pons.

The vestibular nuclei then project to the spinal cord (to mediate postural responses to linear and angular acceleration and to coordinate head movements with eye movements) and to the abducens, trochlear (not shown), and oculomotor nuclei (to mediate eye movements compensating for head movements—the vestibuloocular reflex).

Abundant interconnections between the vestibular nuclei and the cerebellum (particularly the flocculonodular lobe and parts of the vermis) assist in these tasks. Finally, there is a projection (not shown) from the vestibular nuclei to the thalamus through which changes in head position or motion reach consciousness.

The lateral and medial vestibulospinal tracts arise primarily from the lateral and medial vestibular nuclei, respectively. Other vestibular connections are shared, however, among all the nuclei; the apparently exclusive connections in Figure 8–8B are merely a mechanism for minimizing the number of lines in the figure.

Figure 8–8 (Continued)   **B,** The vestibular system, continued.

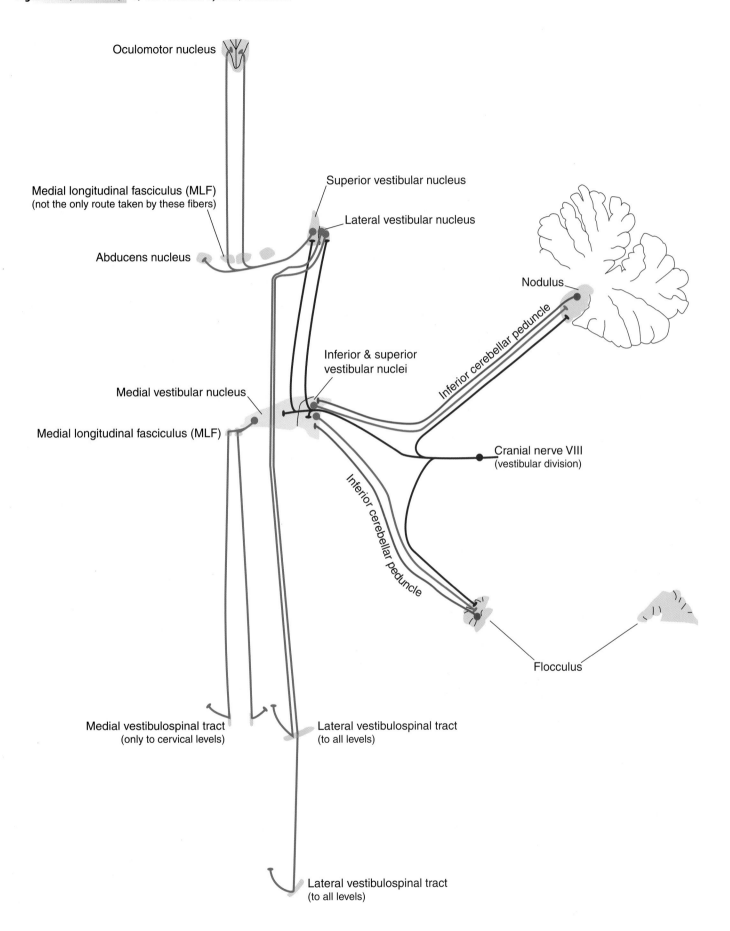

Oculomotor nucleus

Medial longitudinal fasciculus (MLF)
(not the only route taken by these fibers)

Superior vestibular nucleus

Lateral vestibular nucleus

Abducens nucleus

Nodulus

Inferior & superior
vestibular nuclei

Inferior cerebellar peduncle

Medial vestibular nucleus

Medial longitudinal fasciculus (MLF)

Cranial nerve VIII
(vestibular division)

Inferior cerebellar peduncle

Flocculus

Medial vestibulospinal tract
(only to cervical levels)

Lateral vestibulospinal tract
(to all levels)

Lateral vestibulospinal tract
(to all levels)

Figure 8–9 A, The visual system.

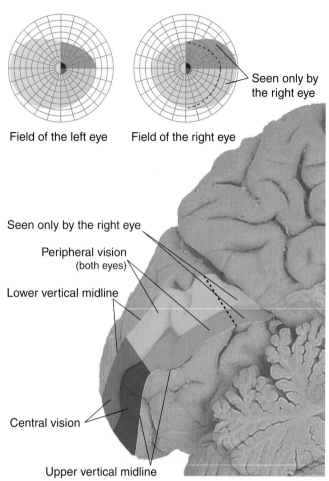

Field of the left eye   Field of the right eye

Seen only by the right eye

Seen only by the right eye
Peripheral vision (both eyes)
Lower vertical midline
Central vision
Upper vertical midline

1, The map of the right visual field (of both eyes) in primary visual cortex of the left occipital lobe. The foveal representation is most posterior and extends over the occipital pole. (Most visual cortex is actually in the walls of the calcarine sulcus.) *(Modified from Nolte J: The human brain, ed 5, St. Louis, 2000, Mosby.)*

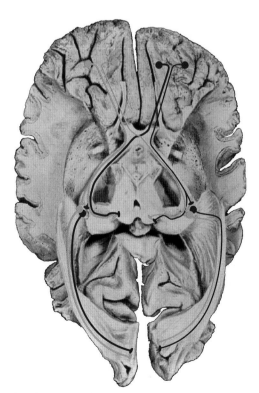

2, The visual pathway, shown over a dissection of the ventral surface of the brain. *(Modified from Ludwig E, Klingler J:* Atlas cerebri humani, *Boston, 1956, Little, Brown.)*

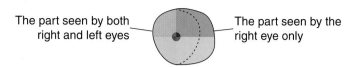

The part seen by both right and left eyes   The part seen by the right eye only

3, The visual field of the right eye.

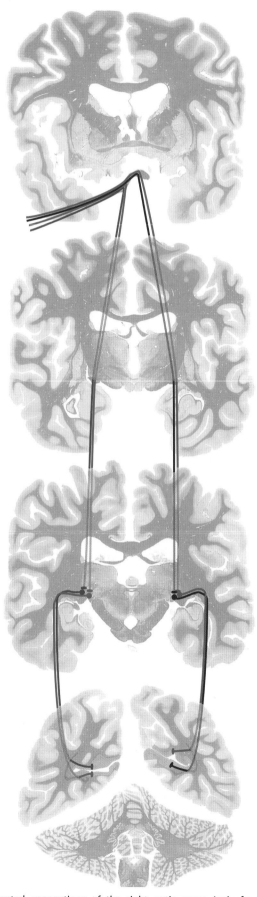

4, The central connections of the right optic nerve (only foveal fibers shown).

Figure 8–9 (Continued) **B,** The visual system, continued.

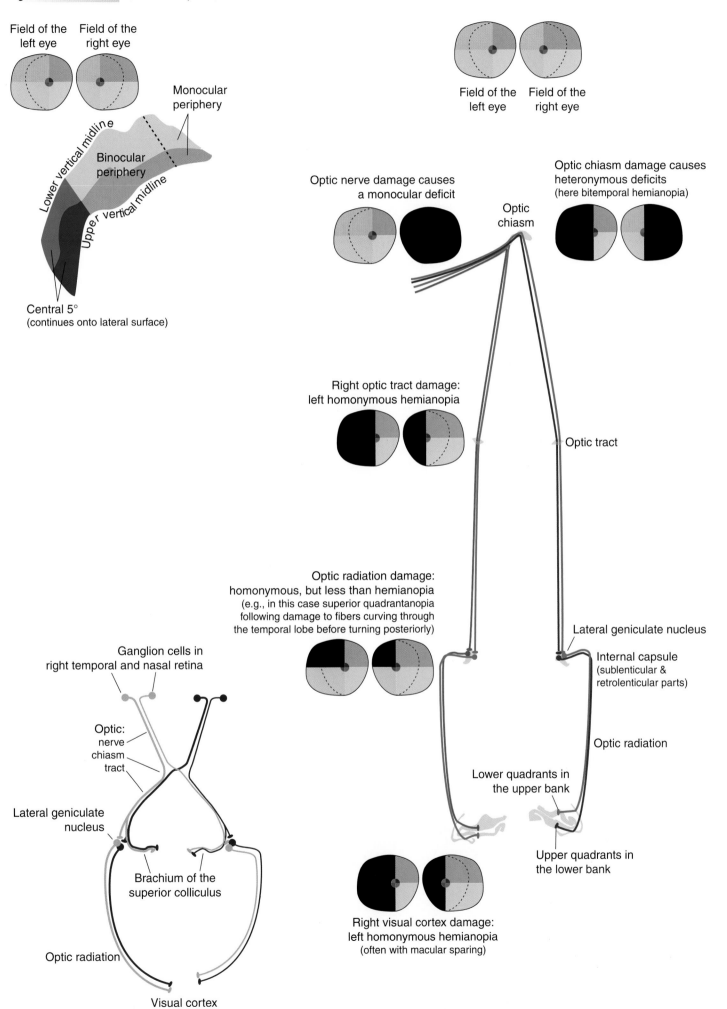

Figure 8-10   Cranial nerve nuclei that innervate ordinary skeletal muscle.

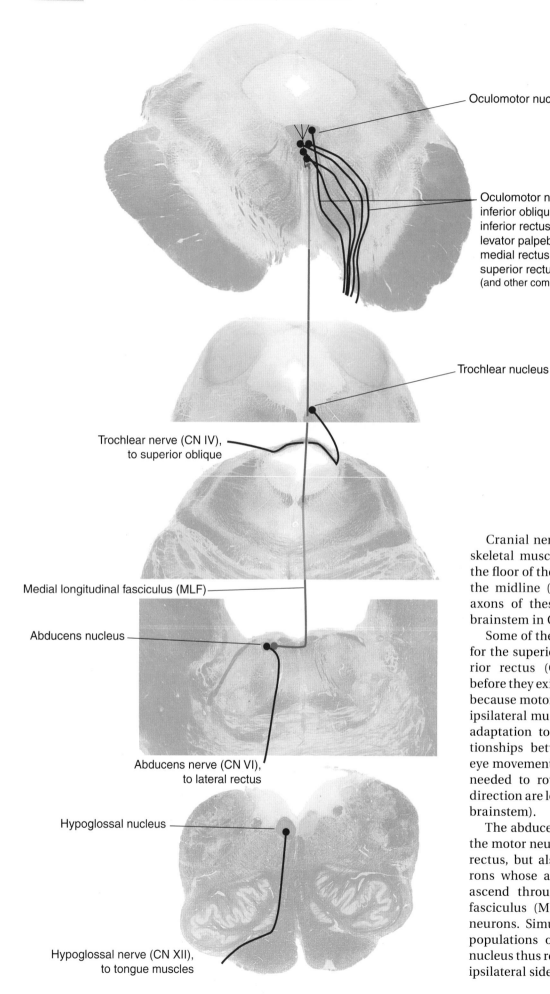

Oculomotor nucleus

Oculomotor nerve (CN III), to:
inferior oblique
inferior rectus
levator palpebrae superioris
medial rectus
superior rectus
(and other components shown in Figure 8-13)

Trochlear nucleus

Trochlear nerve (CN IV),
to superior oblique

Medial longitudinal fasciculus (MLF)

Abducens nucleus

Abducens nerve (CN VI),
to lateral rectus

Hypoglossal nucleus

Hypoglossal nerve (CN XII),
to tongue muscles

Cranial nerve motor nuclei for ordinary skeletal muscle typically are located near the floor of the ventricular system and near the midline (see Figs. 3–3 and 3–4). The axons of these motor neurons leave the brainstem in CN III, IV, VI, and XII.

Some of these axons—specifically, those for the superior oblique (CN IV) and superior rectus (CN III)—cross the midline before they exit. This is an unusual situation because motor neurons generally innervate ipsilateral muscles. It is presumed to be an adaptation to maintain certain interrelationships between head movements and eye movements (e.g., all the motor neurons needed to rotate both eyes in the same direction are located on the same side of the brainstem).

The abducens nucleus contains not only the motor neurons for the ipsilateral lateral rectus, but also a population of interneurons whose axons cross the midline and ascend through the medial longitudinal fasciculus (MLF) to medial rectus motor neurons. Simultaneous activation of both populations of neurons in the abducens nucleus thus results in conjugate gaze to the ipsilateral side.

Figure 8–11   Cranial nerve nuclei that innervate skeletal muscle of branchial arch origin.

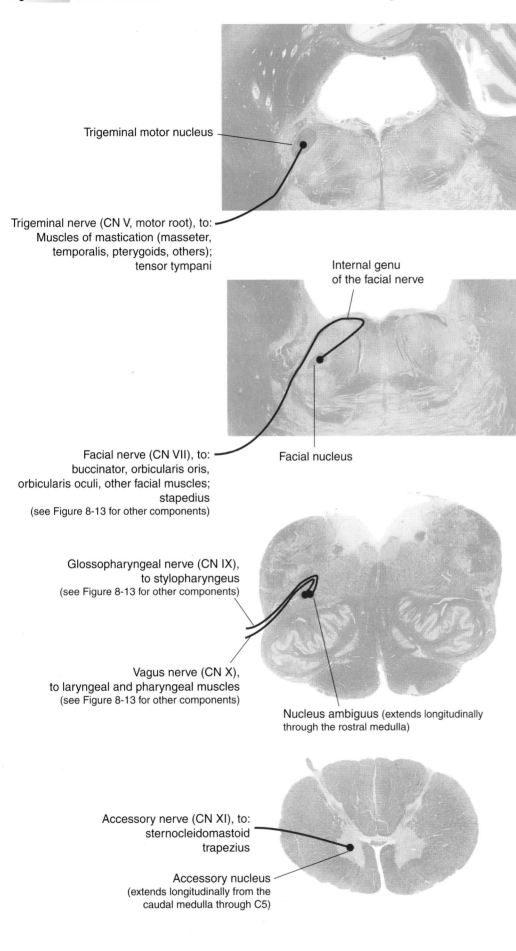

Trigeminal motor nucleus

Trigeminal nerve (CN V, motor root), to:
Muscles of mastication (masseter,
temporalis, pterygoids, others);
tensor tympani

Internal genu
of the facial nerve

Facial nerve (CN VII), to:
buccinator, orbicularis oris,
orbicularis oculi, other facial muscles;
stapedius
(see Figure 8-13 for other components)

Facial nucleus

Glossopharyngeal nerve (CN IX),
to stylopharyngeus
(see Figure 8-13 for other components)

Vagus nerve (CN X),
to laryngeal and pharyngeal muscles
(see Figure 8-13 for other components)

Nucleus ambiguus (extends longitudinally
through the rostral medulla)

Accessory nerve (CN XI), to:
sternocleidomastoid
trapezius

Accessory nucleus
(extends longitudinally from the
caudal medulla through C5)

Cranial nerve motor nuclei for skeletal muscle derived embryologically from branchial arches typically are located farther from both the midline and the floor of the ventricular system than are their counterparts for ordinary skeletal muscle (see Figs. 3–3 and 3–6).

The axons of these motor neurons leave the brainstem in CN V, VII, IX, X, and XI. Many of them make an odd, hairpin turn before their exit. Axons leaving the facial motor nucleus provide the most striking example, hooking around the abducens nucleus in an internal genu (accounting for the facial colliculus in the floor of the fourth ventricle—see Fig. 1–11A).

Figure 8–12   **A,** The corticobulbar tract.

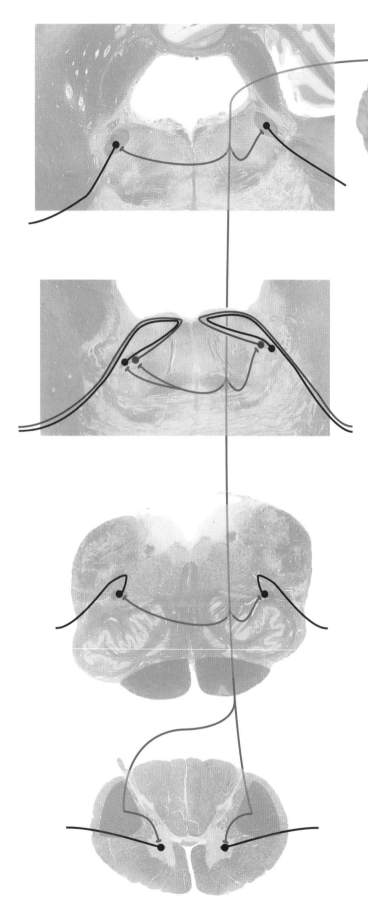

Commands for the initiation of voluntary movements mediated by cranial nerves are conveyed to the brainstem via the corticobulbar tract, which includes not only fibers originating in the precentral gyrus, but also fibers originating in premotor, supplementary motor (not shown), and somatosensory cortex. Corticobulbar axons descend through the internal capsule, cerebral peduncle, basal pons, and medullary pyramids in company with corticopontine and corticospinal fibers. At the levels of the motor nuclei of CN V, VII, IX, X, XI, and XII, contingents of these fibers peel off and terminate on motor neurons there (or, more often, on nearby interneurons). In contrast to the corticospinal tract, which mostly crosses in the pyramidal decussation, the corticobulbar fibers from each hemisphere are distributed bilaterally. This corresponds to the way in which muscles on both sides of the face and head are typically used simultaneously (e.g., chewing, swallowing). As a result of this bilateral distribution, unilateral damage to the internal capsule or corticobulbar tract typically does not cause substantial, lasting weakness of these muscles. The major exception is the muscles of the lower face, whose motor neurons receive a predominantly crossed corticobulbar input (corresponding to the way in which we can make asymmetrical lower facial expressions). Hence, weakness of one lower quadrant of the face is an important clinical sign of contralateral corticobulbar damage. (The nuclei of CN III, IV, and VI receive no direct corticobulbar inputs because cortical projections instead reach brainstem pattern generators that drive coordinated movements of the two eyes.)

Figure 8–12 (Continued)   **B,** The corticobulbar tract, continued.

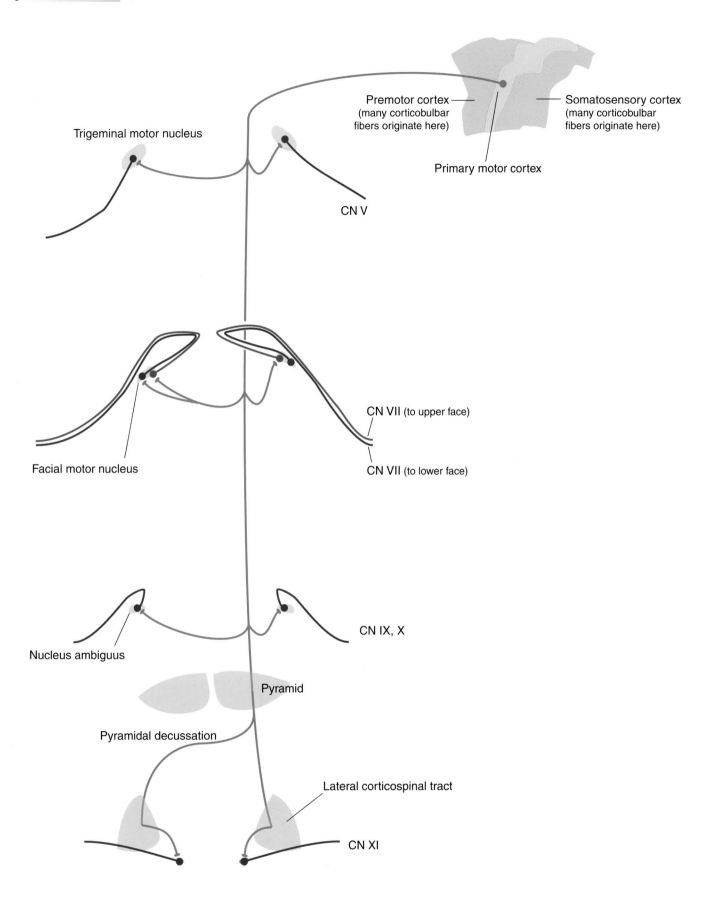

Figure 8–13   A, Visceral and gustatory afferents (right side of the figure); preganglionic sympathetic and parasympathetic neurons (left side of the figure). Relatively minor elements (e.g., visceral afferents in the facial nerve) and some elements lacking a distinct CNS nucleus (e.g., preganglionic parasympathetics mediating lacrimation and salivation via the facial and glossopharyngeal nerves) were omitted.

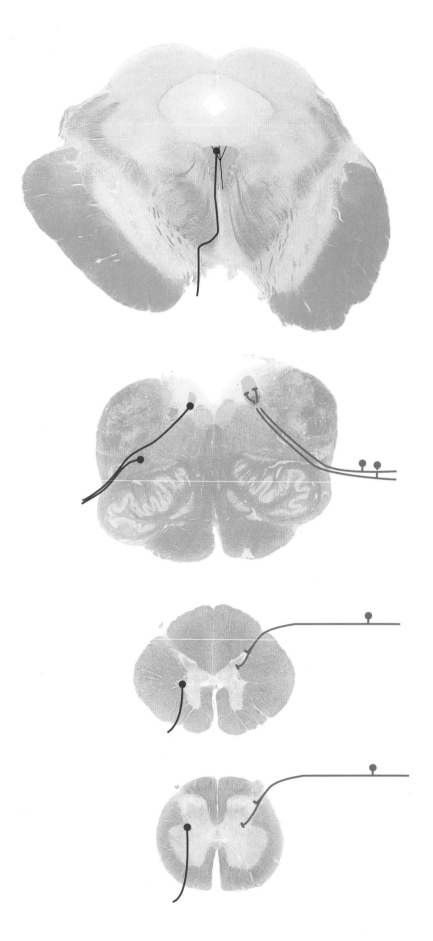

Figure 8–13 (Continued   **B,** Visceral afferents and efferents, continued.

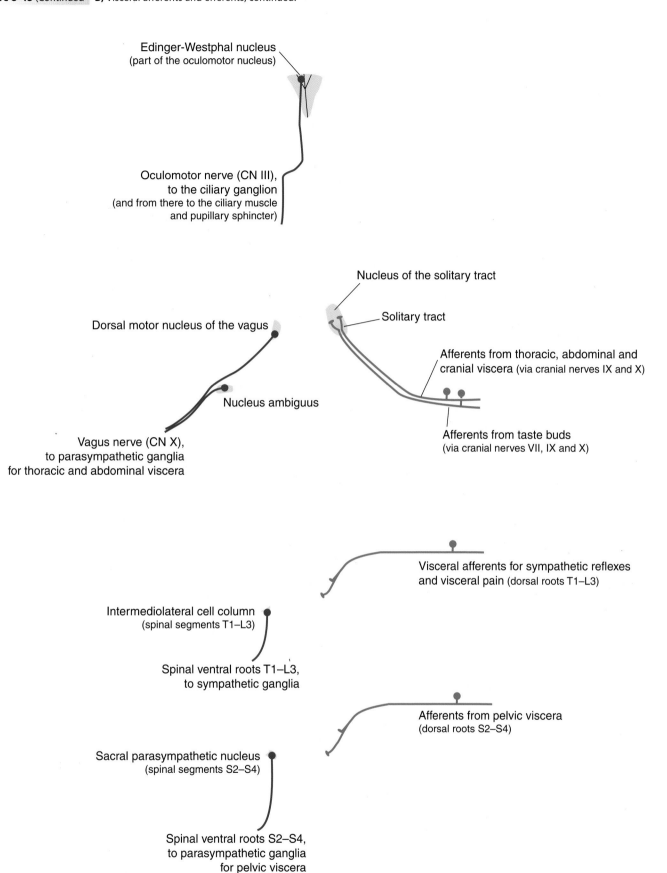

Edinger-Westphal nucleus
(part of the oculomotor nucleus)

Oculomotor nerve (CN III),
to the ciliary ganglion
(and from there to the ciliary muscle
and pupillary sphincter)

Nucleus of the solitary tract

Solitary tract

Dorsal motor nucleus of the vagus

Afferents from thoracic, abdominal and
cranial viscera (via cranial nerves IX and X)

Nucleus ambiguus

Vagus nerve (CN X),
to parasympathetic ganglia
for thoracic and abdominal viscera

Afferents from taste buds
(via cranial nerves VII, IX and X)

Visceral afferents for sympathetic reflexes
and visceral pain (dorsal roots T1–L3)

Intermediolateral cell column
(spinal segments T1–L3)

Spinal ventral roots T1–L3,
to sympathetic ganglia

Afferents from pelvic viscera
(dorsal roots S2–S4)

Sacral parasympathetic nucleus
(spinal segments S2–S4)

Spinal ventral roots S2–S4,
to parasympathetic ganglia
for pelvic viscera

Figure 8–14   The principal circuit of the basal ganglia, shown for the putamen (left side of the figure) and caudate nucleus (right side of the figure). Excitatory connections are shown in green, inhibitory connections in red.

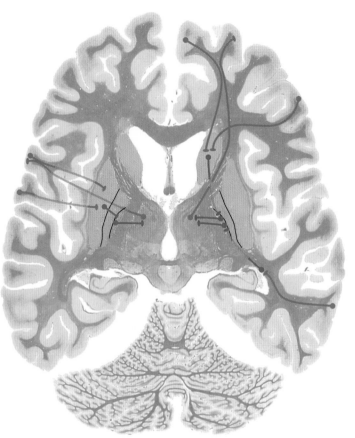

The basal ganglia, which include the striatum,[1] globus pallidus, subthalamic nucleus, and substantia nigra, are prominently involved in motor control (and in cognitive functions as well, in ways less well understood). They affect movement not by projecting to motor neurons in the spinal cord or brainstem, but rather by influencing the output of the cerebral cortex. The principal anatomical circuit underlying this influence is a series of parallel loops of the type indicated in the inset below: A relatively widespread area of cerebral cortex projects to a particular region of the striatum, which by way of the globus pallidus and thalamus feeds back to the cerebral cortex (typically to a frontal or limbic area).

Most parts of the cerebral cortex, and the hippocampus and amygdala as well, participate in such loops. Association areas of cortex are related most prominently to the caudate nucleus, somatosensory and motor cortex to the putamen, and limbic areas to the ventral striatum.

The substantia nigra and subthalamic nucleus form parts of additional basal ganglia circuitry, as indicated in Figures 8–17 and 8–18.

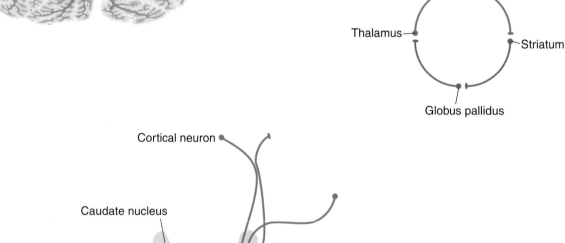

---

[1]Striatum refers to the combination of caudate nucleus, putamen, and ventral striatum (itself a combination of nucleus accumbens and adjacent parts of the caudate, putamen, and basal forebrain).

Figure 8–15 Connections of the striatum; afferents on the left, efferents on the right. Excitatory connections are shown in green, inhibitory connections in red. (Inputs from the compact part of the substantia nigra are shown in a third color because they excite some striatal neurons and inhibit others.)

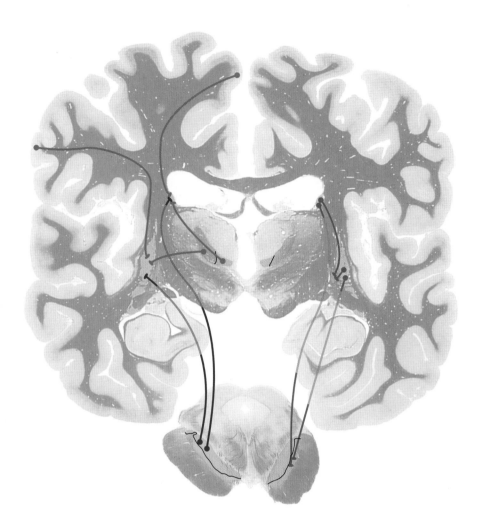

The most prominent afferents to the striatum arise in the cerebral cortex, substantia nigra (compact part), and intralaminar nuclei of the thalamus (especially the centromedian and parafascicular nuclei). Although not shown in this figure, cortical inputs are topographically organized: Association areas project mainly to the caudate nucleus, somatosensory and motor areas to the putamen, and limbic areas (including the hippocampus and amygdala) to the ventral striatum. The implication of these differing inputs, borne out by other aspects of basal ganglia connections and by behavioral studies, is that the different parts of the striatum have distinct functions.

Striatal efferents form the next stage in the path back to cerebral cortex by projecting to both segments of the globus pallidus and to the reticular part of the substantia nigra, which in most respects may be considered an extension of the globus pallidus (internal segment).

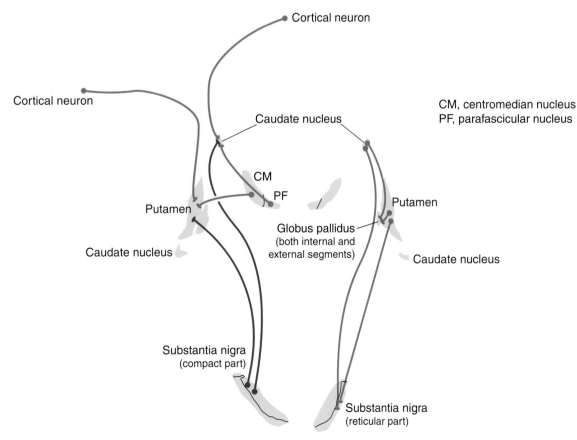

Figure 8–16   Connections of the globus pallidus; afferents on the left, efferents on the right. Excitatory connections are shown in green, inhibitory connections in red.

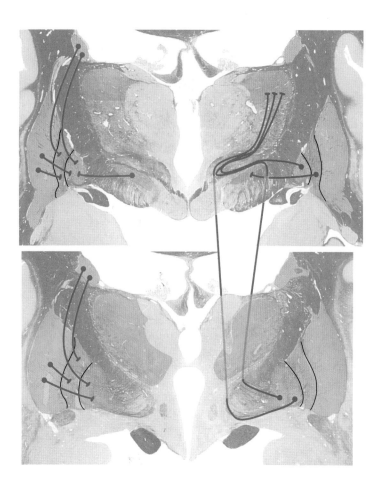

The globus pallidus is prominently subdivided over most of its extent into an external segment (adjacent to the putamen) and an internal segment. Both segments (as well as the reticular part of the substantia nigra [SNr]) receive inputs from the striatum. The subthalamic nucleus provides a prominent excitatory input to the internal segment, through fibers that penetrate the internal capsule as a series of small bundles collectively called the subthalamic fasciculus.

The external (GPe) and internal (GPi) segments of the globus pallidus have distinct efferent projections. GPe projects to the subthalamic nucleus through the subthalamic fasciculus. GPi and SNr, in contrast, form the next stage in the path back to cerebral cortex, by projecting to the thalamus. Some efferents from GPi penetrate the internal capsule as a series of small fiber bundles collectively called the lenticular fasciculus; others emerge from the inferior surface of GPi and hook around the internal capsule in the ansa lenticularis. The ansa lenticularis and lenticular fasciculus join cerebellar efferents underneath the thalamus to form the thalamic fasciculus.

Although pallidal efferents in this figure are shown as ending in the ventral lateral nucleus, many actually end in the ventral anterior nucleus. Others reach more widespread thalamic sites (as might be expected in view of the striatal inputs from diverse cortical areas), such as the dorsomedial nucleus.

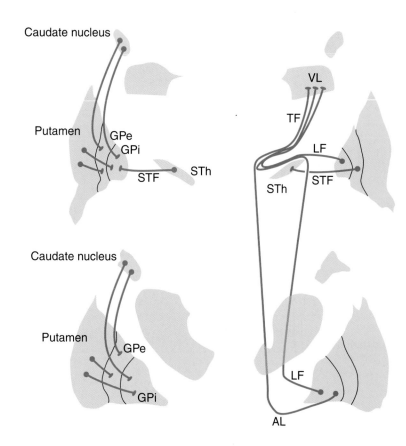

Abbreviations:
AL, ansa lenticularis
GPe, globus pallidus (external segment)
GPi, globus pallidus (internal segment)
LF, lenticular fasciculus
STF, subthalamic fasciculus
STh, subthalamic nucleus
TF, thalamic fasciculus
VL, ventral lateral nucleus of the thalamus

Figure 8–17 Connections of the substantia nigra. Excitatory connections are shown in green, inhibitory connections in red. (Projections from the compact part of the substantia nigra are shown in a third color because they excite some striatal neurons and inhibit others.) *(Histological section from Nolte J: The human brain, ed 5, St. Louis, 2002, Mosby.)*

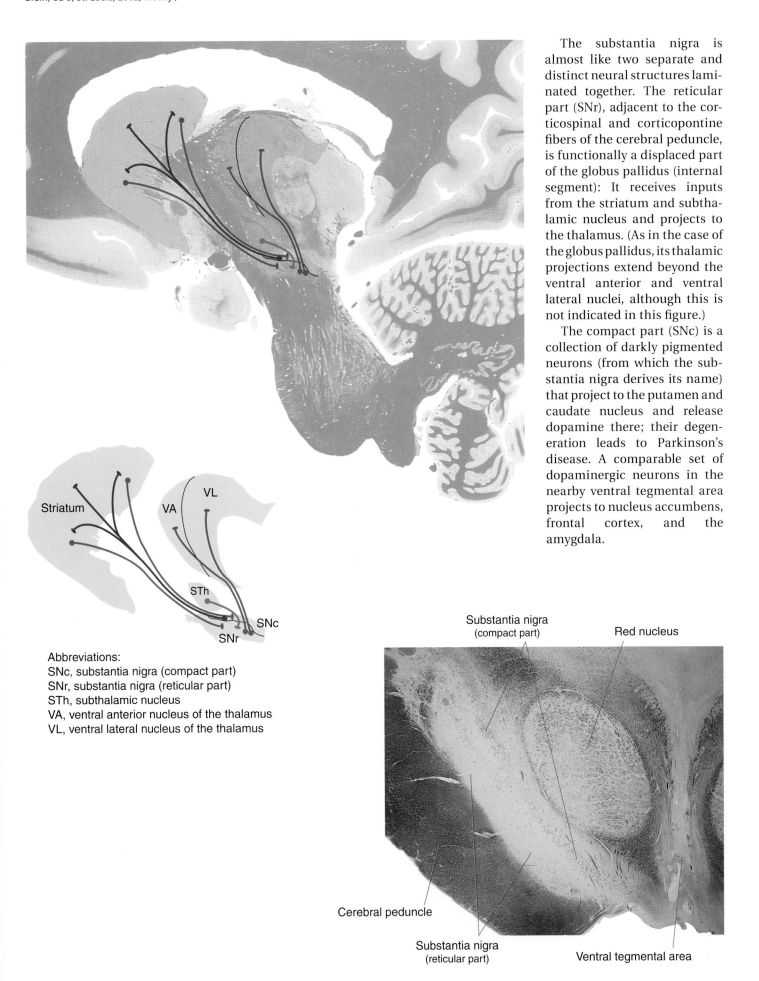

Abbreviations:
SNc, substantia nigra (compact part)
SNr, substantia nigra (reticular part)
STh, subthalamic nucleus
VA, ventral anterior nucleus of the thalamus
VL, ventral lateral nucleus of the thalamus

The substantia nigra is almost like two separate and distinct neural structures laminated together. The reticular part (SNr), adjacent to the corticospinal and corticopontine fibers of the cerebral peduncle, is functionally a displaced part of the globus pallidus (internal segment): It receives inputs from the striatum and subthalamic nucleus and projects to the thalamus. (As in the case of the globus pallidus, its thalamic projections extend beyond the ventral anterior and ventral lateral nuclei, although this is not indicated in this figure.)

The compact part (SNc) is a collection of darkly pigmented neurons (from which the substantia nigra derives its name) that project to the putamen and caudate nucleus and release dopamine there; their degeneration leads to Parkinson's disease. A comparable set of dopaminergic neurons in the nearby ventral tegmental area projects to nucleus accumbens, frontal cortex, and the amygdala.

Figure 8–18   Connections of the subthalamic nucleus. Excitatory connections are shown in green, inhibitory connections in red.

Despite its relatively small size, the subthalamic nucleus has surprisingly widespread connections, with inputs from the cerebral cortex (especially motor cortex) and interconnections with the thalamus, reticular formation, and several nuclei of the basal ganglia. The most important of these connections from a functional standpoint may be inputs from the external segment of the globus pallidus and outputs to the internal segment of the globus pallidus (and to the reticular part of the substantia nigra). These form part of an indirect route through the basal ganglia (see inset below). One general strategy used by the basal ganglia may be to facilitate some cortical activities by means of signals conveyed in the direct route (described in Fig. 8–14), while simultaneously suppressing competing cortical activities by means of signals in this indirect route.

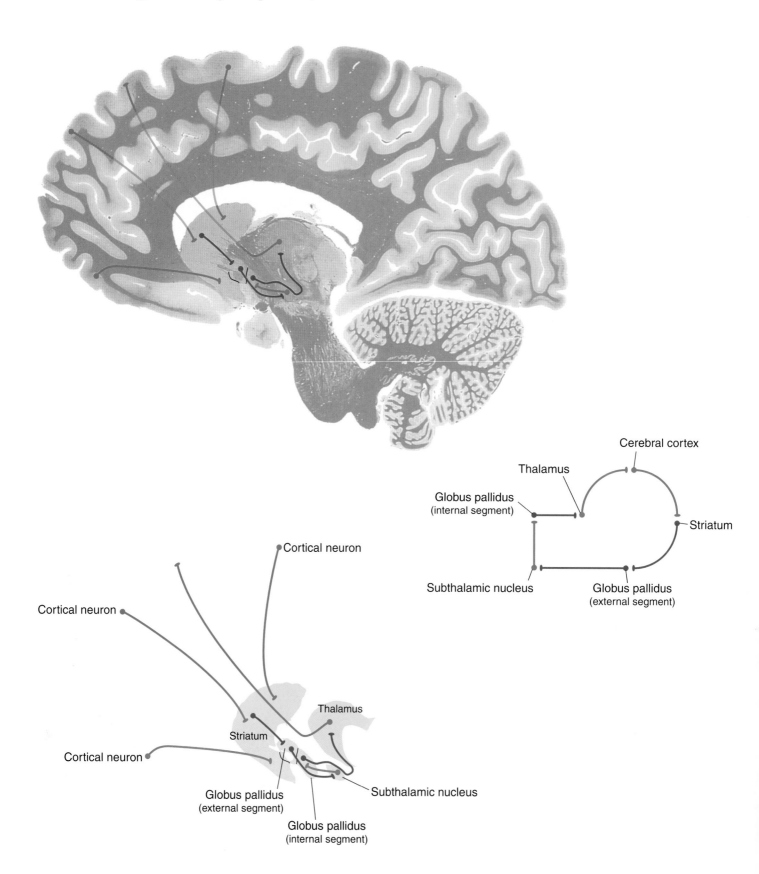

Figure 8–19 Gross anatomy of the cerebellum (see Fig. 1–9 for additional views of the same cerebellum).

The cerebellum is even more highly convoluted than the cerebral hemispheres; this makes room for a large expanse of uniformly organized cerebellar cortex (see Fig. 8–21). Its fissures are mostly oriented transversely, and prominent ones are used as landmarks to divide the cerebellum into lobes and lobules. Thus, the very deep primary fissure separates the anterior and posterior lobes, and the posterolateral fissure separates the posterior and flocculonodular lobes. Along lines roughly at right angles to the fissures, the entire cerebellum is divided into a narrow vermis that straddles the midline and a much larger hemisphere on each side.

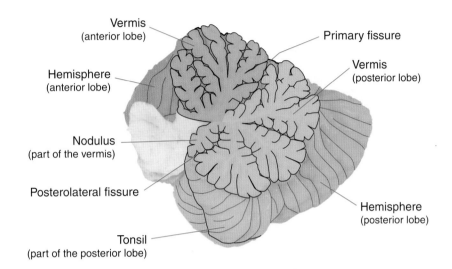

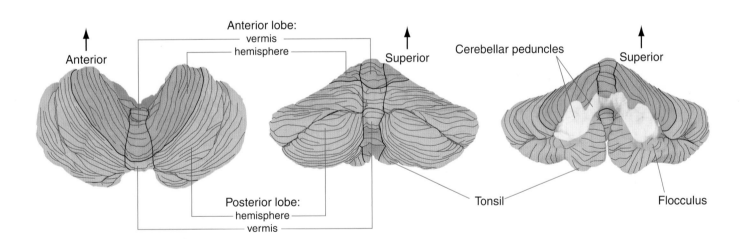

Figure 8–20   Routes into and out of the cerebellum: the cerebellar peduncles.

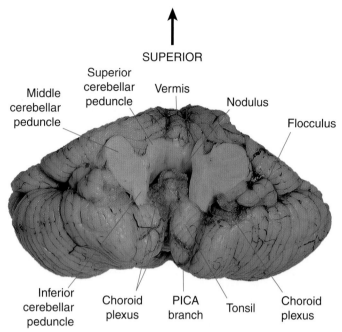

SUPERIOR

Middle cerebellar peduncle · Superior cerebellar peduncle · Vermis · Nodulus · Flocculus · Inferior cerebellar peduncle · Choroid plexus · PICA branch · Tonsil · Choroid plexus

A, Ventral surface of a cerebellum that had been removed from the brainstem by severing the cerebellar peduncles. The view is as if one were looking dorsally from the floor of the fourth ventricle toward its roof. (*A from Nolte J:* The human brain, *ed 5, St. Louis, 2002, Mosby.*)

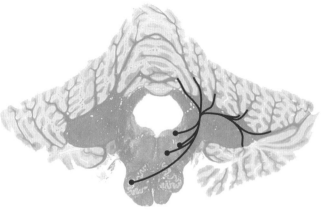

B, The inferior cerebellar peduncle is the major input route for fibers from the inferior olivary nucleus, vestibular nuclei, trigeminal nuclei, reticular formation, and spinal cord. (The inferior peduncle also contains some cerebellar efferents, particularly those bound for vestibular nuclei.)

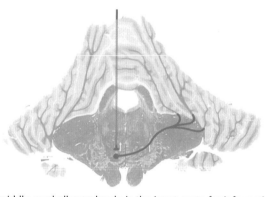

C, The middle cerebellar peduncle is the input route for information from cerebral cortex. Corticopontine fibers traverse the internal capsule and cerebral peduncle and terminate in pontine nuclei. Pontocerebellar fibers then project through the contralateral middle cerebellar peduncle to nearly all areas of the cerebellar cortex.

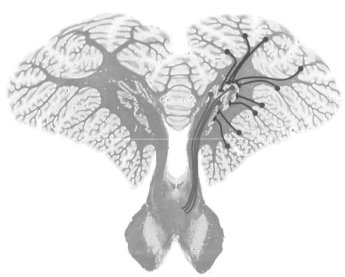

D, The superior cerebellar peduncle is the major output route from the cerebellum. Cerebellar cortex projects to a series of deep cerebellar nuclei, whose axons leave the cerebellum through this peduncle. (A few spinocerebellar afferents also travel through the superior peduncle.)

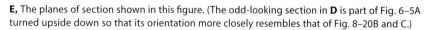

E, The planes of section shown in this figure. (The odd-looking section in **D** is part of Fig. 6–5A turned upside down so that its orientation more closely resembles that of Fig. 8–20B and C.)

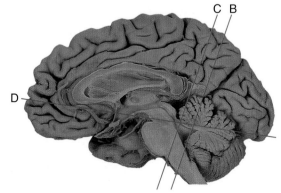

C   B

D

Figure 8–21 The structure of cerebellar cortex. **A,** Cross section of a single folium (as indicated in the *inset*). **B,** Oblique longitudinal section of a folium. **C,** Longitudinal section of a folium. **D,** Cross section of a single folium from a human cerebellum, stained with hematoxylin and eosin. *(A-C modified from Ramón y Cajal S: Histologie du système nerveux de l'homme et des vertébres, Paris, 1909-1911, Norbert Maloine. **D** provided by Dr. Nathaniel T. McMullen, Department of Cell Biology and Anatomy, The University of Arizona College of Medicine.)*

The lobes and lobules of the cerebellum are subdivided further by smaller sulci into numerous folia. Each folium is covered by a remarkably uniform and precisely ordered cortex. Most of the various cell types contained in this cortex are indicated in Figure 8–21A, but the basic organization is one in which two types of afferent fibers (mossy fibers and climbing fibers) enter the cortex, and one type of axon (Purkinje cell axons) leaves to convey information to the deep cerebellar nuclei.

The climbing fibers all come from one place—the contralateral inferior olivary nucleus—and wrap around the proximal dendrites of Purkinje cells, forming powerful excitatory synapses.

All other cerebellar afferents enter the cerebellum as mossy fibers and terminate on the vast numbers of tiny granule cells in the granular layer. Granule cell axons ascend toward the cerebellar surface and bifurcate in the molecular layer to form parallel fibers, which run parallel to the long axis of a given folium. In so doing, the parallel fibers intersect the flattened, transversely oriented dendritic trees of Purkinje cells, where they make excitatory synapses.

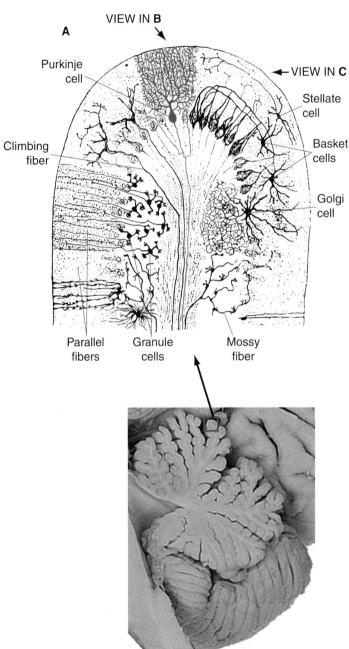

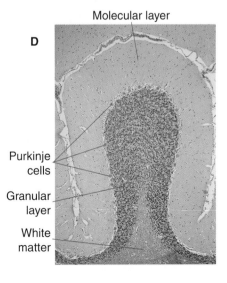

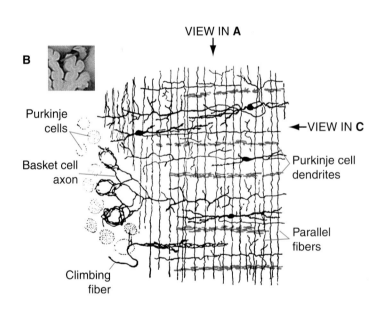

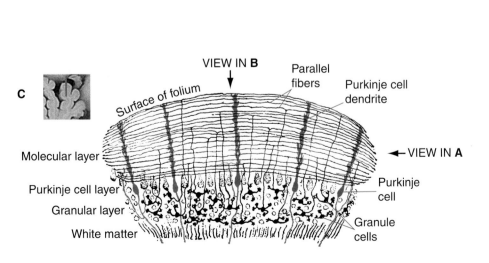

Figure 8–22   A, Afferents to the cerebellum.

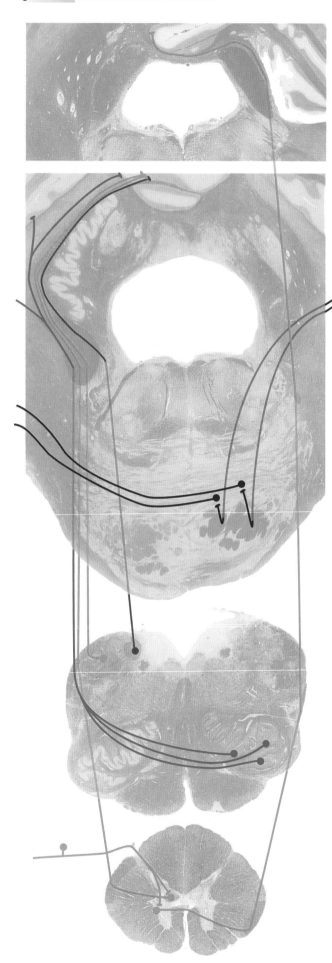

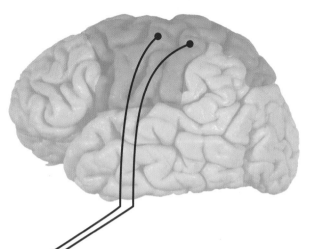

The cerebellum receives afferent inputs of three broad categories: (1) afferents conveying information from the cerebral cortex, (2) afferents conveying sensory information from a variety of subcortical sites, and (3) climbing fibers from the contralateral inferior olivary nucleus.

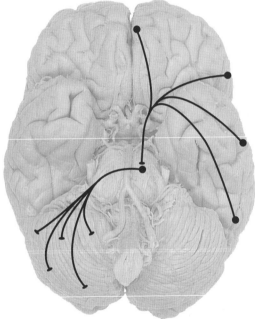

Cerebral cortical input (mostly, but not entirely, from motor and somatosensory areas) reaches the cerebellum through the middle cerebellar peduncle after a relay in the pontine nuclei. Most sensory information, arising most prominently in the spinal cord and vestibular nuclei, arrives via the inferior cerebellar peduncle (although a small amount traverses the superior peduncle). Axons leaving each inferior olivary nucleus travel through the contralateral inferior cerebellar peduncle before ending in the cerebellum as climbing fibers.

(The connections of the cerebellum are actually more widespread than this simple account would indicate, and it may have correspondingly broader functions. For example, interconnections between the cerebellum and the hypothalamus have been described, and the cerebellum may play a role in coordinating autonomic functions. Cortical inputs from association areas, such as prefrontal cortex, suggest that the cerebellum, like the basal ganglia, is also involved in higher cognitive functions.)

Figure 8-22 (Continued) **B,** Afferents to the cerebellum, continued.

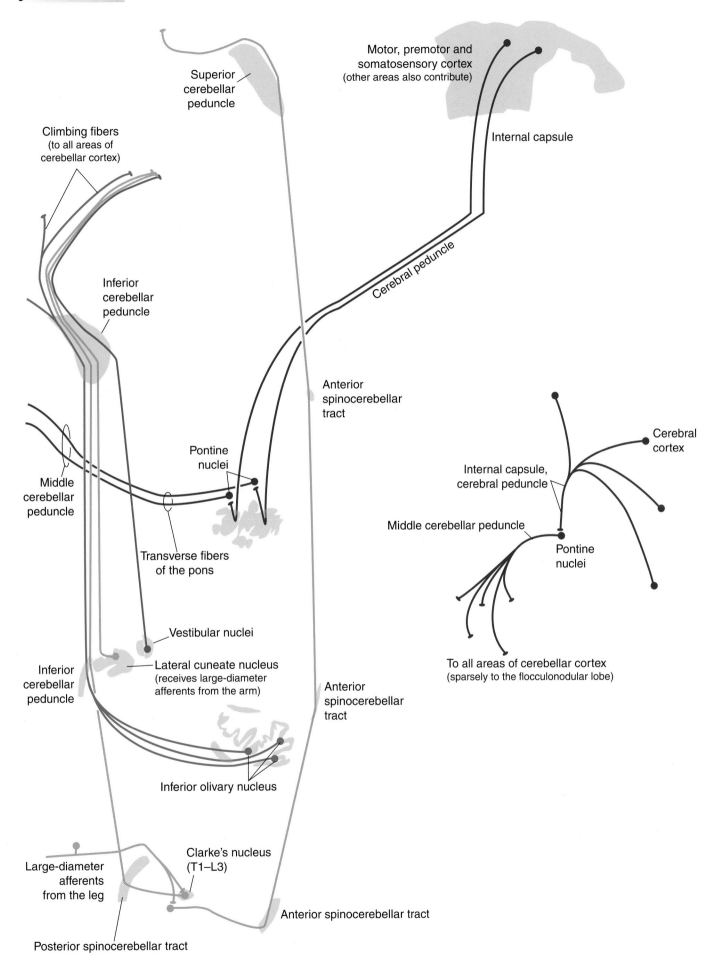

Superior cerebellar peduncle

Motor, premotor and somatosensory cortex (other areas also contribute)

Internal capsule

Climbing fibers (to all areas of cerebellar cortex)

Inferior cerebellar peduncle

Cerebral peduncle

Anterior spinocerebellar tract

Pontine nuclei

Cerebral cortex

Internal capsule, cerebral peduncle

Middle cerebellar peduncle

Middle cerebellar peduncle

Pontine nuclei

Transverse fibers of the pons

To all areas of cerebellar cortex (sparsely to the flocculonodular lobe)

Vestibular nuclei

Lateral cuneate nucleus (receives large-diameter afferents from the arm)

Anterior spinocerebellar tract

Inferior cerebellar peduncle

Inferior olivary nucleus

Large-diameter afferents from the leg

Clarke's nucleus (T1-L3)

Anterior spinocerebellar tract

Posterior spinocerebellar tract

Figure 8–23   A, Efferents from the cerebellum to the cerebrum.

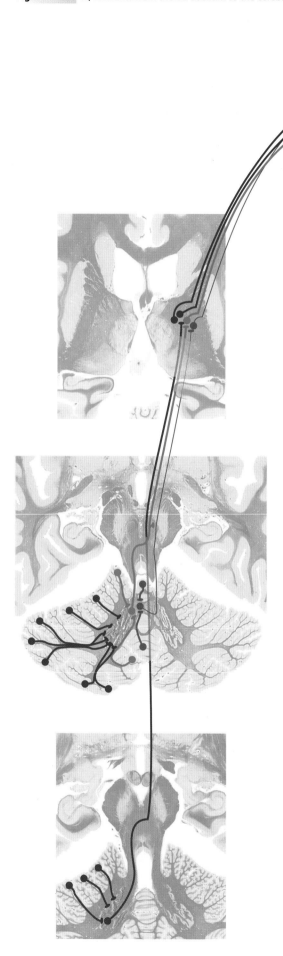

Purkinje cell axons are the sole output from cerebellar cortex. Some leave the cerebellum entirely, through the inferior cerebellar peduncle, to reach the vestibular nuclei. Most, however, project to a series of deep cerebellar nuclei in the roof of the fourth ventricle, which in turn provide most of the output from the cerebellum.

There are three deep cerebellar nuclei on each side, arranged in a lateral-to-medial sequence: the dentate, interposed,[2] and fastigial nuclei. This arrangement of the nuclei corresponds to three longitudinal zones of cerebellar cortex: (1) the large, lateral part of the hemisphere; (2) a smaller, medial part of the hemisphere (also called the intermediate zone); and (3) the vermis most medially. The pairing of deep nuclei and longitudinal zones of cortex is a reflection of functional subdivisions within the cerebellum that are also reflected in cerebellar inputs and outputs.

The lateral part of each cerebellar hemisphere receives its major inputs from the cerebral cortex (motor, somatosensory, and other, more widespread areas) via pontine nuclei. Its outputs then influence the activity of motor and premotor cortex through a pathway involving the dentate nucleus and contralateral thalamus (primarily the ventral lateral nucleus). It is thought to play a role in planning skilled movements.

The medial part of each cerebellar hemisphere receives information about the limbs from two major sources—motor cortex (via the pons) and the spinal cord (via spinocerebellar tracts). It is thus strategically positioned to compare intended and actual movements and to assist with moment-to-moment correction of movement, by way of connections with the interposed nucleus and motor cortex (via the thalamus).

The vermis receives information about axial muscles and body position from the vestibular nuclei and spinal cord and, through the fastigial nucleus, is involved in the maintenance and adjustment of posture. Most of this is accomplished at the level of the brainstem (see Fig. 8–24), and the connections of the fastigial nucleus with the thalamus are relatively minor.

Finally, the flocculonodular lobe (which does not fit comfortably into this longitudinal zonation scheme) is critically involved in eye movements, by way of its connections with the vestibular nuclei.

---

[2]The interposed nucleus is itself a combination of the more lateral emboliform nucleus and more medial globose nucleus.

Figure 8–23 (Continued) B, Efferents from the cerebellum to the cerebrum, continued. (*Histological section modified from Nolte J: The human brain, ed 5, St. Louis, 2002, Mosby.*)

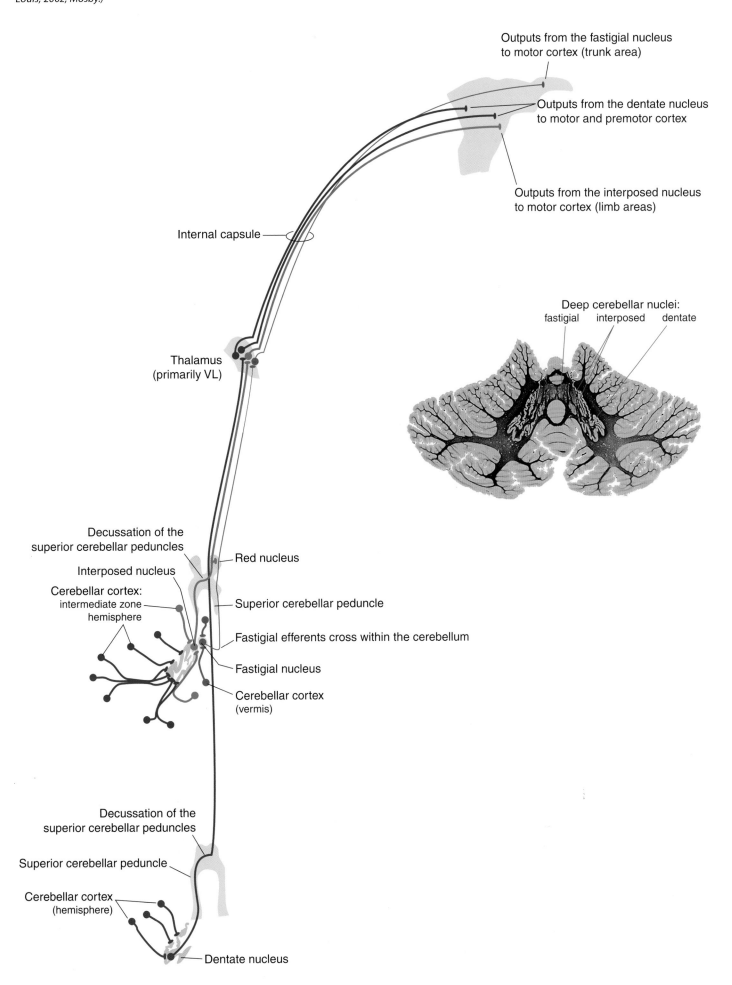

Figure 8–24   A, Efferents from the cerebellum to the brainstem.

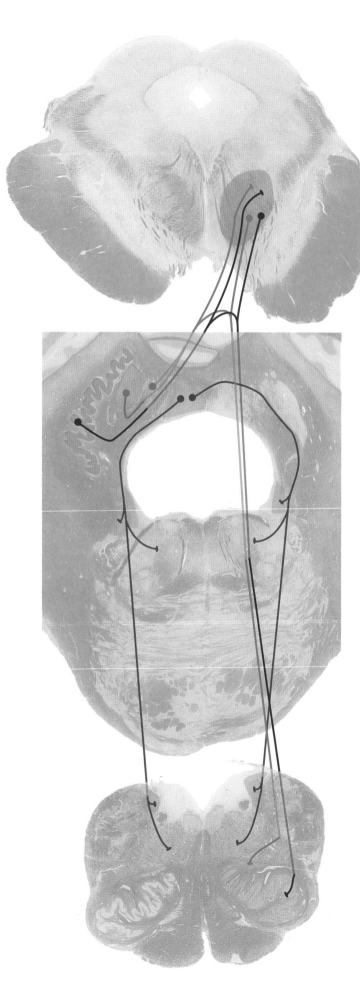

Each of the deep cerebellar nuclei also has outputs to sites in the brainstem; in the case of the fastigial nucleus, these represent its major connections.

As the superior cerebellar peduncle passes through or around the red nucleus, some of its fibers synapse on rubral neurons (*nucleus ruber* is Latin for "red nucleus"). A relatively small part of the red nucleus gives rise to the rubrospinal tract, which decussates and proceeds to the spinal cord. This is one route through which the cerebellum helps make corrections to ongoing movements, but it is relatively unimportant in humans. Most neurons of the red nucleus project instead to the ipsilateral inferior olivary nucleus. In addition, some fibers leave the superior cerebellar peduncle as it traverses the brainstem, turn caudally, cross as the descending limb of the superior cerebellar peduncle, and reach the inferior olivary nucleus directly. The functional significance of these cerebellum–(red nucleus)–inferior olivary nucleus connections is uncertain, but they may play a role in motor learning.

The fastigial nucleus, consistent with its role in postural adjustments, projects bilaterally to the vestibular nuclei and reticular formation. Some of its efferents leave the cerebellum uncrossed through the inferior cerebellar peduncle. Others cross the midline within the cerebellum, hook over the top of the superior cerebellar peduncle (as the uncinate fasciculus), and join the contralateral inferior cerebellar peduncle.

Figure 8–24 (Continued)   **B,** Efferents from the cerebellum to the brainstem, continued.

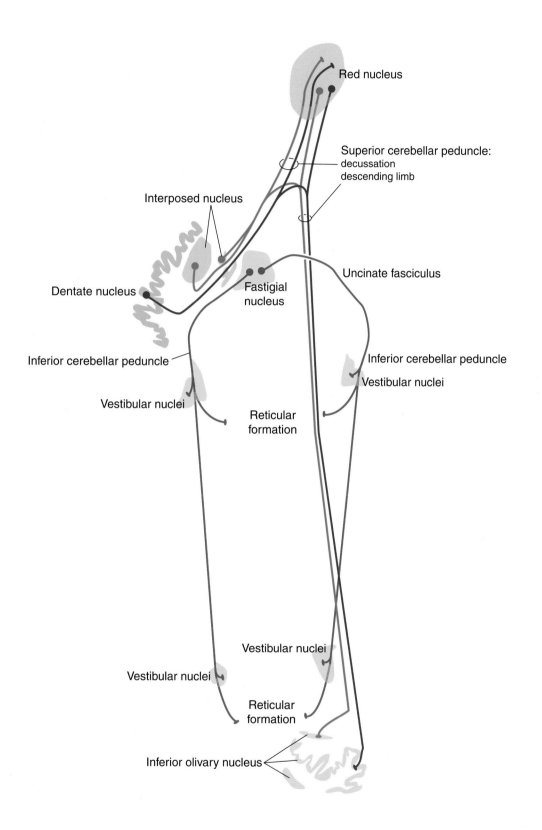

Figure 8–25   A, Projections of thalamic relay nuclei to the cerebral cortex (*not shown:* gustatory projections from VPM to the insula).

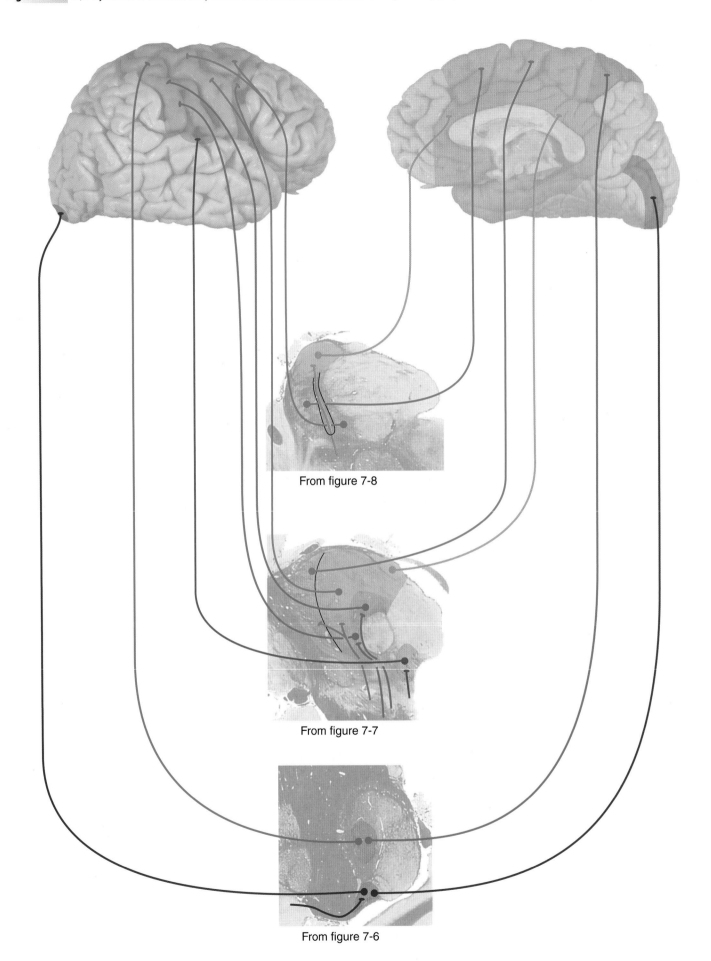

From figure 7-8

From figure 7-7

From figure 7-6

Figure 8–31 (Continued)   **B,** Afferents to the amygdala, continued.

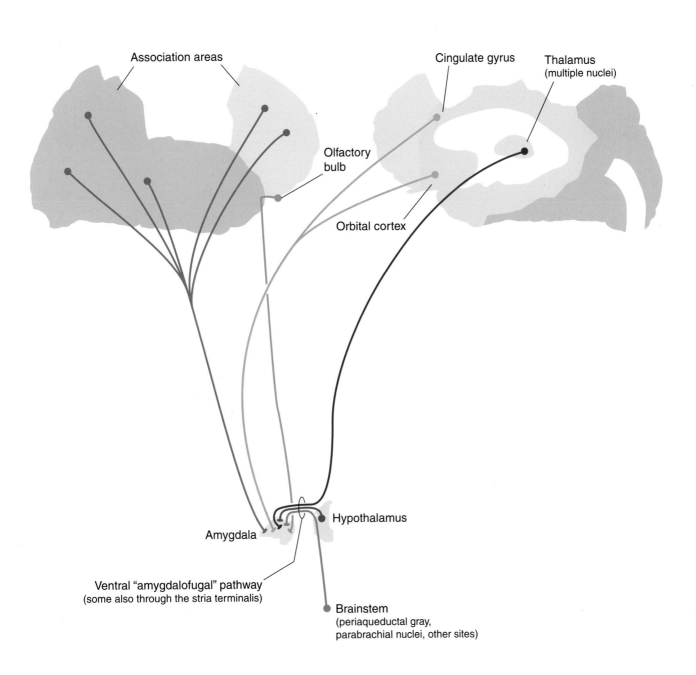

Association areas

Cingulate gyrus

Thalamus
(multiple nuclei)

Olfactory
bulb

Orbital cortex

Amygdala

Hypothalamus

Ventral "amygdalofugal" pathway
(some also through the stria terminalis)

Brainstem
(periaqueductal gray,
parabrachial nuclei, other sites)

Figure 8–32   A, Efferents from the amygdala.

The efferents from the amygdala for the most part reciprocate its afferents, although there are none to the olfactory bulb. Efferents reach more widespread cortical areas than those in which afferents to the amygdala arise, even extending to primary sensory areas. Projections to the hippocampus help ensure that emotionally significant events are remembered, and those to the hypothalamus and brainstem nuclei help regulate autonomic and behavioral responses to such events. In addition, efferents from the amygdala to nucleus accumbens and other parts of the ventral striatum are presumed to play a role in initiating behavioral responses to emotionally significant stimuli.

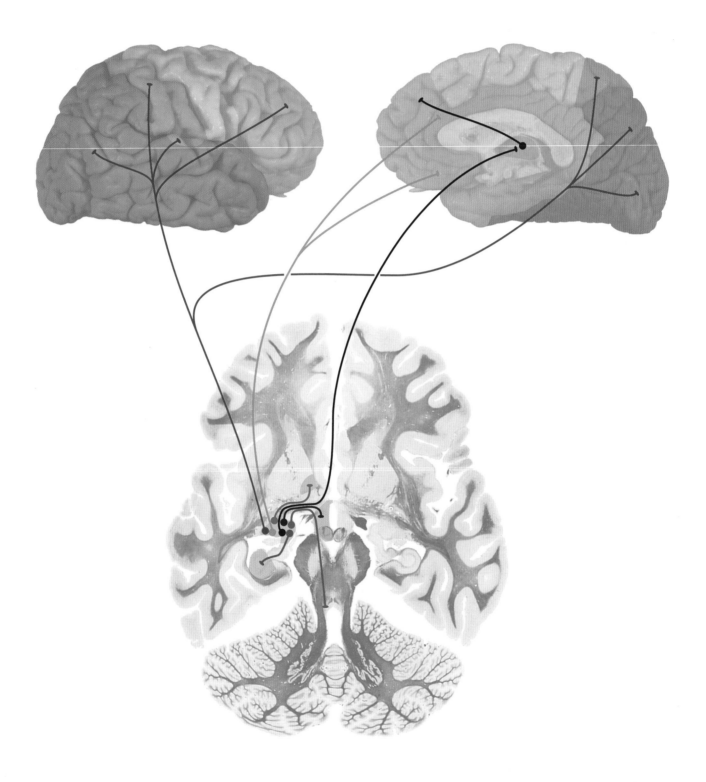

Figure 8–32 (Continued) **B,** Efferents from the amygdala, continued.

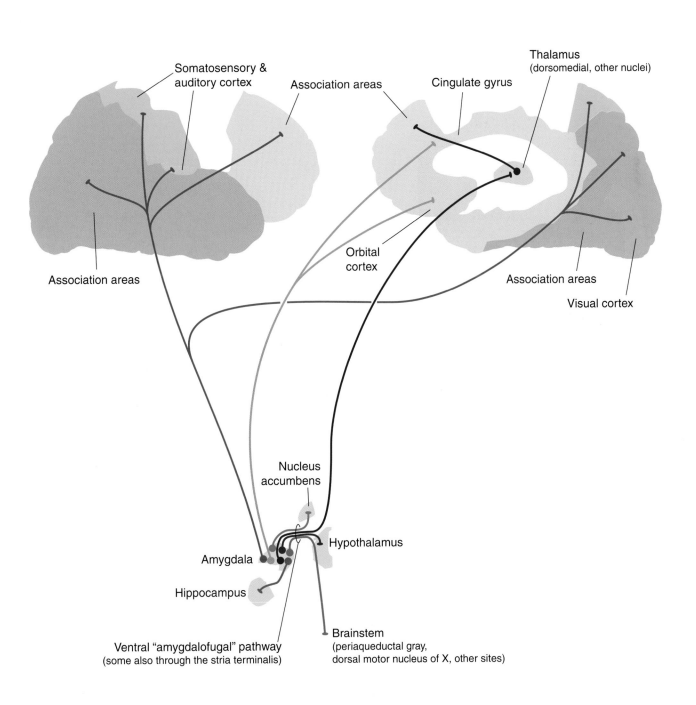

Figure 8–33   A, Afferents to the hippocampus.

The hippocampus is a specialized area of cerebral cortex (see inset in Figure 8–33B)—conceptually, the edge of the cortical sheet—rolled into the medial temporal lobe. It extends in the wall of the lateral ventricle from an enlarged anterior end that overlaps the amygdala underneath the uncus to a tapering posterior end near the splenium of the corpus callosum.[3] Formally, it consists of the dentate gyrus, the hippocampus proper (also called *Ammon's horn* or *cornu ammonis*), and the subiculum, which merges with the cerebral cortex of the parahippocampal gyrus.

As in the case of the amygdala, the hippocampus is connected anatomically like a bridge between the diencephalon and widespread areas of cerebral cortex, in this case as the substrate for its critical role in consolidation of new memories of facts and events.

Cholinergic afferents from the septal nuclei reach the hippocampus directly by traveling "backward" through the fornix, but most other afferents are relayed by adjacent parts of the parahippocampal gyrus (the entorhinal cortex). Afferents to entorhinal cortex from posterior parts of the cingulate gyrus travel through the cingulum, a curved fiber bundle underlying the gyrus; afferents from association areas and the amygdala travel through the white matter of the temporal lobe. To simplify this figure, all cortical afferents are shown as projecting to entorhinal cortex, and all afferents from the amygdala are shown as projecting directly to the hippocampus itself; in fact, each does both in complex patterns.

_____
[3]The hippocampus continues over the top of the corpus callosum as a thin, apparently rudimentary, band of tissue—the indusium griseum, which is not indicated in this atlas. The hippocampus, strictly defined, extends along the entire edge of the cortical mantle.

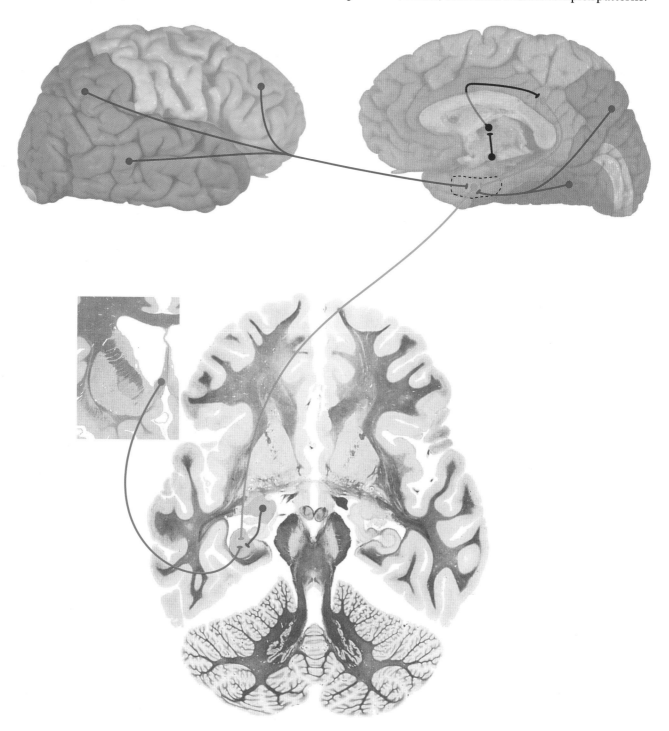

Figure 8–33 (Continued)   **B,** Afferents to the hippocampus, continued. *(Inset provided by Pamela Eller, University of Colorado Health Sciences Center.)*

In cross section, the hippocampus is made up of two interlocking C-shaped strips of cortex (the dentate gyrus and the hippocampus proper) and the subiculum, which is continuous laterally with the hippocampus proper and medially with entorhinal cortex. The hippocampus proper is itself subdivided further into four longitudinal strips called *CA fields* (*CA* for *cornu ammonis*). Abbreviations: C, tail of the caudate nucleus; CA, hippocampus proper (cornu ammonis); D, dentate gyrus; F, fimbria; LGN, lateral geniculate nucleus; LV, inferior horn of the lateral ventricle; ST, stria terminalis; Sub, subiculum.

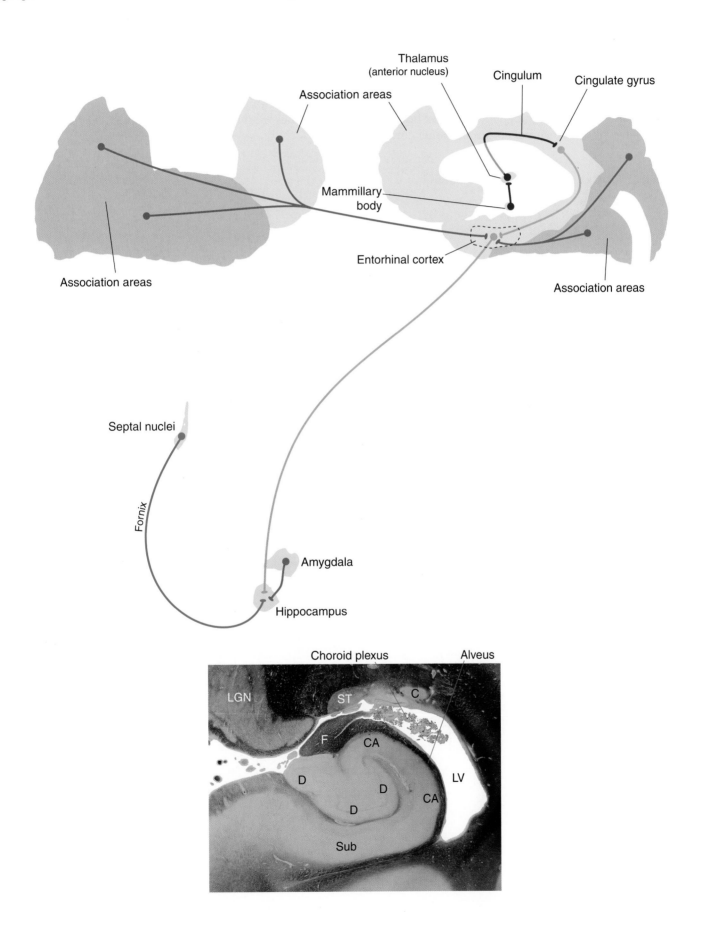

Figure 8–34   A, Efferents from the hippocampus.

The anatomically most prominent efferent pathway from the hippocampus is the fornix (see Fig. 8–30), through which hippocampal pyramidal cells project to the septal nuclei, and subicular neurons project to the septal nuclei, mammillary bodies, ventral striatum, and some cortical areas. At the level of the interventricular foramen, fornix fibers begin to splay out as they move toward their final destinations. Some pass in front of the anterior commissure (the precommissural fornix) to reach the septal nuclei and parts of the frontal lobe. Others turn posteriorly and end directly in the anterior nucleus of the thalamus. A large number descend through the hypothalamus in the column of the fornix, mostly directed toward the mammillary body.

Numerous subicular efferents bypass the fornix, however, and project directly to entorhinal cortex and other cortical areas. (This is presumably part of the reason why bilateral damage to the hippocampus causes a much more severe memory deficit than does bilateral damage to the fornix.) As in the case of afferents to the hippocampus, more than one hippocampal component may project in parallel to the same structure (e.g., both subiculum and entorhinal cortex to other cortical areas).

The fundamental pattern of information flow in the hippocampus is unidirectional: afferents (mostly from entorhinal cortex) → granule cells of the dentate gyrus → CA3 pyramidal cells → CA1 pyramidal cells → pyramidal cells of the subiculum → output targets. Thus, most of the output of the hippocampus comes from the subiculum, although some comes from hippocampal pyramidal cells.

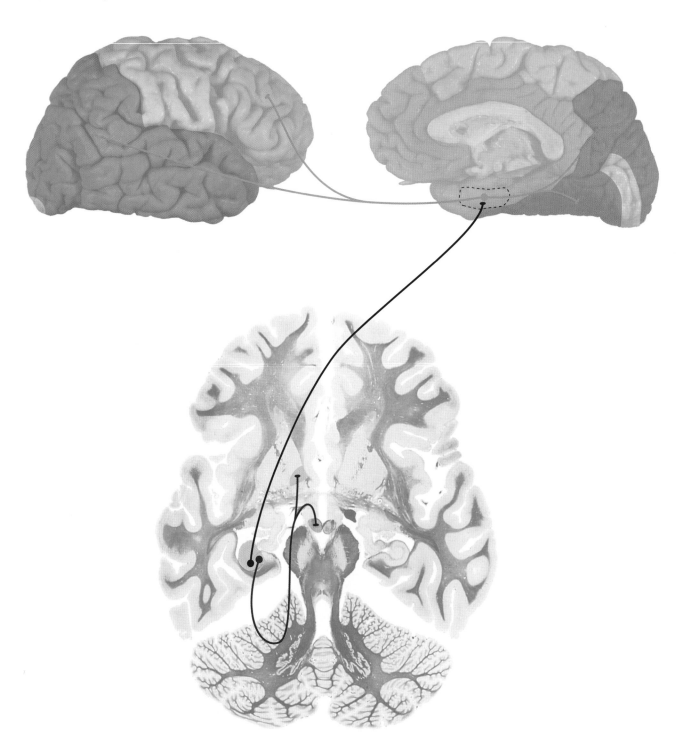

Figure 8–34 (Continued)   **B,** Efferents from the hippocampus, continued. *(Inset from Nolte J: The human brain, ed 5, St. Louis, 2002, Mosby.)*

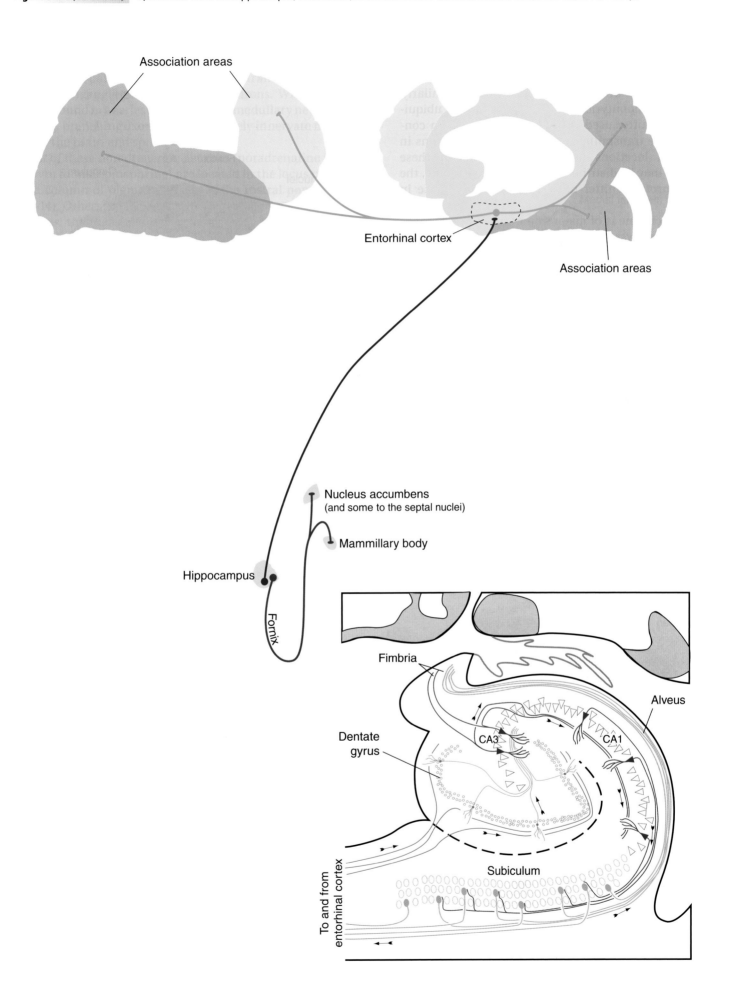

Figure 9-6 A series of seven CT images from the same patient shown in Figure 9-5. In this case, an iodinated intravenous contrast agent was administered before the CT study, making blood vessels visible. (*Provided by Dr. Raymond F. Carmody.*)

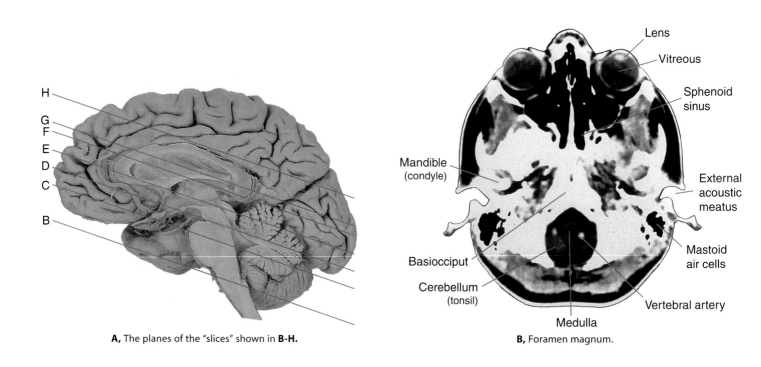

A, The planes of the "slices" shown in **B-H.**

B, Foramen magnum.

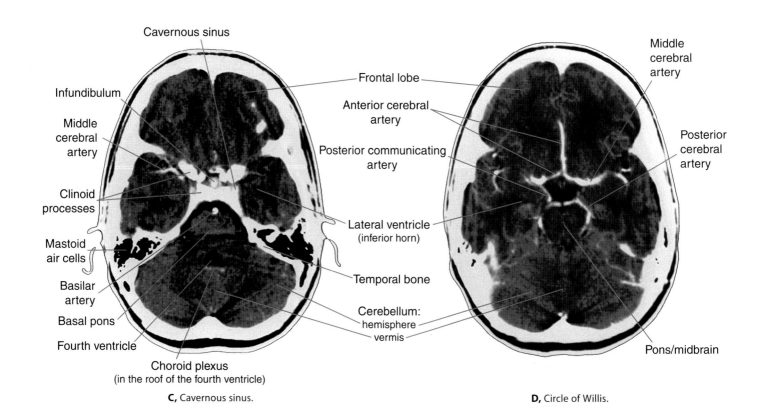

C, Cavernous sinus.

D, Circle of Willis.

Figure 9–6 (Continued)   **E-H,** Contrasted CT images.

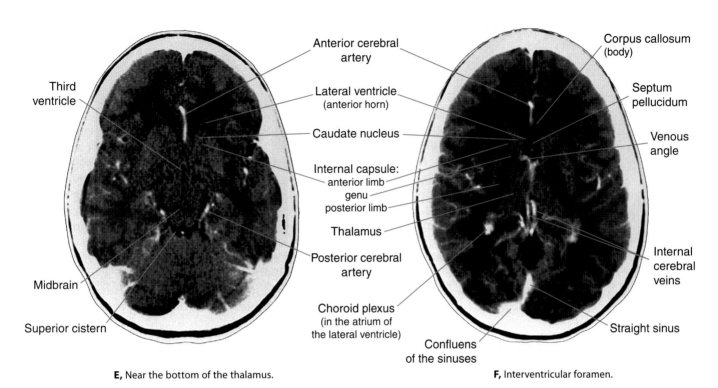

Third ventricle

Anterior cerebral artery

Lateral ventricle (anterior horn)

Caudate nucleus

Internal capsule:
anterior limb
genu
posterior limb

Thalamus

Posterior cerebral artery

Midbrain

Superior cistern

Choroid plexus (in the atrium of the lateral ventricle)

Corpus callosum (body)

Septum pellucidum

Venous angle

Internal cerebral veins

Straight sinus

Confluens of the sinuses

E, Near the bottom of the thalamus.

F, Interventricular foramen.

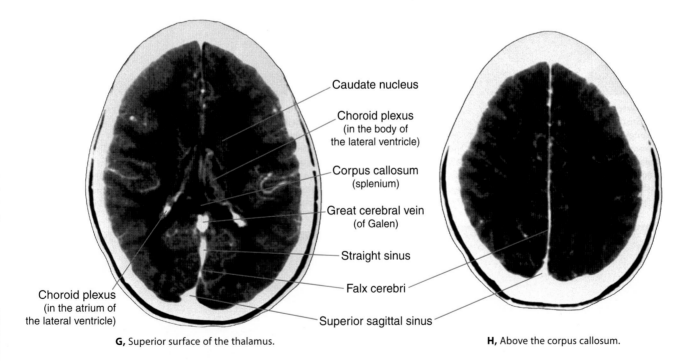

Caudate nucleus

Choroid plexus (in the body of the lateral ventricle)

Corpus callosum (splenium)

Great cerebral vein (of Galen)

Straight sinus

Falx cerebri

Superior sagittal sinus

Choroid plexus (in the atrium of the lateral ventricle)

G, Superior surface of the thalamus.

H, Above the corpus callosum.

Figure 9–10   A-O, T1-weighted coronal MRI of the brain of a young man. (The brain was remapped into Talairach space [i.e., morphed to match a standard brain], which is commonly done in preparation for functional imaging studies, making the data obtained from different subjects comparable.) The same brain is shown in different planes in Figures 9–10 through 9–12, with the planes of "section" indicated in three-dimensional reconstructions. *(Provided by Dr. Elena M. Plante.)*

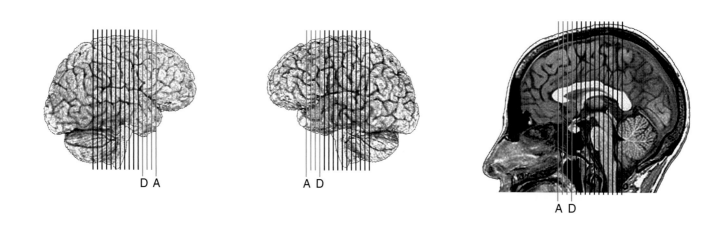

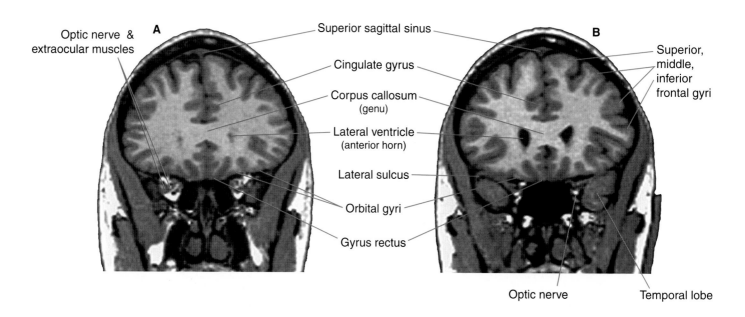

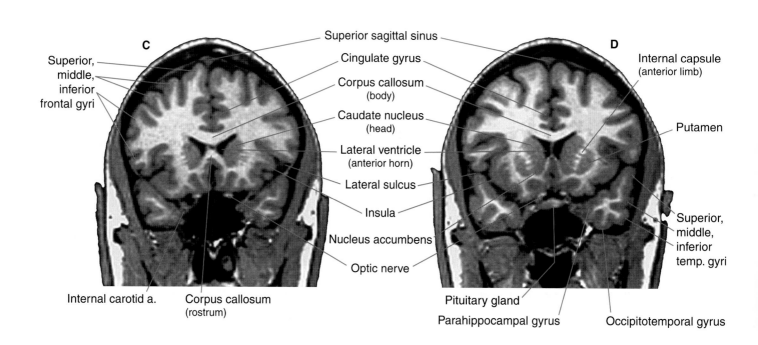

Figure 9–10 (Continued)   T1-weighted coronal MR images.

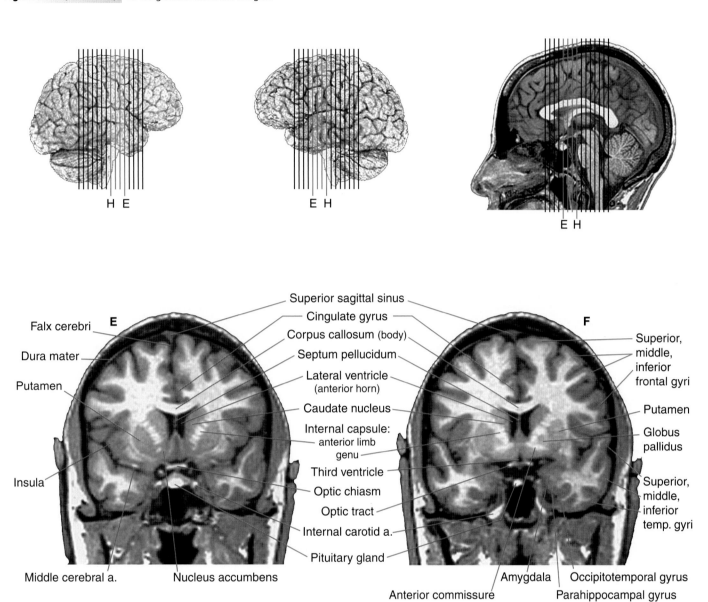

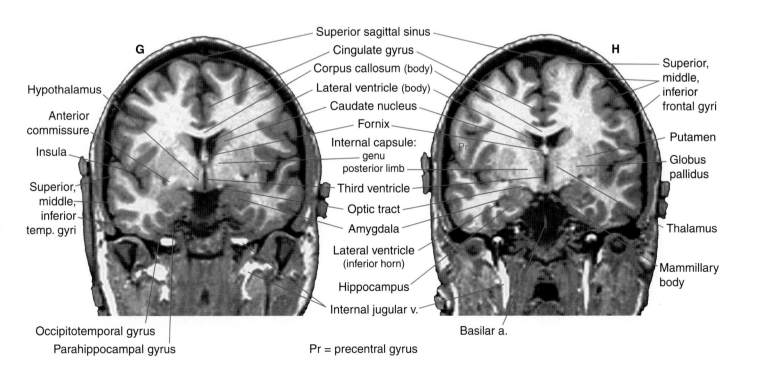

Pr = precentral gyrus

Figure 9–10 (Continued)   T1-weighted coronal MR images.

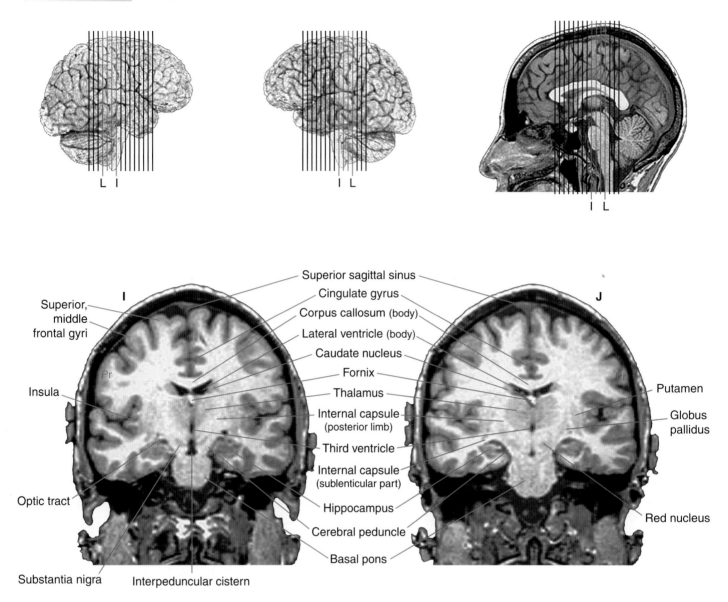

I

- Superior sagittal sinus
- Cingulate gyrus
- Corpus callosum (body)
- Lateral ventricle (body)
- Caudate nucleus
- Fornix
- Thalamus
- Internal capsule (posterior limb)
- Third ventricle
- Internal capsule (sublenticular part)
- Hippocampus
- Cerebral peduncle
- Basal pons

- Superior, middle frontal gyri
- Insula
- Optic tract
- Substantia nigra
- Interpeduncular cistern

J

- Putamen
- Globus pallidus
- Red nucleus

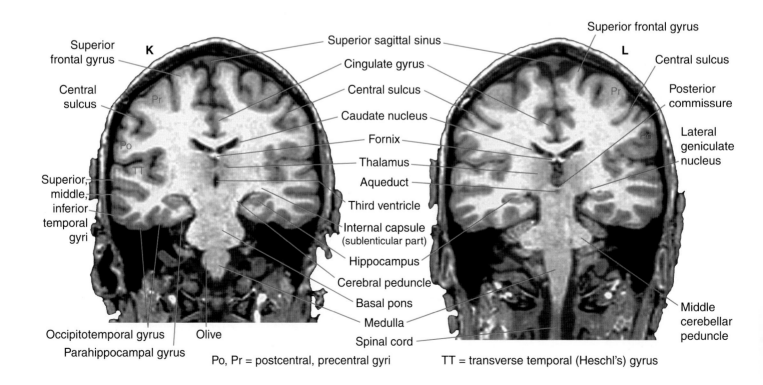

K

- Superior frontal gyrus
- Central sulcus
- Superior, middle, inferior temporal gyri
- Occipitotemporal gyrus
- Parahippocampal gyrus
- Olive

- Superior sagittal sinus
- Cingulate gyrus
- Central sulcus
- Caudate nucleus
- Fornix
- Thalamus
- Aqueduct
- Third ventricle
- Internal capsule (sublenticular part)
- Hippocampus
- Cerebral peduncle
- Basal pons
- Medulla
- Spinal cord

Po, Pr = postcentral, precentral gyri

L

- Superior frontal gyrus
- Central sulcus
- Posterior commissure
- Lateral geniculate nucleus
- Middle cerebellar peduncle

TT = transverse temporal (Heschl's) gyrus

Figure 9–10 (Continued) T1-weighted coronal MR images.

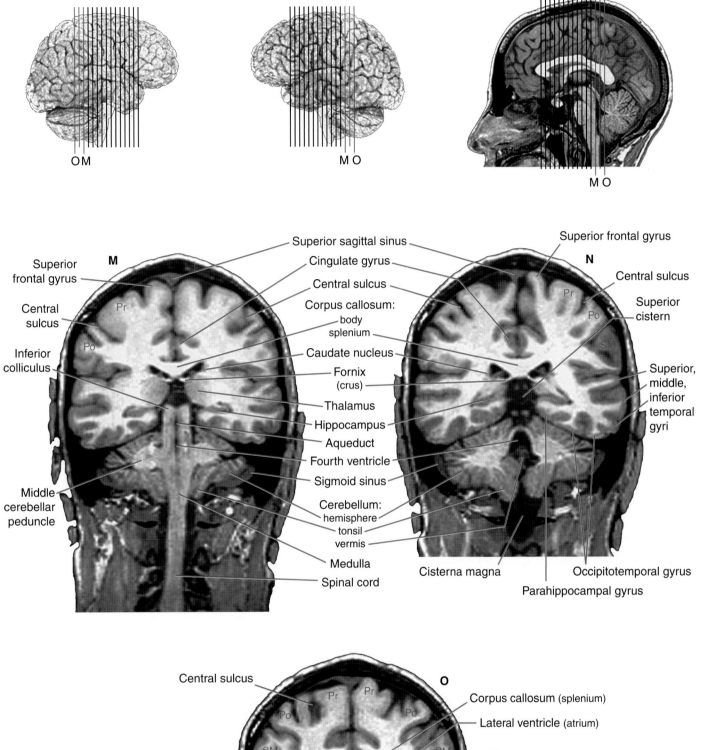

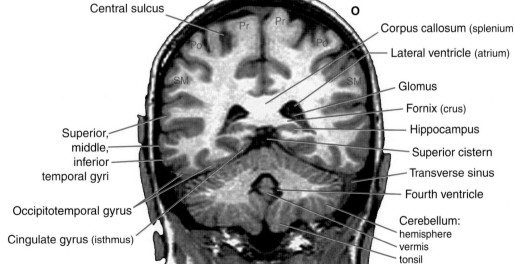

Po, Pr = postcentral, precentral gyri; SM = supramarginal gyrus

Figure 9–11   A-O, T1-weighted axial (horizontal) MRI of the brain of a young man. The same brain is shown in different planes in Figures 9–10 through 9–12, with the planes of "section" indicated in three-dimensional reconstructions. *(Provided by Dr. Elena M. Plante.)*

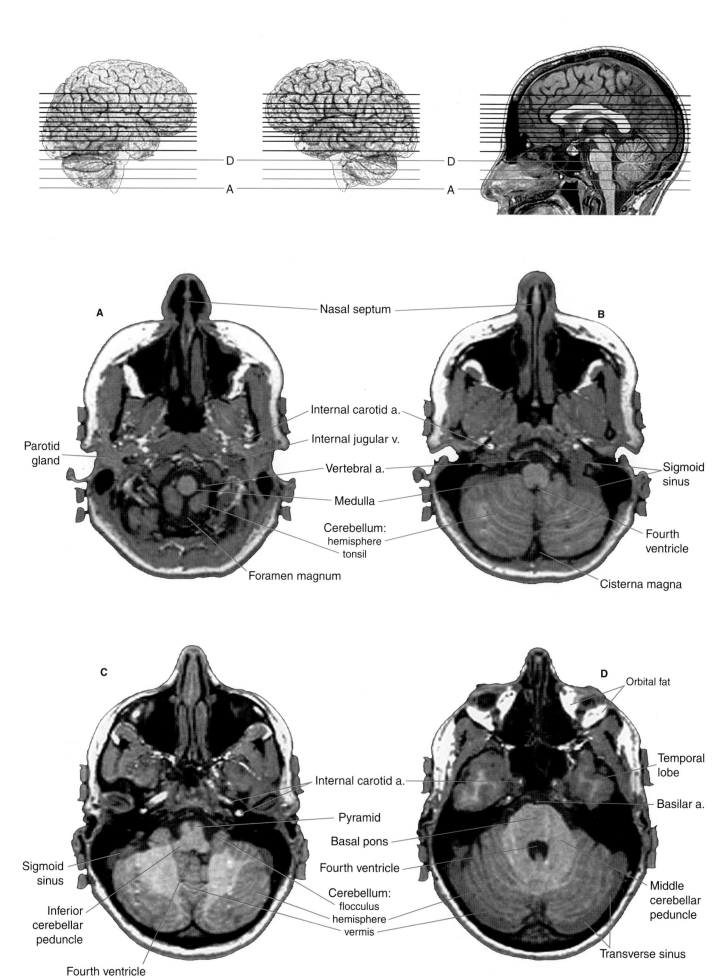

Figure 9–11 (Continued)   T1-weighted axial (horizontal) MR images.

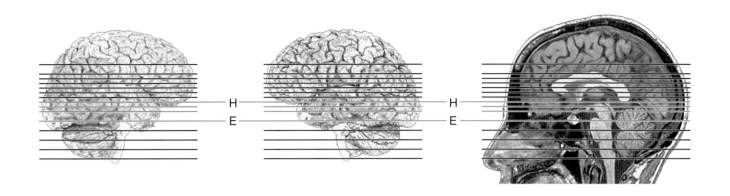

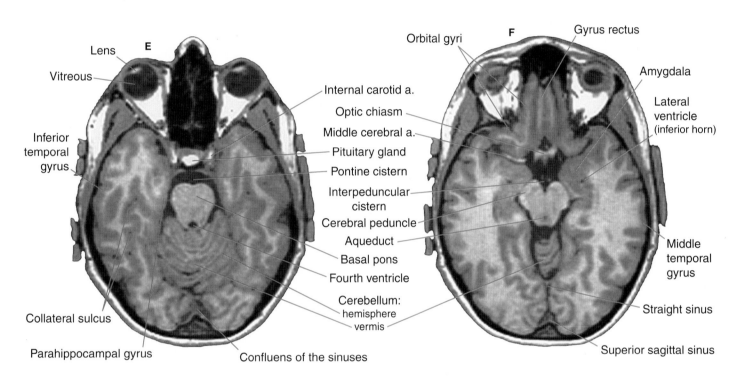

E

Lens
Vitreous
Inferior temporal gyrus
Collateral sulcus
Parahippocampal gyrus

Internal carotid a.
Optic chiasm
Middle cerebral a.
Pituitary gland
Pontine cistern
Interpeduncular cistern
Cerebral peduncle
Aqueduct
Basal pons
Fourth ventricle
Cerebellum:
  hemisphere
  vermis
Confluens of the sinuses

Orbital gyri
F
Gyrus rectus
Amygdala
Lateral ventricle (inferior horn)
Middle temporal gyrus
Straight sinus
Superior sagittal sinus

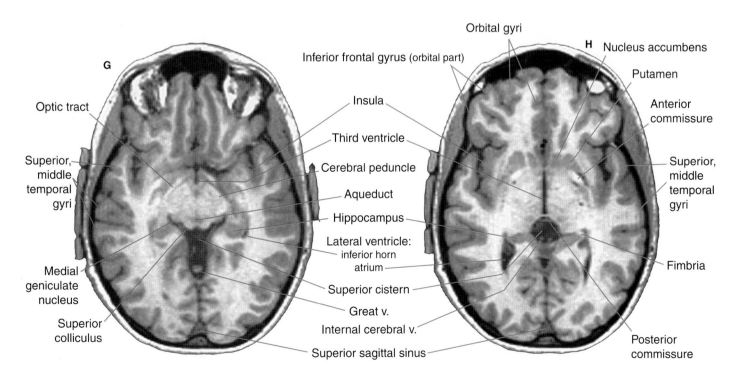

G
Optic tract
Superior, middle temporal gyri
Medial geniculate nucleus
Superior colliculus

Orbital gyri
Inferior frontal gyrus (orbital part)
Insula
Third ventricle
Cerebral peduncle
Aqueduct
Hippocampus
Lateral ventricle:
  inferior horn
  atrium
Superior cistern
Great v.
Internal cerebral v.
Superior sagittal sinus

H
Nucleus accumbens
Putamen
Anterior commissure
Superior, middle temporal gyri
Fimbria
Posterior commissure

Figure 9–11 (Continued)   T1-weighted axial (horizontal) MR images.

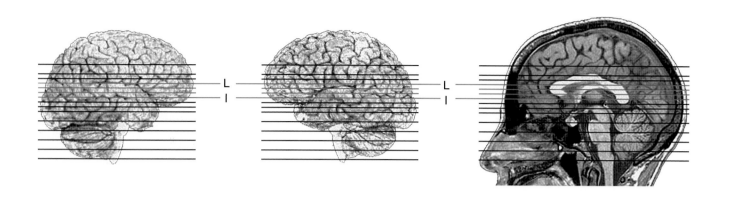

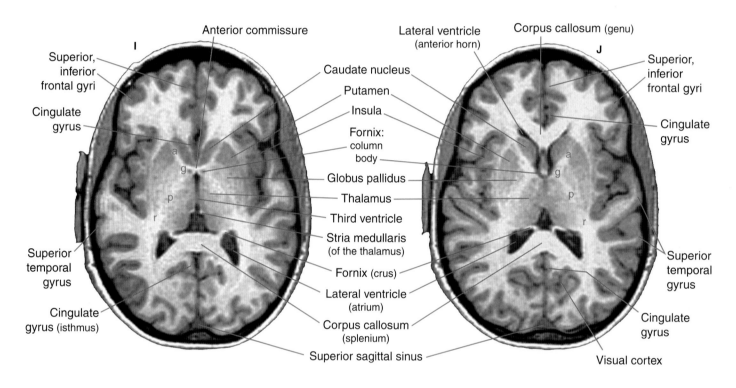

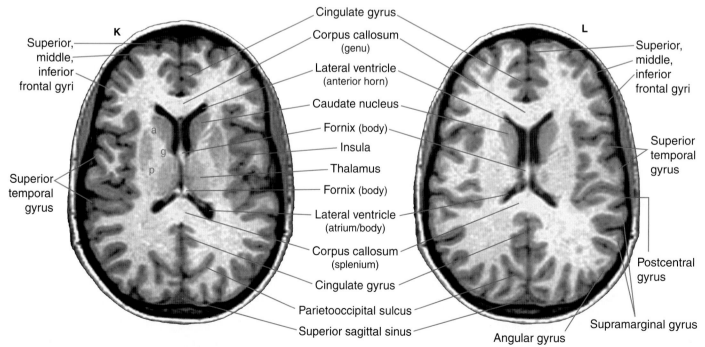

a, g, p, r = anterior limb, genu, posterior limb, retrolenticular part of the internal capsule

Figure 9–11 (Continued) T1-weighted axial (horizontal) MR images.

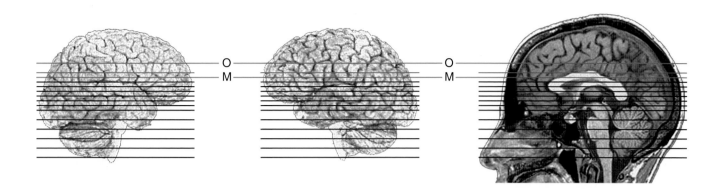

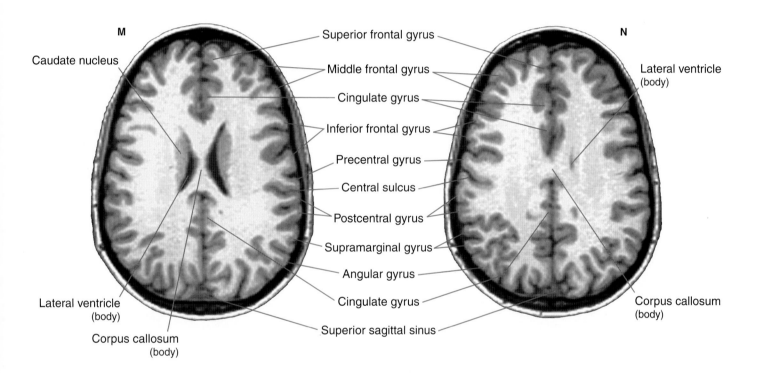

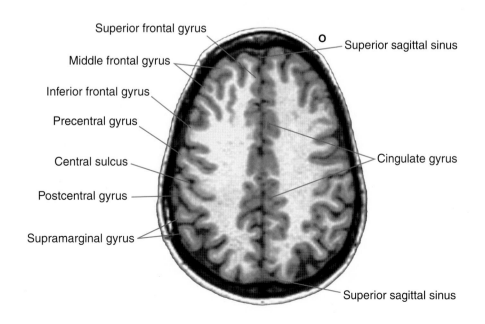

Figure 9–12   A-G, T1-weighted sagittal and parasagittal MRI of the brain of a young man. The same brain is shown in different planes in Figures 9–10 through 9–12, with the planes of "section" indicated in three-dimensional reconstructions. *(Provided by Dr. Elena M. Plante.)*

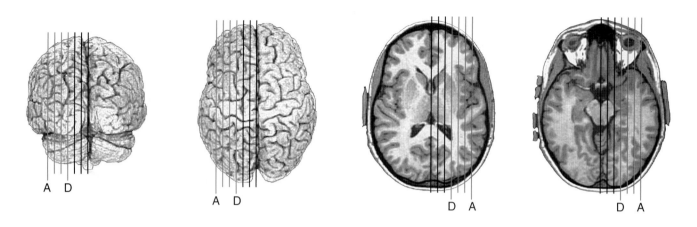

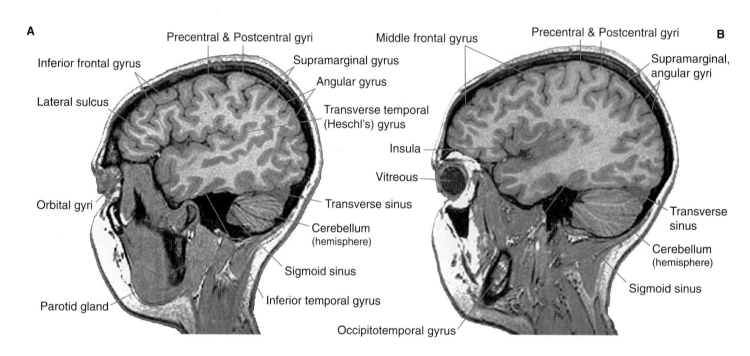

A

Inferior frontal gyrus

Precentral & Postcentral gyri

Middle frontal gyrus

Precentral & Postcentral gyri

B

Lateral sulcus

Supramarginal gyrus

Angular gyrus

Supramarginal, angular gyri

Transverse temporal (Heschl's) gyrus

Insula

Vitreous

Orbital gyri

Transverse sinus

Transverse sinus

Cerebellum (hemisphere)

Cerebellum (hemisphere)

Sigmoid sinus

Sigmoid sinus

Parotid gland

Inferior temporal gyrus

Occipitotemporal gyrus

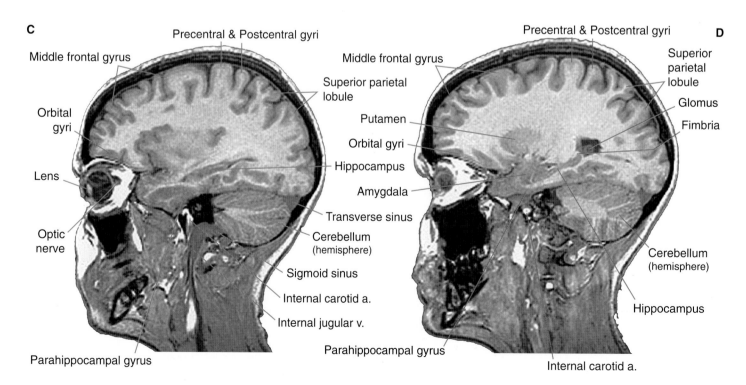

C

Middle frontal gyrus

Precentral & Postcentral gyri

Precentral & Postcentral gyri

D

Middle frontal gyrus

Superior parietal lobule

Orbital gyri

Superior parietal lobule

Putamen

Glomus

Lens

Orbital gyri

Fimbria

Hippocampus

Amygdala

Optic nerve

Transverse sinus

Cerebellum (hemisphere)

Cerebellum (hemisphere)

Sigmoid sinus

Internal carotid a.

Hippocampus

Internal jugular v.

Parahippocampal gyrus

Parahippocampal gyrus

Internal carotid a.

Figure 9–12 (Continued) **A-G,** T1-weighted sagittal and parasagittal MR images.

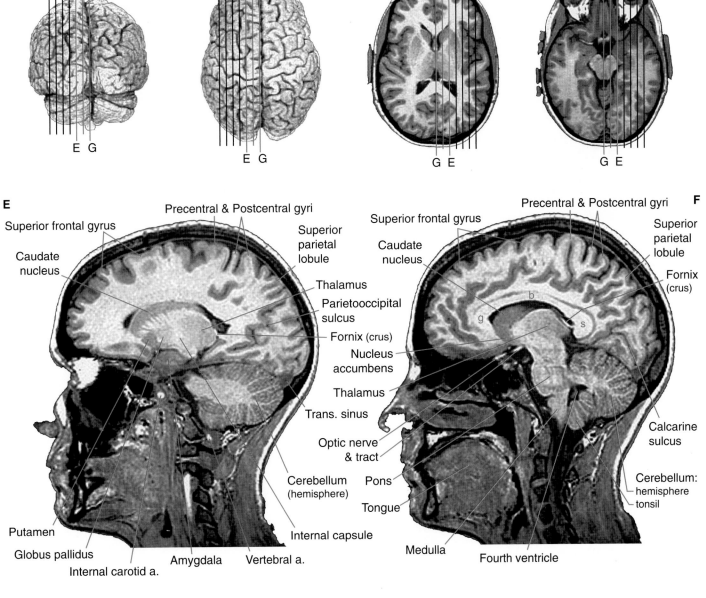

E
Superior frontal gyrus
Precentral & Postcentral gyri
Superior parietal lobule
Caudate nucleus
Thalamus
Parietooccipital sulcus
Fornix (crus)
Nucleus accumbens
Thalamus
Trans. sinus
Optic nerve & tract
Cerebellum (hemisphere)
Pons
Tongue
Putamen
Globus pallidus
Amygdala
Internal capsule
Vertebral a.
Internal carotid a.

F
Superior frontal gyrus
Precentral & Postcentral gyri
Superior parietal lobule
Caudate nucleus
Fornix (crus)
b
g
s
Calcarine sulcus
Cerebellum: hemisphere tonsil
Medulla
Fourth ventricle

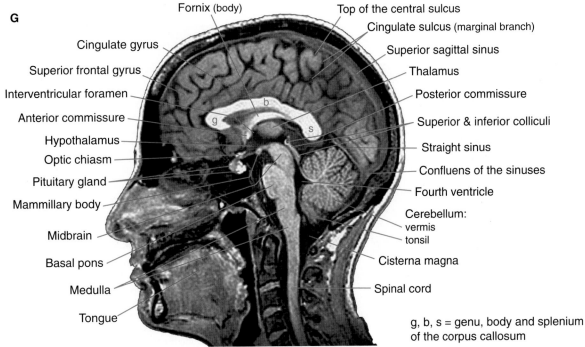

G
Fornix (body)
Top of the central sulcus
Cingulate sulcus (marginal branch)
Cingulate gyrus
Superior sagittal sinus
Superior frontal gyrus
Thalamus
Interventricular foramen
Posterior commissure
Anterior commissure
Superior & inferior colliculi
Hypothalamus
Straight sinus
Optic chiasm
Confluens of the sinuses
Pituitary gland
Fourth ventricle
Mammillary body
Cerebellum: vermis tonsil
Midbrain
Basal pons
Cisterna magna
Medulla
Spinal cord
Tongue
b
g
s

g, b, s = genu, body and splenium of the corpus callosum

Figure 9–13   The use of MRI to show intracranial pathology. *(Provided by Dr. Raymond F. Carmody.)*

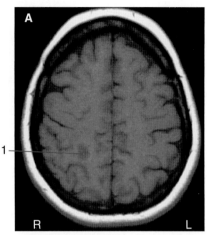

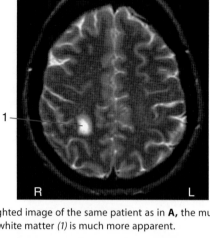

A, This T1-weighted image shows a slight change in signal in the cerebral white matter *(1)* of a patient with multiple sclerosis.

B, In a T2-weighted image of the same patient as in **A,** the multiple sclerosis plaque in the white matter *(1)* is much more apparent.

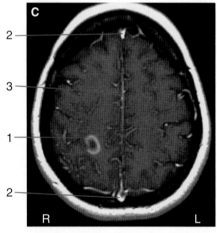

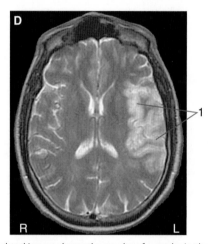

C, The same patient as in **A** and **B**. A contrast agent (gadolinium) effective in MRI studies was injected intravenously before this MRI, revealing a rim around the edge of the plaque *(1)* where the blood-brain barrier had broken down. Blood vessels, including the superior sagittal sinus *(2),* also can be seen, as can the falx cerebri *(3)* (because the dura mater is outside the blood-brain barrier).

D, This T2-weighted image shows the results of a stroke in the territory of the left middle cerebral artery. The damaged cerebral cortex *(1)* is edematous, and the increased water concentration makes it appear lighter than neighboring cortex.

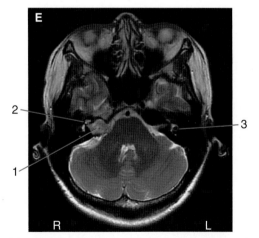

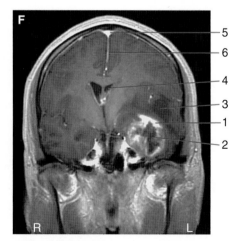

E, A T2-weighted image showing a tumor *(1)* of the eighth nerve (a vestibular schwannoma, often referred to as an acoustic neuroma). Because fluids are bright in T2-weighted images, the cochlea *(2)* and semicircular canals *(3)* also can be seen.

F, A T1-weighted image of a patient with a tumor (*1* and *2,* a glioblastoma multiforme) in the left temporal lobe. The tumor has a disrupted blood-brain barrier around its edges that allows contrast material to leak into it *(1)* and a necrotic core *(2)*. Adjacent areas *(3)* appear darker than normal because of edema. The tumor has compressed the left lateral ventricle *(4)* and shifted parts of the left hemisphere to the right. Structures normally made visible by contrast agents include the superior sagittal sinus *(5)* and the falx cerebri *(6)*.

Blood vessels can be visualized with most imaging techniques by finding a way to make the blood contained within them differ in some way from surrounding structures. Cerebral angiography uses the intravenous injection of iodinated dyes to make blood much more opaque than brain to x-rays (Figure 9–14). More recently, MRI techniques that depend on the intrinsic properties of flowing blood have been developed (Figure 9–15). Magnetic resonance angiography (MRA) has the advantage of being completely noninvasive—no intravenous contrast material is required—but the resulting images are not as detailed as those produced by traditional angiography.

A cerebral angiogram typically is produced by introducing a catheter into the femoral artery, threading it (under fluoroscopic control) up the aorta and into the aortic arch, then steering the catheter tip into the artery of interest. In this way, the contrast material can be introduced into a single vertebral or internal carotid artery. Once the dye has been introduced, a rapid series of radiographs can follow it as it flows through the artery, into capillaries, and then into veins (see Fig. 9–14). Finally, photographic* (as in Fig. 9–14) or digital (Figure 9–20) techniques can be used to remove bone images and reveal blood vessels in relative isolation.

---

*A radiographic image is made before injection of the iodinated dye, and its contrast is reversed (i.e., a positive image is made, so that bone is dark). The reverse-contrast image is stacked on top of the image made after dye injection, and a print is made of both together. The reciprocally contrasting portions of the two images provide a relatively uniform background from which the blood vessels stand out.

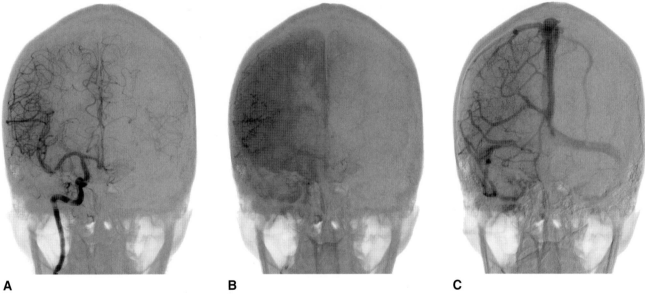

A **B** **C**

Figure 9–14 Movement of contrast material through the intracranial vasculature, as seen in a series of anteroposterior (A-P) views (as though you were looking at the patient's forehead) after injection of the right internal carotid artery. **A,** About 2 seconds after injection, the arteries are filled. **B,** About 5 seconds after injection, the contrast agent has moved out of arteries and into capillary beds. **C,** About 7 seconds after injection, the contrast agent has moved into veins and venous sinuses. *(Provided by Dr. Joachim F. Seeger.)*

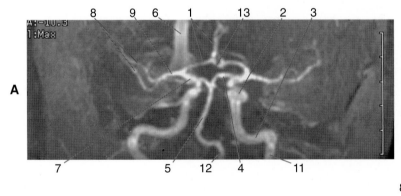

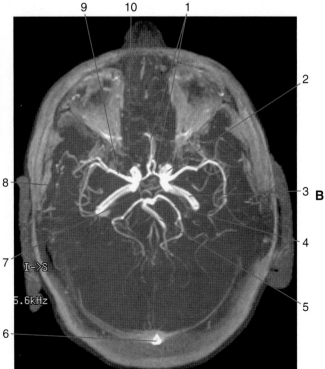

Figure 9–15 Magnetic resonance angiography uses some of the intrinsic properties of flowing blood to create images of parts of the vasculature; appropriate adjustments of technical parameters can emphasize arteries or veins. The views in these images are as though you were looking from the front **(A)** or looking up from below **(B)** at the entire arterial supply of the brain. The internal carotid artery can be seen ascending through the neck *(11)*, traversing the temporal bone *(3)*, and passing through the cavernous sinus *(2)*. The other arteries of the circle of Willis also can be seen—the anterior cerebral *(1)*, posterior cerebral *(4)*, and anterior *(13)* and posterior *(7)* communicating arteries—in addition to the middle cerebral artery *(9)*, its branches on the surface of the insula *(8)*, the vertebral *(12)* and basilar *(5)* arteries, the superior sagittal sinus *(6)*, and even the ophthalmic artery *(10)*. *(Provided by Dr. Raymond F. Carmody.)*

Figure 9–16   The arterial phase of a right internal carotid angiogram. **A,** A lateral view; the patient's face is to the right. **B,** An anteroposterior projection; the view is as though you were looking at the patient's forehead.

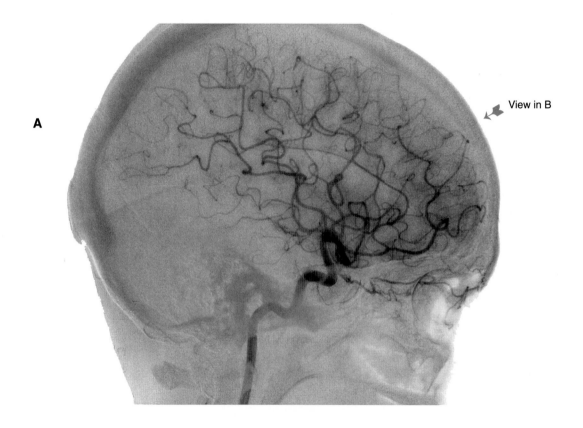

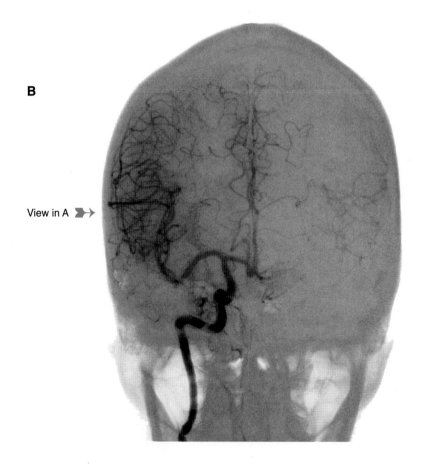

Figure 9–16 (Continued) **C,** The internal carotid artery bifurcates into the anterior and middle cerebral arteries. The anterior cerebral artery gives rise to two prominent branches, the pericallosal *(dark blue arrows)* and callosomarginal *(light blue arrows)* arteries, which curve around above the corpus callosum and supply most of the medial surface of the cerebral hemisphere. Branches of the middle cerebral artery traverse the insula *(green arrows)*, emerge from the lateral sulcus *(purple arrows)*, and supply the lateral surface of the hemisphere. **D,** In an anteroposterior projection, the separation between anterior and middle cerebral territories can be seen more easily. *(Provided by Dr. Joachim F. Seeger.)*

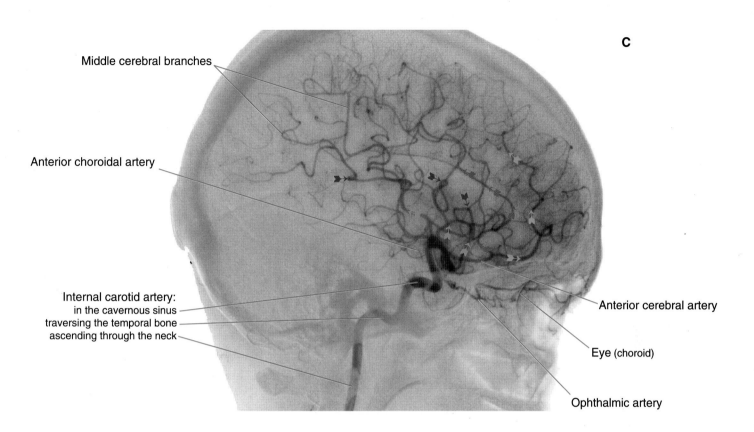

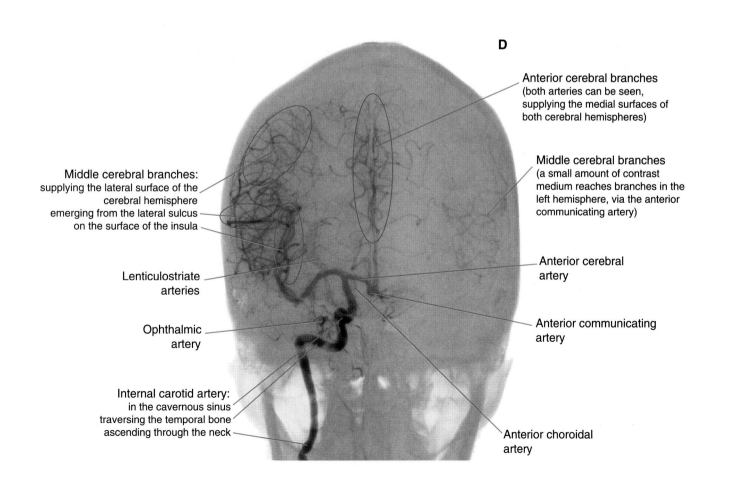

Figure 9–17   The venous phase of a right internal carotid angiogram. **A,** A lateral view; the patient's face is to the right. **B,** An anteroposterior projection; the view is as though you were looking at the patient's forehead. Flow into the transverse sinuses is typically asymmetrical; in this patient, most blood from the superior sagittal sinus flows into the left transverse sinus (more commonly it flows to the right).

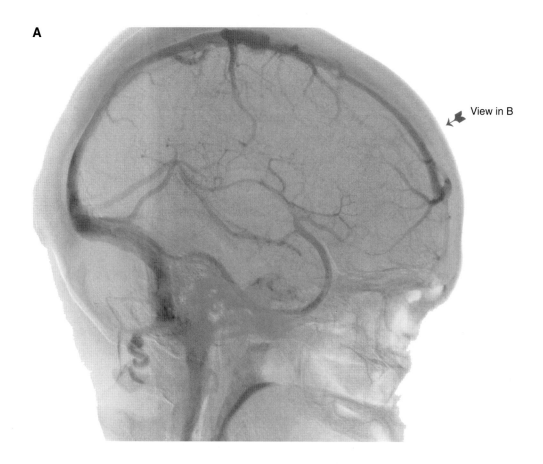

A

View in B

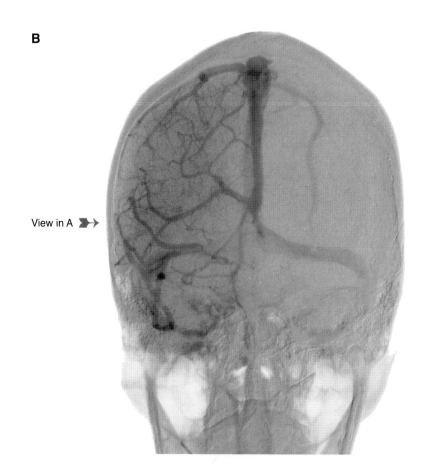

B

View in A

Figure 9–17 (Continued)   **C,** Blood flows through a system of deep veins *(blue arrows)* to the straight and transverse sinuses and through a system of superficial veins *(purple arrows)* to the superior sagittal sinus; both systems meet at the confluens of the sinuses. **D,** In an anteroposterior view, the superior sagittal sinus occupies much of the midline, obscuring other vessels. *(Provided by Dr. Joachim F. Seeger.)*

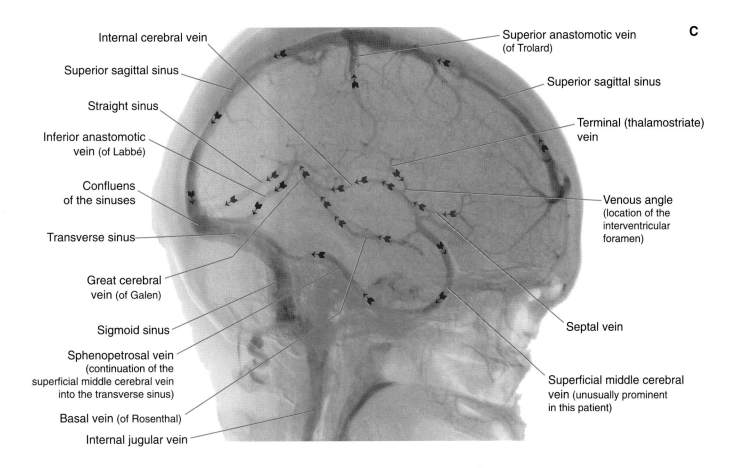

C

Internal cerebral vein

Superior sagittal sinus

Straight sinus

Inferior anastomotic vein (of Labbé)

Confluens of the sinuses

Transverse sinus

Great cerebral vein (of Galen)

Sigmoid sinus

Sphenopetrosal vein (continuation of the superficial middle cerebral vein into the transverse sinus)

Basal vein (of Rosenthal)

Internal jugular vein

Superior anastomotic vein (of Trolard)

Superior sagittal sinus

Terminal (thalamostriate) vein

Venous angle (location of the interventricular foramen)

Septal vein

Superficial middle cerebral vein (unusually prominent in this patient)

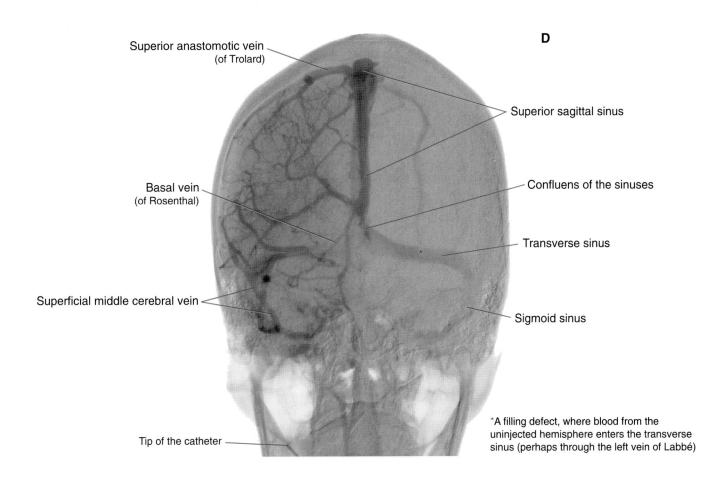

D

Superior anastomotic vein (of Trolard)

Basal vein (of Rosenthal)

Superficial middle cerebral vein

Tip of the catheter

Superior sagittal sinus

Confluens of the sinuses

Transverse sinus

Sigmoid sinus

*A filling defect, where blood from the uninjected hemisphere enters the transverse sinus (perhaps through the left vein of Labbé)

Figure 9–18   The arterial phase of a left vertebrobasilar angiogram. **A,** A lateral view; the patient's face is to the right. **B,** An anteroposterior projection; the view is as though you were looking at the patient's forehead. In **B,** the basilar artery appears shorter than it really is because of the angle of view—you are looking almost longitudinally along it. (The right vertebral artery is visible because the pressure of the injection propelled some contrast material into it.)

A

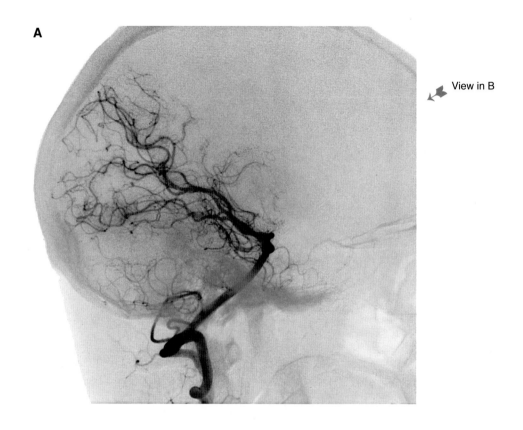

View in B

B

View in A

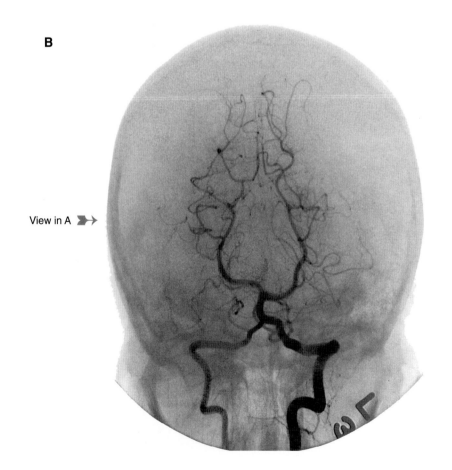

Figure 9–18 (Continued) **C,** The vertebral and basilar arteries and their branches supply areas below the tentorium cerebelli (location indicated by *red asterisks*), and the posterior cerebral arteries supply parts of the midbrain and supratentorial structures (including much of the thalamus). **D,** The two vertebral arteries *(blue arrows)* join to form a single, midline basilar artery *(green arrow),* which gives rise to a series of branches as it courses along the anterior surface of the pons, finally bifurcating at the level of the midbrain to form the two posterior cerebral arteries *(red arrows). (Provided by Dr. Joachim F. Seeger.)*

C

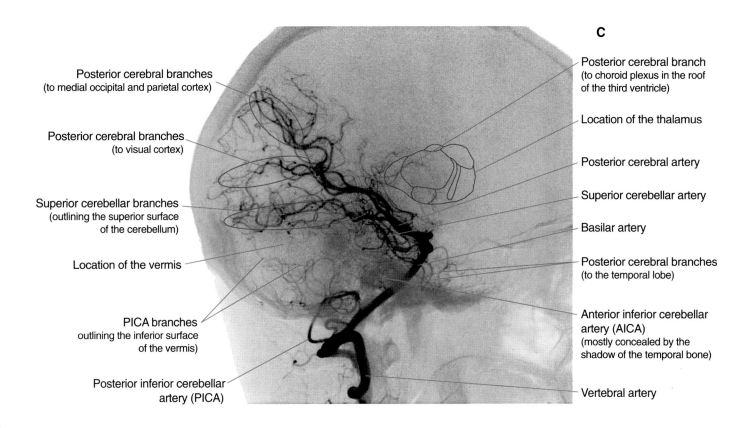

Posterior cerebral branches
(to medial occipital and parietal cortex)

Posterior cerebral branches
(to visual cortex)

Superior cerebellar branches
(outlining the superior surface
of the cerebellum)

Location of the vermis

PICA branches
outlining the inferior surface
of the vermis)

Posterior inferior cerebellar
artery (PICA)

Posterior cerebral branch
(to choroid plexus in the roof
of the third ventricle)

Location of the thalamus

Posterior cerebral artery

Superior cerebellar artery

Basilar artery

Posterior cerebral branches
(to the temporal lobe)

Anterior inferior cerebellar
artery (AICA)
(mostly concealed by the
shadow of the temporal bone)

Vertebral artery

D

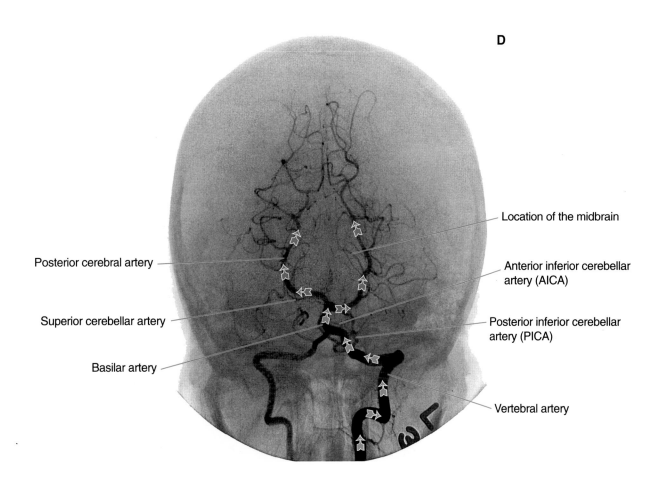

Posterior cerebral artery

Superior cerebellar artery

Basilar artery

Location of the midbrain

Anterior inferior cerebellar
artery (AICA)

Posterior inferior cerebellar
artery (PICA)

Vertebral artery

Figure 9–20 The use of angiography to show intracranial pathology. (*Provided by Dr. Raymond F. Carmody.*)

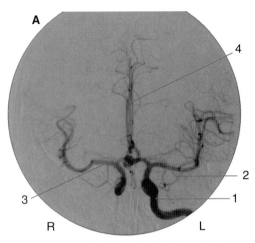

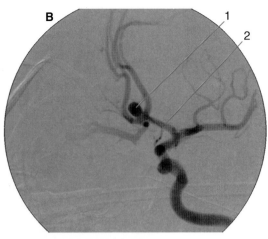

A, An anteroposterior view of a patient who had subarachnoid bleeding from a ruptured aneurysm (a balloonlike swelling of the wall of an artery). The internal carotid artery (1) was injected, and the left (2) and right (3) middle cerebral arteries and the anterior cerebral arteries (4) can be seen.

B, The same patient as in **A.** Rotating the point of view by about 45 degrees makes the aneurysm (1) apparent, at a branch point of the anterior cerebral artery (2).

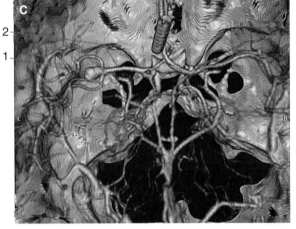

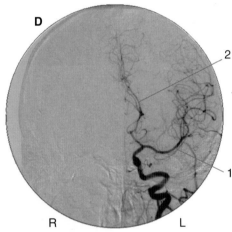

C, A 38-year-old woman with an aneurysm. A three-dimensional reconstruction based on contrast-enhanced CT scans shows the shape of the aneurysm (1), at a branch point of the middle cerebral artery (2).

D, An angiogram of a 78-year-old man who complained of a headache reveals that the left middle (1) and anterior (2) cerebral arteries were bowed outward, as though something were distorting them.

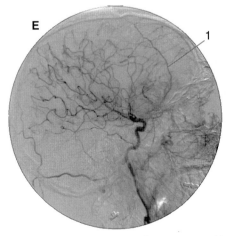

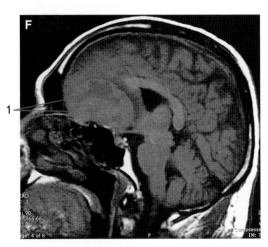

E, The same patient as in **D.** A lateral view shows an upward bowing of the anterior cerebral artery (1).

F, The same patient as in **D.** T1-weighted MRI reveals a large meningioma (1).

Glossary

This glossary provides brief descriptions and definitions of the neuroanatomical structures labeled in the preceding chapters (except for the bones and muscles indicated in Chapter 9). Within each entry, terms discussed further in their own entries elsewhere in the glossary are italicized. Additional details can be found in standard neuroscience texts.

Although all of these definitions were written specifically for this atlas, many are adapted from passages in Nolte's *The Human Brain,* fifth edition.[1] Some others derive, with modifications, from a text by Jay B. Angevine, Jr. (with Carl W. Cotman), *Principles of Neuroanatomy.*[2] We thank Jeffrey House of Oxford University Press for permission to draw on the latter source.

We have illustrated many of the glossary terms in this edition, placing adaptations of figures in the atlas and some from Nolte[1] below relevant entries. Space did not permit doing this for all entries, however, so alternative terms that may be consulted for an illustration are indicated by an asterisk (*).

Abducens nerve. The 6th cranial nerve, which emerges anteriorly from the *brainstem* between the *pons* and *medulla.* It innervates the lateral rectus muscle of the ipsilateral eye, producing abduction (hence its name).

Abducens nucleus. Contains the motor neurons for the ipsilateral lateral rectus muscle, as well as interneurons that project through the contralateral *medial longitudinal fasciculus* (MLF) to medial rectus motor neurons; this feature provides for conjugate horizontal eye movements.

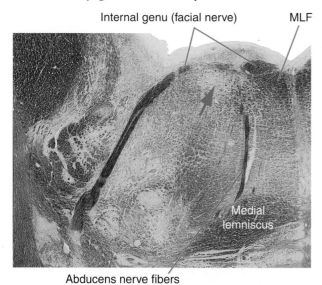

Internal genu (facial nerve)   MLF

Medial lemniscus

Abducens nerve fibers

[1]Nolte J: *The human brain,* ed 5, St. Louis, 2002, Mosby.
[2]Angevine JB Jr, Cotman CW: *Principles of neuroanatomy,* New York, 1981, Oxford University Press.

Accessory nerve. The 11th cranial nerve, which emerges laterally from the upper cervical spinal cord and innervates the sternocleidomastoid and trapezius muscles to mediate turning the head and elevating the shoulder. (The accessory nerve used to be described as having both cranial and spinal parts. The spinal part corresponded to the accessory nerve as defined here, and the cranial part corresponded to a series of rootlets that emerge laterally from the caudal *medulla,* join the vagus, and run to the palate, pharynx, and larynx with the *vagus nerve.)*

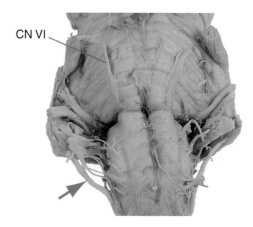

CN VI

Alveus. A layer of white matter on the ventricular surface of the *hippocampus**, mostly conveying efferents from this structure.

Ambient cistern. The combination of the *superior cistern* and sheetlike extensions from it that partially encircle the *midbrain.*

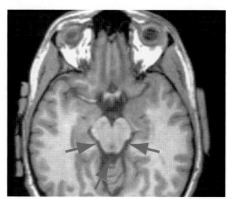

Provided by
Dr. Elena Plante,
University of Arizona

Amygdala. A collection of nuclei in the anteromedial part of the *temporal lobe,* just beneath the *uncus,* forming the core of one of the two major limbic circuits. (The core of the other is the *hippocampus*.)

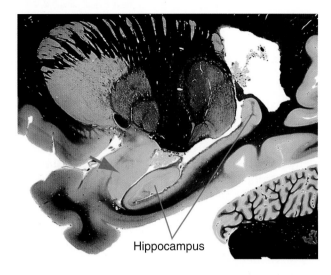

Hippocampus

Angular gyrus. The part of the *inferior parietal lobule** formed by the cortex surrounding the upturned end of the superior temporal sulcus; although variable in size and shape, this region is important in language function.

Ansa lenticularis. Part of the projection from the *globus pallidus* to the *thalamus*. It has fewer axons than the other part (the *lenticular fasciculus*). It forms a compact, conspicuous cable of myelinated fibers running beneath the *internal capsule* and hooking around its medial edge.

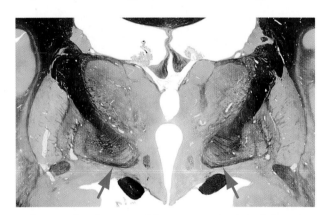

Anterior cerebral artery. The more anterior of the two terminal branches of the *internal carotid artery*. It curves around the *corpus callosum* with branches supplying *gyrus rectus* and *orbital gyri*, the medial surface of the *frontal* and *parietal lobes*, and an adjoining narrow band of cortex along their superior surfaces.

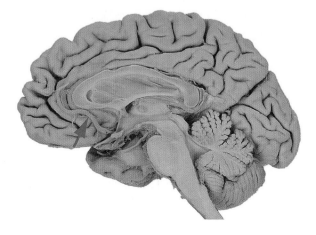

Anterior choroidal artery. A long, thin branch of the *internal carotid artery* that accompanies the *optic tract* and supplies many structures along the way: the *optic tract*, *choroid plexus* of the inferior horn of the *lateral ventricle*, part of the *cerebral peduncle*, deep regions of the *internal capsule*, and parts of the *thalamus* and *hippocampus*. The anterior choroidal artery is a particularly large example of the numerous penetrating arteries that arise from all arteries around the base of the brain and supply nearby deep structures.

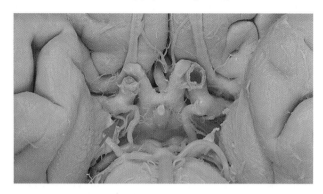

Anterior commissure. A small, sharply defined bundle of commissural fibers just beneath and behind the rostrum of the *corpus callosum*, to which it is closely related developmentally; a few inconspicuous anterior fibers interconnect olfactory structures, whereas its many large posterior fibers link the two *temporal lobes*.

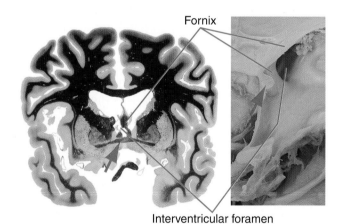

Fornix

Interventricular foramen

Anterior communicating artery. A short vessel at the anterior end of the circle of Willis interconnecting the two *anterior cerebral arteries* just anterior to the *optic chiasm*; a common site of aneurysm formation.

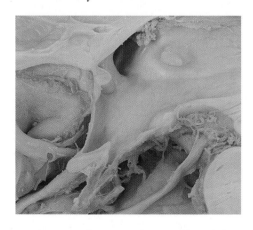

Anterior corticospinal tract. The smaller of the two *corticospinal tracts*. It consists of the fibers (about 15%) in each medullary *pyramid* that continue directly into the *anterior funiculus* of the spinal cord without decussating; many fibers eventually cross in the anterior white commissure of the cord before terminating, but some end ipsilaterally. Fibers of the anterior corticospinal tract end (mainly in the cervical and thoracic spinal cord) on spinal motor neurons or nearby interneurons.

Anterior funiculus. One of the three major divisions of the spinal white matter, the others being the *lateral* and *posterior* funiculi. (*Funiculus* is Latin for "string" or "cord," as in the term "funicular" for cable-car) The anterior funiculus is located between the anterior median fissure and the exiting *ventral roots* and contains various tracts (mostly descending), including the *anterior corticospinal tract.*

Anterior horn. One of the three general divisions of the spinal gray matter, the others being the *posterior horn* and the *intermediate gray;* contains numerous local-circuit neurons, cell bodies of alpha motor neurons, axons of which enter the ventral (anterior) spinal nerve roots and end on skeletal muscle, and cell bodies of gamma motor neurons that regulate muscle spindles.

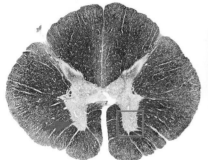 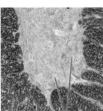

Motor neurons

Anterior inferior cerebellar artery. A long, circumferential branch of the *basilar artery* arising just above the union of the two *vertebral arteries.* It supplies anterior regions of the inferior surface of the *cerebellum,* including the *flocculus,* and parts of the caudal *pons;* often referred to by the acronym *AICA.*

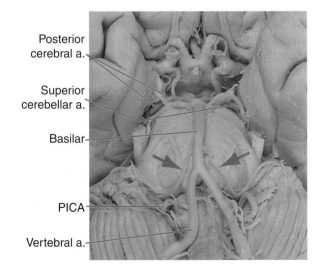

Posterior cerebral a.

Superior cerebellar a.

Basilar

PICA

Vertebral a.

Anterior nucleus. See *thalamus*.*

Anterior perforated substance. The inferior surface of the forebrain, roughly between the *orbital gyri* and the *hypothalamus.* So named because numerous *lenticulostriate* and other small penetrating branches enter the brain here.

Anterior root. See *ventral root*.*

Anterior spinal artery. A single midline vessel that originates rostrally as two arteries (one from each *vertebral artery*), which shortly join and then course within the anterior median fissure along the entire spinal cord. It receives additional blood from the thoracic/abdominal aorta through numerous anastomoses with radicular arteries below the upper cervical region and gives rise to hundreds of central and circumferential branches that supply the anterior two thirds of the cord.

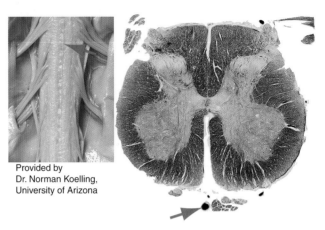

Provided by
Dr. Norman Koelling,
University of Arizona

Anterior spinocerebellar tract. Crossed fibers from lumbosacral spinal gray matter, carrying mechanoreceptive and other information related to leg movement. The anterior spinocerebellar tract stays in a lateral position along the spinal cord and *brainstem* until the rostral *pons,* and there moves over the *superior cerebellar peduncle* and enters the *cerebellum,* where it largely recrosses.

Anterolateral system. An umbrella term for the *spinothalamic tract* and closely related ascending fibers, all of which deal with pain, temperature, and to some extent tactile/pressure sensation. Many do not reach the *thalamus,* ending instead at higher spinal levels or in *brainstem* sites, such as the *reticular formation.*

Aqueduct (of Sylvius). The narrow channel (a remnant of the lumen of the embryonic mesencephalon) through the *midbrain* connecting the *third* and *fourth ventricles.* The aqueduct lacks a *choroid plexus* and serves only as a conduit for cerebrospinal fluid descending through the ventricular system (its stenosis or obstruction is the most common cause of congenital hydrocephalus).

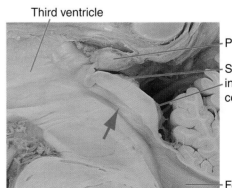

Third ventricle

Pineal gland

Superior & inferior colliculi

Fourth ventricle

Arachnoid. The middle layer of the three layers of meninges, named for its cobweblike appearance. The arachnoid is loosely adherent to the dura mater and connected to the pia mater by fine strands of connective tissue (arachnoid

Genu. The kneelike sharp anterior bend, containing fibers that lead to the *frontal lobes.*

Rostrum. The slender, narrow part beneath the genu, resembling the prow of the (overturned) boat; interconnects *orbital gyri.*

Splenium. The thick, rounded posterior bend (similar to a rolled bandage), containing fibers to the *occipital* and *temporal lobes.*

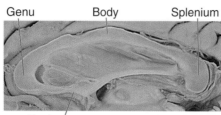

Genu   Body   Splenium

Rostrum

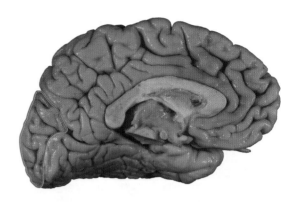

Corticobulbar tract. Strictly defined, a large collection of fibers originating in the cerebral cortex and descending through the *internal capsule* (immediately anterior to the closely related *corticospinal* fibers) to terminate (via numerous, often intricate routes) in the "bulb" (an old term for the *medulla* or, by extension, for the entire *brainstem*) on neurons of sensory relay nuclei, the *reticular formation,* and motor nuclei of cranial nerves. In common usage, the term refers only to the last fibers of this group. Basically, the equivalent of the *corticospinal tract* for cranial nerve nuclei.

Corticopontine tract. A very large collection of fibers originating in the *frontal, parietal, occipital, temporal,* and even *limbic lobes* and descending through the *internal capsule* (anterior and posterior to the *corticospinal/corticobulbar* projections) to nuclei in the *basal pons,* from which axons pass to the contralateral *cerebellar hemispheres* through the *middle cerebellar peduncles.*

Corticospinal tract. A collection of about a million axons that originate in the cerebral cortex, descend through the *internal capsule, cerebral peduncle, basal pons,* and medullary *pyramid,* then reach the spinal cord, where they terminate, via the *lateral* and *anterior corticospinal tracts.* Roughly a third of them originate in primary motor cortex, the rest arising from premotor and supplementary motor areas and the *parietal lobe* (especially somatosensory cortex). Corticospinal axons end in the spinal cord on cells of the *posterior horn, intermediate gray,* and *anterior horn,* where some synapse directly on alpha and gamma motor neurons. A single functional role is difficult to specify, but this is the principal pathway on which skilled volitional movements depend.

Cuneate tubercle. A subtle swelling on the dorsolateral aspect of the lower *medulla* overlying *nucleus cuneatus,* which mediates the part of the *posterior column–medial lemniscus* pathway carrying tactile and proprioceptive information from the arm and upper body.

Cuneus. The wedge-shaped area of the medial surface of the *occipital lobe* between the *calcarine* and *parietooccipital sulci.* Includes the upper half of primary visual cortex and parts of visual association cortex.

Dentate nucleus. The largest and most lateral of the deep cerebellar nuclei, featuring a highly convoluted narrow band of neurons arranged like a bag, with an anteriorly directed opening (hilus) from which efferents emerge to form most of the *superior cerebellar peduncle.*

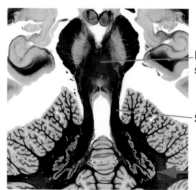

Decussation of superior cerebellar peduncles

Superior cerebellar peduncle

Denticulate ligament. A thickened, lateral, serrated sheet of pia mater on each side of the spinal cord, with periodic extensions that attach to the *arachnoid* and *dura mater,* supporting the weight and stabilizing the position of the cord within the dural sac.

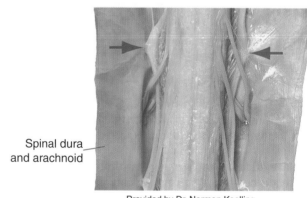

Spinal dura and arachnoid

Provided by Dr. Norman Koelling, University of Arizona

Diencephalon. Literally, the "in-between brain," the caudal subdivision of the embryonic forebrain, giving rise to the *pineal gland, habenula, thalamus, subthalamic nucleus,* retina, *optic nerve* and *tract, hypothalamus, infundibulum* (pituitary stalk), and neurohypophysis.

Dorsal cochlear nucleus. See *cochlear nuclei*.*

Dorsal longitudinal fasciculus. Ascending and descending fibers connecting the *hypothalamus* directly and indirectly to visceral sensory neurons and preganglionic autonomic neurons, traveling through the *periaqueductal* and periventricular gray matter.

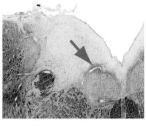

Dorsal motor nucleus of the vagus. A prominent autonomic efferent nucleus containing most of the preganglionic parasympathetic neurons for thoracic and abdominal viscera.

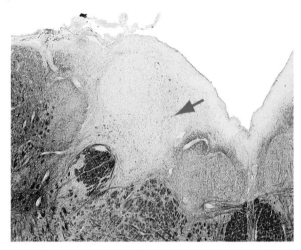

Dorsal root. The posterior (sensory) root of a spinal nerve, which divides into a variable number of regularly spaced rootlets that enter the spinal cord along its posterolateral sulcus.

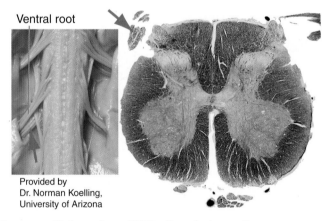

Ventral root

Provided by
Dr. Norman Koelling,
University of Arizona

Dorsomedial nucleus (DM). See *thalamus**.

Dura mater. The outermost of the three layers of meninges, providing crucial mechanical support for the CNS. Cranial dura mater is continuous with the periosteum of the inner surface of the skull, whereas in the vertebral canal it forms a dural sac within which the spinal cord is suspended by *denticulate ligaments**.

Edinger-Westphal nucleus. A column of small nerve cell bodies near the midline of the *oculomotor nucleus*. Its neurons form the efferent arm of the direct and consensual pupillary light reflexes: preganglionic parasympathetic neurons effect (via postganglionic neurons in the ciliary

ganglion) contraction of the pupillary sphincter to constrict the pupil. Also part of the efferent arm of the near reflex: it mediates (again via postganglionic neurons in the ciliary ganglion) ciliary muscle contraction to thicken the lens and pupillary constriction to increase depth of focus.

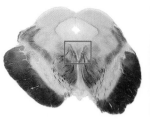
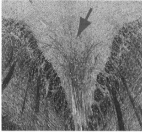

Entorhinal cortex. The cortex covering the anterior part of the *parahippocampal gyrus*, near the *uncus*. Entorhinal cortex receives inputs from the *amygdala*, *olfactory bulb*, *limbic lobe*, and other cortical areas, and is the major source of afferents to the *hippocampus*.

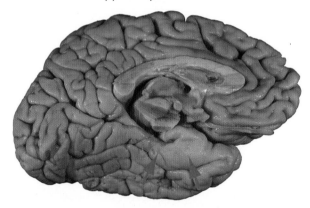

External capsule. A thin layer of white matter interposed between the *claustrum** and *putamen*, containing association fibers that interconnect various cortical areas and modulatory fibers from sites such as the *basal nucleus*.

External medullary lamina (of the thalamus). A thin, curved sheet of myelinated fibers (afferent and efferent), in places fenestrated and in others dense, surrounding the lateral surface of the *thalamus**; enclosed by a thin shell of gray matter, the *reticular nucleus*, which intervenes between it and the *internal capsule*.

Extreme capsule. A thin layer of white matter interposed between the *claustrum** and *insula*. The extreme capsule is the subcortical white matter of the *insula*, but also contains association fibers that interconnect various other cortical areas.

Facial colliculus. A swelling in the floor of the fourth ventricle, caused by the underlying internal genu of the *facial nerve* looping around the *abducens nucleus*.

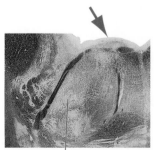
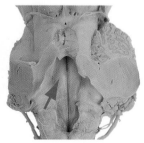

Facial nucleus

Facial nerve. The 7th cranial nerve, which emerges antero-laterally from the *brainstem* along the groove between the *basal pons* and the *medulla*. The facial nerve serves nasopharyngeal, taste, and external ear sensation; controls muscles of facial expression; and regulates secretion by the submandibular, sublingual, and lacrimal glands.

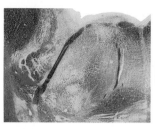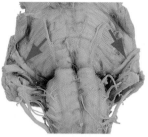

Facial nucleus. A group of motor neurons in the caudal pontine tegmentum that innervate muscles of the ipsilateral half of the face. Their axons travel just beneath the floor of the *fourth ventricle* in the *facial colliculus** before leaving the *brainstem*.

Fasciculus cuneatus. Uncrossed, large, myelinated, primary afferents entering the *posterior column* of the spinal cord rostral to T6 and carrying tactile and proprioceptive information from the arm; many of these fibers ascend to the *medulla* to terminate in *nucleus cuneatus*.

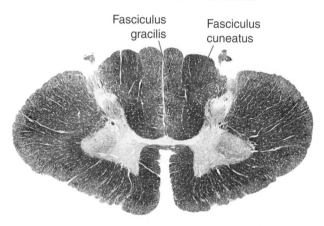

Fasciculus gracilis   Fasciculus cuneatus

Fasciculus gracilis. Uncrossed, large, myelinated, primary afferents entering the *posterior column* of the spinal cord caudal to T6 and carrying tactile and proprioceptive information from the leg; many of these fibers ascend to the medulla, medial to *fasciculus cuneatus**, to terminate in *nucleus gracilis*.

Fastigial nucleus. The most medial of the deep cerebellar nuclei. Its afferents come mainly from the *cerebellar vermis*, and its efferents project bilaterally to the *vestibular nuclei* and *reticular formation*.

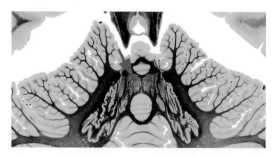

Filum terminale. A thin strand of connective tissue that anchors the caudal end of the spinal cord to the coccyx. It begins as a pial extension from the *conus medullaris*, extends through the lumbar cistern surrounded by the *cauda equina**, picks up a dural covering at about vertebral level S2 (where the spinal dural sac ends), and merges with the periosteum of the coccyx.

Fimbria. Literally, the "fringe", a prominent band of white matter along the medial edge of the *hippocampus*. The fimbria is an accumulation of myelinated axons (mostly efferent) that first collect on the ventricular surface of the *hippocampus** as the *alveus* (a thin layer resembling an inverted trough). Near the splenium of the *corpus callosum*, the fimbria separates from the *hippocampus* as the crus of the *fornix**.

Flocculus. The hemispheral component of the flocculonodular lobe, the part of the *cerebellum** particularly concerned with the vestibular system and eye movements.

Foramen of Monro. See *interventricular foramen**.

Fornix. A prominent paired fiber bundle, mostly containing hippocampal efferents, that interconnects the *hippocampus* of each cerebral hemisphere and the ipsilateral *septal nuclei* and *hypothalamus*.

Body. Upper arched cable formed by the union of the crura beneath the *septa pellucida* in the midline.

Column. One of the two bundles that diverge from the body, then pass down and back toward the *mammillary bodies*.

Crus. One of the two origins (legs) of the body, formed by detachment of the *fimbria* from the *hippocampus*.

Fimbria. Hippocampal efferents that have assembled from the *alveus* on their way into the crus.

Precommissural fornix. Fornix fibers that leave the columns just above the *anterior commissure*, bound for the *septal nuclei, ventral striatum*, and some nearby cortical areas.

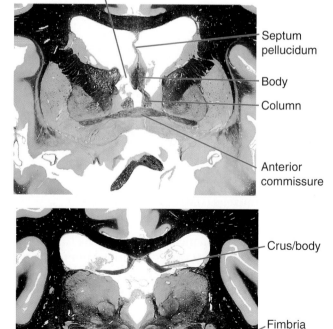

Interventricular foramen

Septum pellucidum

Body

Column

Anterior commissure

Crus/body

Fimbria

Alveus

Hippocampus

Fourth ventricle. The most caudal of the brain ventricles, shaped like a tent with a peaked roof protruding into the overlying *cerebellum* and a diamond-shaped floor formed by the upper surface of the *pons* and rostral *medulla;* confluent with the *third ventricle* via the cerebral *aqueduct* and open to the subarachnoid space through three foramina: one median aperture and two lateral apertures.

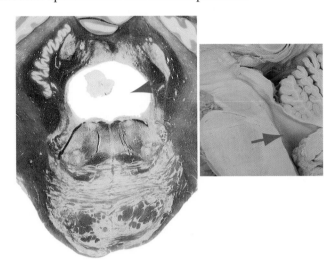

Frontal lobe. The most anterior lobe of each cerebral hemisphere. The frontal lobe includes motor, premotor, and supplementary motor cortex; an extensive prefrontal region; and a large expanse of *orbital* cortex. The latter two regions have access via long association fibers to all other lobes and also to the limbic system; they are important (in a poorly understood way) in regulating emotional tone, prioritizing bodily/environmental demands, and stabilizing short-range and long-range goal-directed activity.

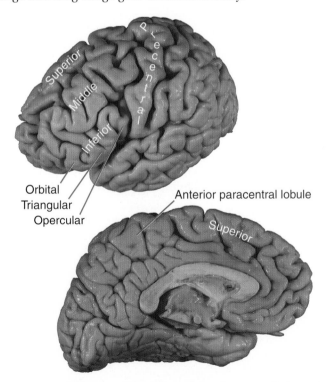

Globus pallidus. A wedge-shaped nucleus medial to the *putamen* that gives rise to most of the efferents from the basal ganglia.

External segment (GPe). Afferents from the *striatum,* efferents (via the *subthalamic fasciculus*) to the *subthalamic nucleus.*

Internal segment (GPi). Afferents from the *striatum* and *subthalamic nucleus,* efferents (via the *ansa lenticularis* and *lenticular fasciculus*) to the *thalamus.*

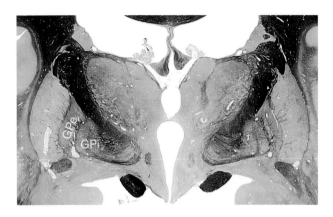

Glomus. An enlarged strand of choroid plexus in the atrium of the *lateral ventricle.* The glomus ("ball of thread") accumulates calcium deposits with age and so can often be seen in CT images.

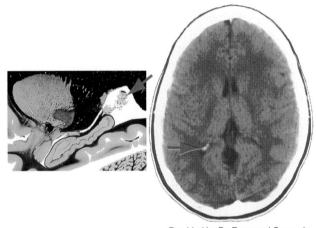

Provided by Dr. Raymond Carmody, University of Arizona

Glossopharyngeal nerve. The 9th cranial nerve. Its rootlets emerge laterally from a shallow groove on the lateral surface of the *medulla,* at the rostral end of the series of filaments that form the *vagus nerve**. This nerve serves nasoooropharyngeal, carotid body/sinus, middle ear, taste, and outer ear sensations; assists with swallowing (stylopharyngeus muscle); and regulates salivation (parotid gland).

Gracile tubercle. A conspicuous swelling, just caudal to the *obex,* located dorsomedially on the lower *medulla* overlying *nucleus gracilis,* which mediates that part of the *posterior column–medial lemniscus* pathway carrying tactile and proprioceptive information from the leg and lower body.

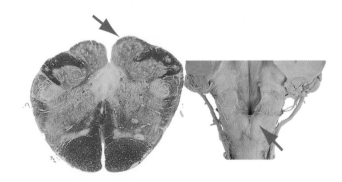

Great vein (great cerebral vein of Galen). A large unpaired vessel arising in the *superior cistern* by union of the two *internal cerebral veins*. During its short course, it receives the *basal veins* (of Rosenthal), then turns superiorly around the splenium of the *corpus callosum* and joins the inferior sagittal sinus to form the *straight sinus*. The *great vein* is a key conduit in the deep venous drainage of the brain.

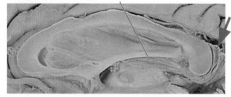

Internal cerebral vein

Gyrus rectus. A slender straight convolution, medial to the *orbital gyri** covering the rest of the inferior surface of the *frontal lobe*. Gyrus rectus has extensive limbic connections, particularly in circuits involving the *amygdala*.

Habenula. A small mound of neurons (derived from the embryonic *diencephalon*) on the dorsomedial surface of the caudal *thalamus*. The habenula receives diverse afferents from the mediobasal forebrain (e.g., *septal nuclei, preoptic area*) that arrive through the superiorly arching *stria medullaris* of the thalamus. Habenular efferents descend to various paramedian *midbrain* reticular nuclei via the *habenulointerpeduncular tract*. Hence, it is anatomically evident that the habenula is a relay in caudally directed limbic projections, although its exact role is poorly understood.

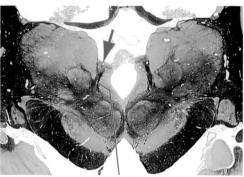

Habenulointerpeduncular tract

Habenulointerpeduncular tract. (Also called *fasciculus retroflexus*, owing to its lordotic curvature.) Conveys output from the superiorly coursing *stria medullaris/habenula** route precipitously down again to the paramedian *midbrain reticular formation* (where all other caudally directed limbic projections arrive more expediently by passing inferiorly through the *hypothalamus*).

Heschl's gyri. See *transverse temporal gyri**.

Hippocampus. A specialized cortical area rolled into the medial *temporal lobe*. The hippocampus plays a critical role in the consolidation of new memories of facts and events. Anatomically, it has three subdivisions (until fairly recently, usually referred to collectively as the hippocampal formation rather than the hippocampus), from within outward as follows:

Dentate gyrus. In cross section, one of two interlocking C-shaped strips of cortex (the hippocampus proper is the other). Afferents from *entorhinal cortex*, efferents to hippocampal pyramidal cells.

Hippocampus proper. Afferents from the dentate gyrus and *septal nuclei*, efferents to the subiculum and *septal nuclei*. (Also called cornu ammonis, or Ammon's horn.)

Subiculum. A transitional zone between the hippocampus proper and *entorhinal cortex*, the subiculum receives afferents from the hippocampus proper and is the principal source of efferents from the hippocampus in general.

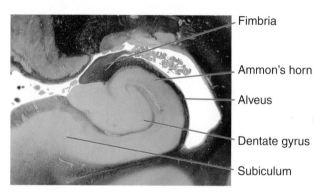

Fimbria
Ammon's horn
Alveus
Dentate gyrus
Subiculum

Hypoglossal nerve. The 12th cranial nerve, whose rootlets emerge from the *medulla* in an anterolateral sulcus between the *pyramid* and the *olive;* it innervates intrinsic and extrinsic skeletal muscles of the tongue.

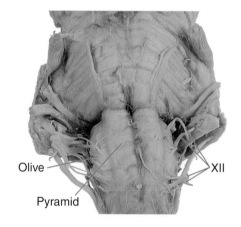

Olive
XII
Pyramid

Hypoglossal nucleus. A group of motor neurons that innervate muscles of the ipsilateral half of the tongue.

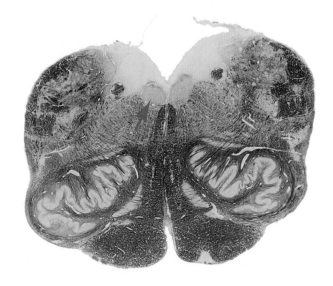

Hypoglossal trigone. A triangular elevation in the floor of the caudal *fourth ventricle* formed by the underlying *hypoglossal nucleus*.

Hypothalamic sulcus. A shallow, curved indentation (convex side down) in the wall of the *third ventricle*, extending from the *interventricular foramen* to the opening of the cerebral *aqueduct*. The hypothalamic sulcus is the boundary between the *thalamus* and the *hypothalamus**.

Hypothalamus. The most inferior of the four longitudinal divisions of the *diencephalon*, the hypothalamus plays a major role in orchestrating visceral and drive-related activities. It has three general zones:

Anterior region. Includes the suprachiasmatic, supraoptic, and paraventricular nuclei and continues anteriorly into the *preoptic region*; projects axons to the neurohypophysis and to caudal sites (including the spinal cord).

Tuberal region. Includes the dorsomedial, ventromedial, and arcuate nuclei. The latter secretes releasing hormones and inhibiting hormones into the pituitary portal system.

Posterior region. Includes the *mammillary* and posterior nuclei and projects to the *thalamus* and *midbrain tegmentum*.

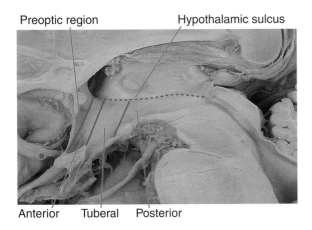

Preoptic region — Hypothalamic sulcus

Anterior — Tuberal — Posterior

Inferior brachium. See *brachium of the inferior colliculus**.

Inferior cerebellar peduncle. A major input route to the *cerebellum*, containing crossed olivocerebellar fibers, the uncrossed *posterior spinocerebellar* and cuneocerebellar tracts, vestibulocerebellar fibers, and other cerebellar afferents. Sometimes referred to as the restiform (Latin for "ropelike") body.

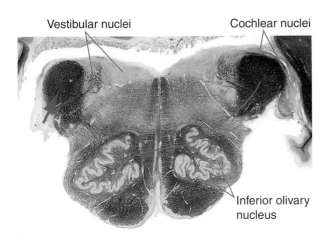

Vestibular nuclei — Cochlear nuclei

Inferior olivary nucleus

Inferior colliculus. A large, rounded mass of gray matter in the roof of the caudal *midbrain*. The inferior colliculus is a major link in the auditory system, receiving the *lateral lemniscus* and giving rise to the *brachium of the inferior colliculus**, which in turn conveys auditory fibers to the *medial geniculate nucleus*.

Inferior frontal gyrus. The most inferior of three longitudinally oriented gyri in the anterior part of the *frontal lobe**. The opercular and triangular parts of this gyrus in the dominant hemisphere form Broca's area, which is a language area important for the production of spoken and written language.

Inferior olivary nucleus. A large nucleus in the anterolateral *medulla*, shaped like a bag, with a convoluted wall of gray matter (like a crumpled, pitted olive). Olivary afferents are diverse (from the spinal cord, *red nucleus*, deep cerebellar nuclei, and other sites), but efferents are all olivocerebellar. They pour out of its medially facing mouth (or hilus), cross the midline as *internal arcuate fibers*, join the *inferior cerebellar peduncle**, and blanket the contralateral *cerebellum* as climbing fibers that powerfully excite Purkinje cells and other neurons.

Inferior parietal lobule. The lower part of the lateral surface of the *parietal lobe*, below the *intraparietal sulcus* and behind the *postcentral gyrus*. The inferior parietal lobule consists of the *angular* and *supramarginal gyri*, which (in the dominant hemisphere) are functionally related to Wernicke's area and thus important in the comprehension of language.

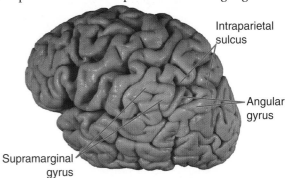

Intraparietal sulcus

Angular gyrus

Supramarginal gyrus

Inferior temporal gyrus. The most inferior of three longitudinally oriented convolutions visible on the lateral aspect of the *temporal lobe**. The inferior temporal gyrus is part of a large region of visual association cortex occupying most of the *occipital lobe* and much of the *temporal lobe*.

Inferior thalamic peduncle. A small bundle of fibers emerging anteriorly from the *thalamus* and curving down toward the *basal forebrain* (just medial to the *ansa lenticularis*). Its fibers include interconnections between the dorsomedial nucleus and *orbital* cortex, but they do not traverse the *internal capsule* like other thalamic connections.

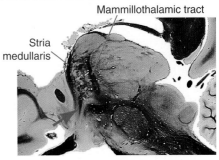

Mammillothalamic tract

Stria medullaris

Infundibulum. The hollow, funnel-like stalk of the pituitary gland descending from the median eminence of the *hypothalamus* to the neurohypophysis. The infundibulum arises during embryonic development as a ventral outgrowth of the floor of the *diencephalon*, and is later joined by the adenohypophysis derived from the roof of the oral cavity.

Insula. The original lateral surface of the embryonic telencephalic vesicle overlying an area of fusion with the *diencephalon*, forming in the adult a central lobe of the cerebral hemisphere, typically convoluted into about three short gyri (located more anteriorly) and two long gyri. With rapid cerebral expansion during fetal development, the insula is overgrown and by birth concealed by frontal, parietal, and temporal *opercula*. It includes gustatory and autonomic areas, but is less well understood than other cortical areas because of its hidden location.

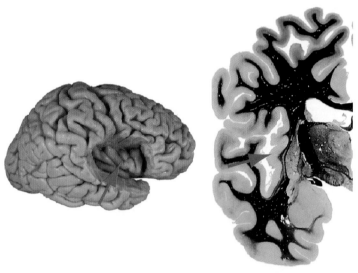

Intermediate gray. The spinal gray matter interposed between the *posterior* and *anterior horns*. It contains interneurons and tract cells of various sensory and motor circuits (including *Clarke's nucleus*), preganglionic sympathetic neurons in thoracic and upper lumbar segments, and preganglionic parasympathetic neurons in segments S2-4.

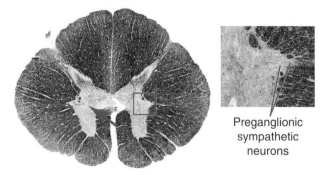

Preganglionic sympathetic neurons

Internal arcuate fibers. A general term for the large collection of axons that arch across the midline of the *medulla*. Many internal arcuate fibers are axons leaving the *posterior column nuclei* to form the contralateral *medial lemniscus*, some are trigeminothalamic fibers leaving the spinal trigeminal nucleus to join the contralateral *spinothalamic tract*, and most others are efferents from the *inferior olivary nucleus* to the contralateral half of the *cerebellum*.

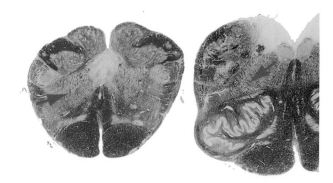

Internal capsule. A compact, curved sheaf of thalamocortical, corticothalamic, and other cortical projection fibers shaped like part of a funnel. The internal capsule is divided into five regions, based on each region's relationship to the *lenticular nucleus*:

Anterior limb. Between the *lenticular nucleus* and the head of the *caudate nucleus*. Connections between the *thalamus* (dorsomedial and anterior nuclei) and prefrontal and anterior *cingulate* cortex, plus many frontopontine fibers.

Genu. At the junction between the anterior and posterior limbs. Connections between the *thalamus* (VA, VL) and motor/premotor cortex, plus some frontopontine fibers.

Posterior limb. Between the *lenticular nucleus* and the *thalamus*. Connections between the *thalamus* (VA, VL, VPL/VPM) and motor, somatosensory, and other parietal cortex, plus *corticobulbar* and *corticospinal* fibers.

Retrolenticular part. Passing posterior to the *lenticular nucleus*. Connections between the *thalamus* (pulvinar, LP) and parietal-occipital-temporal association cortex, plus the upper part of the *optic radiation* (from the lateral geniculate nucleus).

Sublenticular part. Dipping under the posterior part of the *lenticular nucleus*. Projections to and from the *temporal lobe*, including the auditory radiation (from the medial geniculate nucleus) and the lower part of the *optic radiation* (from the lateral geniculate nucleus) before it turns posteriorly toward the *occipital lobe*.

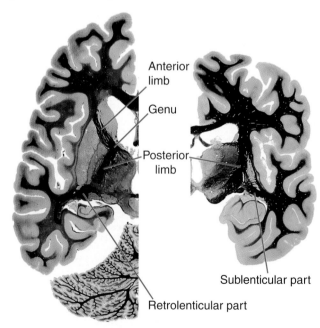

Anterior limb

Genu

Posterior limb

Sublenticular part

Retrolenticular part

Internal carotid artery. A large distributing artery, originating from the bifurcation of the common carotid artery and running cranially in the neck to enter the base of the skull and eventually the cranial vault. The internal carotid artery branches at the circle of Willis into *anterior* and *middle cerebral arteries*. The paired carotids account for 85% of cerebral blood flow and thus supply most of the blood to the brain.

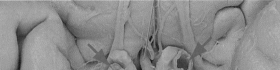

Anterior cerebral arteries

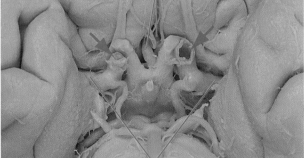

Middle cerebral arteries

Internal cerebral vein. The major deep vein of each cerebral hemisphere, formed at the *interventricular foramen* by the confluence of the smaller septal and *terminal* (thalamostriate) *veins* (the latter receiving the *choroidal vein*, which drains much of the *choroid plexus*). Immediately after its origin, the internal cerebral vein bends sharply posteriorly (through the *venous angle*), proceeds posteriorly in the *transverse fissure,* and fuses with its counterpart in the *superior cistern* to form the unpaired *great vein**.

Internal medullary lamina (of the thalamus). A dense, curved sheet of myelinated fibers within the *thalamus** that divide it into medial and lateral compartments everywhere except posteriorly, where it does not enter the pulvinar, and anteriorly, where it forks into a V-shaped groove for the anterior nuclei. The internal medullary lamina contains several small and two large intralaminar nuclei (the centromedian and parafascicular nuclei).

Interpeduncular fossa. A depression on the anterior aspect of the *midbrain* between the two *cerebral peduncles*. Its surface is penetrated by paramedian branches of the *basilar artery* and therefore is termed the posterior perforated substance. Rootlets of the *oculomotor nerve* exit here.

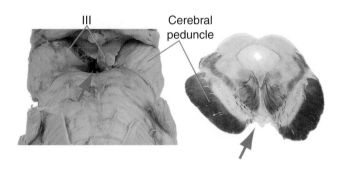

III   Cerebral peduncle

Interposed nucleus. The deep cerebellar nucleus interposed between the *dentate* and *fastigial nuclei*. The interposed nucleus has two distinct subdivisions, the globose nucleus medially and emboliform nucleus laterally (looks

like an embolus in the hilus of the adjoining *dentate nucleus*). Both subdivisions receive input from the paravermal (intermediate) zone of cerebellar cortex, both project (via the *superior cerebellar peduncle*, like the *dentate nucleus*) to the *red nucleus* and VL of the *thalamus*. (The projection of the interposed nucleus differs mainly in emphasis, favoring the *red nucleus* over VL, whereas the dentate projection is just the opposite.)

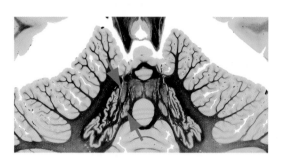

Interthalamic adhesion (massa intermedia). A small, ovoid area of continuity between the two *thalami* resulting from expansion and fusion of the walls of the *third ventricle* during development. The interthalamic adhesion is mainly gray matter, containing neurons and axonal and dendritic processes. (This structure is often reduced in size or absent, especially in the brains of elderly individuals; however, in some mammals, such as rodents, it is massive, reducing the size of the *third ventricle* but anatomically making the *thalamus* almost a single unpaired structure; see *third ventricle**.)

Interventricular foramen (of Monro). The narrow orifice between each *lateral ventricle* and the *third ventricle*.

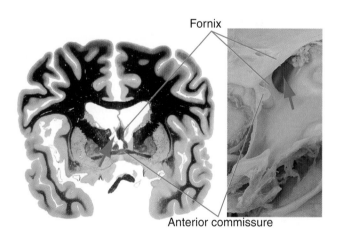

Fornix

Anterior commissure

Intraparietal sulcus. A longitudinally oriented sulcus on the lateral aspect of the *parietal lobe,* separating it into a *superior parietal lobule* above and an *inferior parietal lobule** below.

Lamina terminalis. A thin membrane at the anterior end of the *third ventricle,* curving down from the rostrum of the *corpus callosum* to the *optic chiasm* and corresponding (roughly, if not precisely) to the rostral end of the neural tube. The lamina terminalis connects the two telencephalic vesicles of the embryonic forebrain and provides a route through which commissural fibers that later form the *anterior commissure* and *corpus callosum* begin to grow.

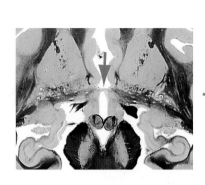
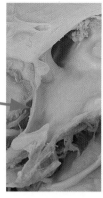

Lateral corticospinal tract. The larger of the two *corticospinal tracts,* comprising the fibers (about 85%) in each medullary *pyramid* that enter the *pyramidal decussation* and cross the midline to the opposite *lateral funiculus.* The axons of this tract end on spinal motor neurons or (more often) on smaller interneurons that in turn synapse on motor neurons. Its fibers are often said to be arranged somatotopically, with those passing to more caudal cord levels located more laterally, but anatomical evidence does not support this view.

Lateral cuneate nucleus. The equivalent for the arm of *Clarke's nucleus* for the leg. Proprioceptive primary afferents travel through *fasciculus cuneatus* to this nucleus, which then gives rise to uncrossed cuneocerebellar fibers that enter the *cerebellum* via the *inferior cerebellar peduncle.*

Lateral dorsal nucleus (LD). See *thalamus*.*

Lateral funiculus. One of the three major divisions of the spinal white matter, the others being the *anterior* and *posterior* funiculi.* The lateral funiculus contains various ascending and descending tracts, including the *anterior* and *posterior spinocerebellar, spinothalamic,* and *lateral corticospinal tracts.*

Lateral geniculate nucleus (LGN). See *thalamus*.*

Lateral horn. A small, pointed lateral extension of the *intermediate spinal gray* noted from T1 through L2 or L3. The lateral horn contains the intermediolateral cell column, a long strand of preganglionic sympathetic neurons serving the entire body. Axons of these preganglionic sympathetic neurons leave through the *ventral roots.*

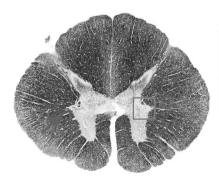

Preganglionic sympathetic neurons

Lateral lemniscus. A flattened ribbon of fibers on the lateral surface of the rostral pontine tegmentum, arising from the *cochlear* and *superior olivary nuclei.* The lateral lemniscus is part of the ascending auditory pathway, conveying information from both ears to the *inferior colliculus.*

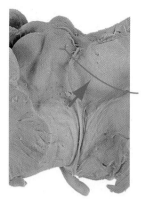
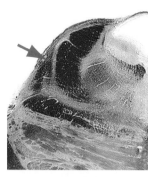

Lateral olfactory tract. A small tract in humans (although much larger in animals that rely more extensively on the sense of smell) through which fibers that originated in the *olfactory bulb* and passed through the *olfactory tract* continue on their way by traveling across the surface of the *basal forebrain* to olfactory cortex and the *amygdala.*

Piriform cortex

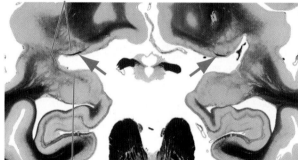

Periamygdaloid cortex

Lateral posterior nucleus (LP). See *thalamus*.*

Lateral sulcus (sylvian fissure). A long, deep fossa on the lateral aspect of each cerebral hemisphere resulting from downward and forward expansion of the *temporal lobe* during fetal development. The *insula* lies hidden within the depths of this sulcus, which separates the temporal lobe from the *frontal* and *parietal lobes* and provides a route by which the *middle cerebral artery* accesses the lateral convexity.

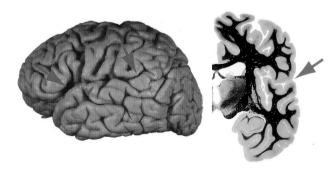

Lateral ventricle. The large central cavity of each cerebral hemisphere, following a C-shaped course throughout its extent and derived from the lumen of the embryonic telencephalic vesicle.

Anterior horn. The frontal horn, in the *frontal lobe* anterior to the *interventricular foramen.*

Body. In the *frontal* and *parietal lobes,* extending posteriorly to the region of the splenium of the *corpus callosum.*

Atrium (or trigone). The region near the splenium of the *corpus callosum* where the body and the posterior and inferior horns meet.

Inferior horn. The temporal horn, curving down and forward into the *temporal lobe.*

Posterior horn. The occipital horn, projecting backward into the *occipital lobe.*

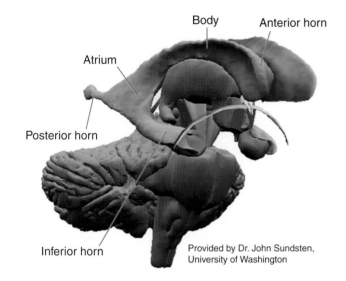

Body
Anterior horn
Atrium
Posterior horn
Inferior horn
Provided by Dr. John Sundsten,
University of Washington

Lenticular fasciculus. Part of the projection from the *globus pallidus* to the *thalamus.* It has more axons than the other part (see *ansa lenticularis*) and is more spread out, forming numerous conspicuous bundles of myelinated fibers running medially through the *internal capsule,* like the teeth of a comb. Medial to the internal capsule, the lenticular fasciculus is joined by the *ansa lenticularis* before both enter the *thalamus* through the *thalamic fasciculus.*

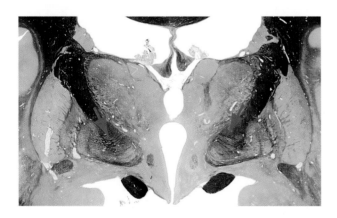

Lenticular nucleus. The *putamen* and *globus pallidus* considered as one anatomical structure.

Lenticulostriate arteries. A collection of about a dozen small branches of the *middle cerebral artery* along its course toward the *lateral sulcus.* They penetrate the overlying brain near their origin and pass upward to supply deep structures *(internal capsule, globus pallidus, putamen).* The lenticulostriate arteries exemplify a large collection of small penetrating vessels that arise from all arteries around the base of the brain; these narrow, thin-walled vessels are involved frequently in strokes that deprive deep cerebral structures

of blood and thus cause neurological deficits out of proportion to their size.

Limbic lobe. The most medial lobe of the cerebral hemisphere, facing the midline and visible grossly only in sagittal section. The limbic lobe consists of a continuous border zone of cortex around the *corpus callosum,* comprising the *cingulate* and *parahippocampal gyri* and their narrow connecting isthmus; this lobe and its many connections, cortical and subcortical, account for a large part of the limbic system and give the latter its name.

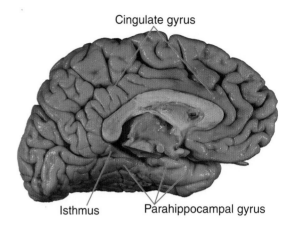

Cingulate gyrus
Isthmus
Parahippocampal gyrus

Limen insulae. *Limen* is Latin for "threshold" and in this case refers to the transition point from *anterior perforated substance* to *insula.* The circular sulcus, which surrounds almost the entire *insula,* ends on either side of the limen insulae, allowing access for the *middle cerebral artery.*

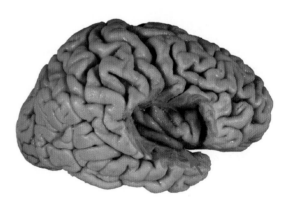

Lingual gyrus. The gyrus forming the inferior bank of the *calcarine sulcus.* The lingual gyrus overlaps the posterior part of the *occipitotemporal gyrus*,* separated from it by the *collateral sulcus.*

Lissauer's tract. A pale-staining area of white matter between the *substantia gelatinosa** (capping the *posterior horn* of the spinal gray matter) and the pial surface of the cord. Lissauer's tract stains more lightly than the rest of the spinal white matter because it contains finely myelinated and unmyelinated pain and temperature fibers (derived from the lateral division of each *dorsal root* filament), which then distribute into the underlying gelatinosa over several segments.

Locus ceruleus. A column of pigmented, blue-black neurons (*locus ceruleus* is Latin for "blue place") near the floor of the *fourth ventricle,* extending through the rostral *pons.* Locus ceruleus neurons provide most of the far-flung noradrenergic innervation of the cerebrum.

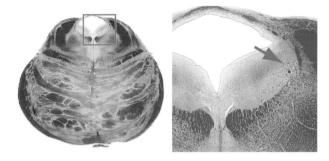

Longitudinal fissure. An extensive vertical cleft, oriented sagittally and occupied by the falx cerebri, separating the two cerebral hemispheres around the margin of the undivided *corpus callosum*.

Mammillary body. A prominent component of the posterior *hypothalamus*. The mammillary body receives afferents from the *hippocampus* (chiefly the subiculum) via the *fornix* and sends efferents to the anterior nucleus of the *thalamus* via the *mammillothalamic tract*. This is part of a historic neural circuit proposed by James Papez in 1937 as an anatomical substrate for emotion. Although derided by some then and viewed as simplistic by others now, the Papez circuit—a grand loop from *hippocampus* through *hypothalamus, thalamus,* and cortex back to *hippocampus* again—was unquestionably the impetus for the decades of research that led to the limbic system concept of today.

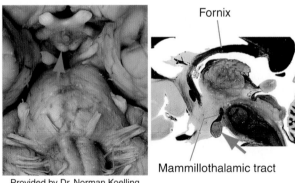

Fornix

Mammillothalamic tract

Provided by Dr. Norman Koelling, University of Arizona

Mammillothalamic tract. The projection from the *mammillary body** to the anterior nucleus of the *thalamus;* part of the Papez circuit.

Medial geniculate nucleus (MGN). See *thalamus*.*

Medial lemniscus. Somatosensory afferents originating from the contralateral *posterior column nuclei* and *trigeminal main sensory nucleus* and ascending through the brainstem to the *thalamus* (VPL/VPM). The medial lemniscus is the principal ascending pathway for tactile and proprioceptive information.

Medial longitudinal fasciculus (MLF). A longitudinal fiber bundle involved in coordinating eye and head movements. The MLF includes fibers from contralateral abducens interneurons to medial rectus motor neurons in the *oculomotor nucleus.* It also is the route of descent for fibers of the medial vestibulospinal tract.

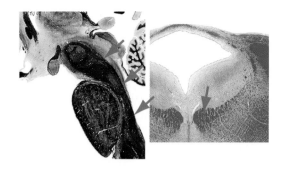

Medial striate artery. A large penetrating branch of the *anterior cerebral artery,* also known as the recurrent artery of Heubner. It supplies the *striatum* and *internal capsule* in the region of *nucleus accumbens,* and some posterior parts of the *orbital gyri.*

Median aperture. One of the three apertures through which the *fourth ventricle* communicates with subarachnoid space. The median aperture (also called the *foramen of Magendie*) opens into *cisterna magna.*

Medulla (medulla oblongata). The most caudal of the three subdivisions of the *brainstem,* continuous rostrally with the *pons* and caudally with the spinal cord. This small structure is important out of proportion to its size: It is crucial to vital functions (respiratory, cardiovascular, visceral activity) and other integrative activities; most sensory and motor tracts of the CNS run up and down through it.

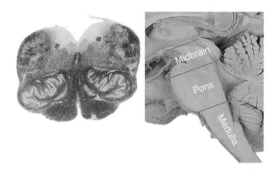

Midbrain (mesencephalon). The most rostral of the three subdivisions of the *brainstem.* The midbrain remains tubular in plan, but features a great variety of structures: the *superior* and *inferior colliculi* in its roof (tectum), *aqueduct* and *periaqueductal gray, oculomotor* and *trochlear nuclei* and *pretectal area,* upper part of the *reticular formation, red nuclei, substantia nigra,* and *cerebral peduncles.* Like the *medulla,* a small region of enormous importance.

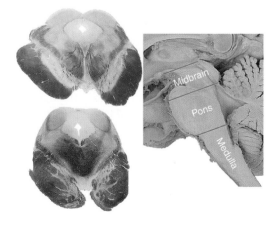

Middle cerebellar peduncle. The largest of the cerebellar peduncles, containing fibers that arise in the *basal pons** from contralateral *pontine nuclei* and end as mossy fibers in almost all areas of cerebellar cortex. Sometimes referred to as the brachium pontis (the "arm of the pons").

Middle cerebral artery. The more posterior of the two terminal branches of the *internal carotid artery**. The middle cerebral artery runs laterally beneath the *basal forebrain* to reach the *lateral sulcus,* where many branches emerge. It supplies the *insula,* most of the lateral surface of the cerebral hemisphere, and the anterior tip of the *temporal lobe.*

Middle frontal gyrus. One of three longitudinally oriented gyri in the anterior part of the *frontal lobe**, situated between the *superior* and *inferior frontal gyri.* It includes part of premotor cortex and the frontal eye field, which is involved in initiating voluntary eye movements to the contralateral side.

Middle temporal gyrus. One of three longitudinally oriented gyri on the lateral surface of the *temporal lobe** between the *superior* and *inferior temporal gyri.* It contains some visual association cortex, as well as multimodal or heteromodal association cortex.

MLF. See *medial longitudinal fasciculus**.

Nucleus accumbens. The most inferior part of the *striatum**, with predominantly limbic connections. Nucleus accumbens was traditionally known as nucleus accumbens septi, but is now recognized as a major component of the *ventral striatum.* (The original, longer name reflects its position immediately lateral to the base of the *septum pellucidum,* as if leaning against it.)

Nucleus ambiguus. A collection of motor neurons for laryngeal and pharyngeal muscles, and preganglionic parasympathetic neurons for the heart. So called because these neurons are somewhat scattered in the *reticular formation* of the rostral *medulla* and do not form a compact, easily seen nucleus.

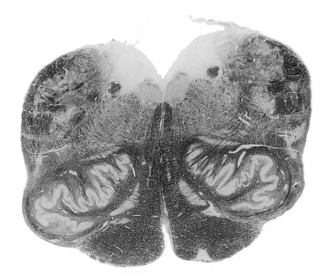

Nucleus cuneatus. The more lateral of the *posterior column nuclei**. Site of termination of *fasciculus cuneatus* and origin of the arm region of the *medial lemniscus.*

Nucleus gracilis. The more medial of the *posterior column nuclei**. Site of termination of *fasciculus gracilis* and origin of the leg region of the *medial lemniscus.*

Nucleus of the solitary tract. The principal visceral sensory nucleus of the *brainstem;* the site of termination of the visceral primary afferents in the *solitary tract,* which it surrounds, doughnutlike, in cross section.

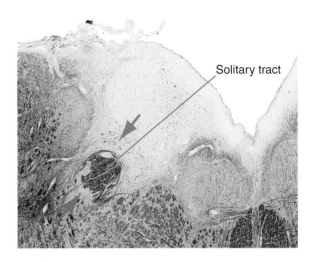

Solitary tract

Obex. Apex of the V-shaped caudal *fourth ventricle,* where the ventricle narrows into the *central canal* of the lower *medulla* and spinal cord.

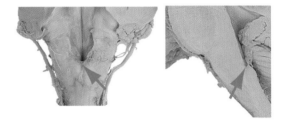

Occipital lobe. The most posterior lobe of each cerebral hemisphere. The occipital lobe includes the primary visual cortex in the banks of the *calcarine sulcus,* as well as adjoining areas of visual association cortex.

Occipitotemporal gyrus (fusiform gyrus). A long gyrus, beginning just lateral to the *uncus* and running posteriorly along the inferior surface of the *temporal lobe* to the *occipital lobe.* Along its course in the *temporal lobe,* the occipitotemporal gyrus is bounded laterally by the *inferior temporal gyrus* and medially by the *parahippocampal gyrus.*

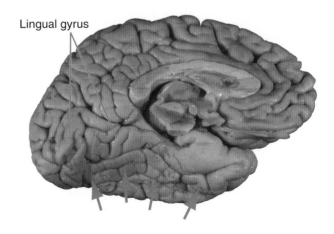

Lingual gyrus

Oculomotor nerve. The 3rd cranial nerve, emerging into the *interpeduncular fossa* of the *midbrain.* The oculomotor nerve innervates most of the extrinsic ocular muscles (see also *oculomotor nucleus*): superior, medial, and inferior recti; inferior oblique; and levator palpebrae superioris. It also conveys preganglionic parasympathetic fibers to the ciliary ganglion, where postganglionic fibers arise to innervate the pupillary sphincter and ciliary muscle.

Oculomotor nucleus. Motor neurons for the ipsilateral medial and inferior recti and inferior oblique, the contralateral superior rectus, and the levator palpebrae of both sides. Preganglionic parasympathetic neurons in one of its columns, the *Edinger-Westphal nucleus**, control the ipsilateral pupillary sphincter and ciliary muscle.

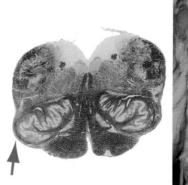

Oculomotor nerves

Olfactory bulb. The knoblike anterior end of the *olfactory tract** on the *orbital* surface of the *frontal lobe*. The olfactory bulb is the site of central termination of incoming olfactory fibers from the olfactory epithelium in the nasal cavity. It is large and well laminated in animals depending heavily on the sense of smell (e.g., rats, dogs), but relatively small and poorly differentiated in the human brain.

Olfactory sulcus. A sulcus on the *orbital* surface of the *frontal lobe*, immediately lateral to *gyrus rectus* and harboring the *olfactory bulb* and *tract**.

Olfactory tract. Projections from *olfactory bulb* neurons (mitral and tufted cells) to *olfactory (piriform) cortex* and the *amygdala*. The olfactory tract also conveys modulatory efferents traveling from deeper olfactory centers back to the *olfactory bulb*.

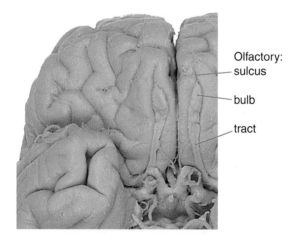

Olfactory:
- sulcus
- bulb
- tract

Olfactory tubercle. A restricted area of the *anterior perforated substance* where some *olfactory tract* fibers terminate. The olfactory tubercle forms a distinct elevation in some animals, but is not very apparent in human brains.

Olive. Protuberance on the lateral aspect of the rostral *medulla*, just dorsolateral to the *pyramid*, caused by the underlying *inferior olivary nucleus*.

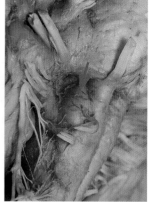

Provided by Dr. Norman Koelling, University of Arizona

Opercula (*singular*, operculum). The parts of the *frontal, parietal*, and *temporal lobes* bordering the *lateral sulcus* and overlying the *insula*, hiding it from view.

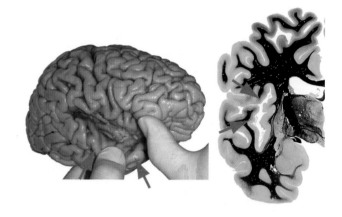

Opercular part (of the inferior frontal gyrus). The most caudal part of the *inferior frontal gyrus*, the most inferior of three longitudinally oriented gyri in the anterior part of the *frontal lobe**. Contains the caudal half of Broca's area.

Optic chiasm. The site at which *optic nerve* fibers from ganglion cells in the nasal half of each retina decussate, so that each *optic tract* contains fibers arising in the temporal retina of the ipsilateral eye and the nasal retina of the opposite eye.

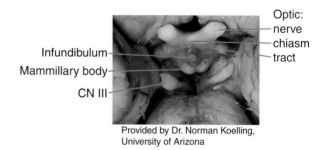

Optic:
- nerve
- chiasm
- tract

Infundibulum
Mammillary body
CN III

Provided by Dr. Norman Koelling, University of Arizona

Optic nerve. The 2nd cranial nerve, containing axons of the various types of retinal ganglion cells projecting to the lateral geniculate nucleus of the *thalamus, the superior colliculus, pretectal area*, suprachiasmatic nucleus of the *hypothalamus*, and a few other sites.

Optic radiation. A conspicuous, sharply defined, and heavily myelinated bundle of visual fibers originating in the lateral geniculate nucleus, departing the *thalamus* through the retrolenticular and sublenticular parts of the *internal capsule,* curving in a broad fan around the atrium and the posterior and inferior horns of the *lateral ventricle,* and terminating in the primary visual cortex in the upper and lower banks of the *calcarine sulcus.*

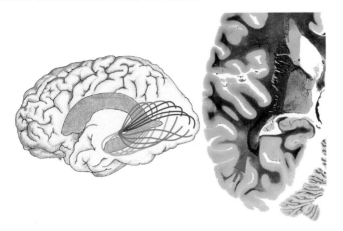

Optic tract. Axons of ganglion cells from corresponding (homonymous) halves of each retina on their way to the lateral geniculate nucleus, *superior colliculus, pretectal area,* and a few other sites.

Orbital gyri. The variably sulcated (in a pattern often resembling the letter H) group of gyri that occupy the orbital surface of the *frontal lobe.* The orbital gyri usually are not named individually, in contrast to the *gyrus rectus* immediately medial to them. (The *gyrus rectus* is on the orbital surface, but is usually not included among the orbital gyri.)

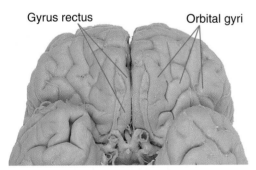

Gyrus rectus   Orbital gyri

Orbital part (of the inferior frontal gyrus). The most anterior of the various frontal folds covering the *insula,* so named because it merges with the *orbital gyri* (see *inferior frontal gyrus**).

Parabrachial nuclei. A collection of nuclei adjacent to the *superior cerebellar peduncle* (brachium conjunctivum) as the latter traverses the rostral *pons.* Various parts of the parabrachial nuclei are involved in transferring visceral, pain, and temperature information to the *hypothalamus* and *amygdala.*

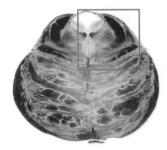
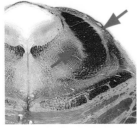

Paracentral lobule. The extensions of the *precentral* and *postcentral gyri* onto the medial surface of the hemisphere, forming a lobule that surrounds the end of the *central sulcus.*

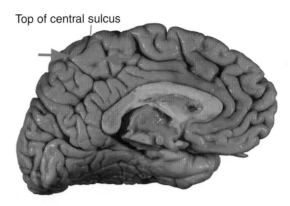

Top of central sulcus

Parafascicular nucleus (PF). See *thalamus*.*

Parahippocampal gyrus. The gyrus immediately adjacent to the *hippocampus,* forming a major part of the *limbic lobe*.* Its anterior region contains the *entorhinal cortex,* a meeting ground for cortical projections from multiple areas and the source of most afferents to the *hippocampus.*

Parietal lobe. A cerebral lobe bounded by the *frontal, temporal,* and *occipital lobes* on the lateral surface of each hemisphere, and by the *frontal, limbic,* and *occipital lobes* on the medial surface. The parietal lobe contains primary somatosensory cortex in the *postcentral gyrus,* areas involved in language comprehension (in the *inferior parietal lobule,* usually on the left), and regions involved in complex aspects of spatial orientation and perception.

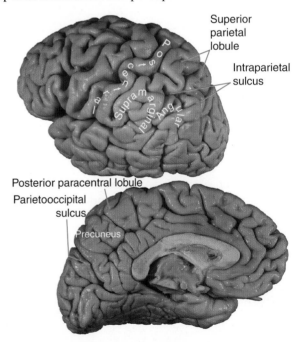

Superior parietal lobule

Intraparietal sulcus

Posterior paracentral lobule

Parietooccipital sulcus

Precuneus

Parietooccipital sulcus. A deep fissure separating the *parietal** and *occipital lobes* on the medial aspect of the cerebral hemisphere. Inferiorly, the parietooccipital sulcus joins the *calcarine sulcus*,* which continues into the *temporal lobe* as a common stem for both these sulci.

Periamygdaloid cortex. A cortical area covering part of the *amygdala* and merging with it; part of primary olfactory cortex. (See *lateral olfactory tract**.)

Periaqueductal gray. An area of gray matter and poorly myelinated fibers surrounding the *aqueduct* in the *midbrain*. The periaqueductal gray is the site of origin of a descending pain-control pathway that relays in nucleus raphe magnus (among other connections).

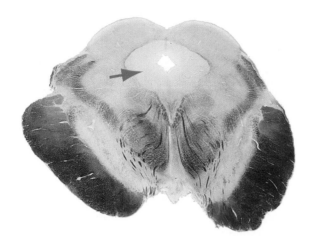

Pineal gland. A dorsal outgrowth of the *diencephalon*, protruding from the *third ventricle* immediately caudal to the paired *habenulae*. The pineal is an endocrine gland important in seasonal cycles of some animals. In humans, it secretes the hormone melatonin, which is involved in the synchronization of circadian rhythms.

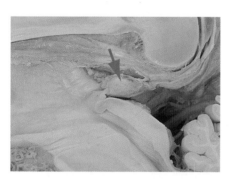

Piriform cortex. A cortical area adjacent to the *lateral olfactory tract** as it moves toward the *temporal lobe;* part of primary olfactory cortex.

Pons. The second of the three parts of the *brainstem*, continuous rostrally with the *midbrain* and caudally with the *medulla*. The pons is overlain by the *cerebellum* and includes an enlarged basal region (see *basal pons*).

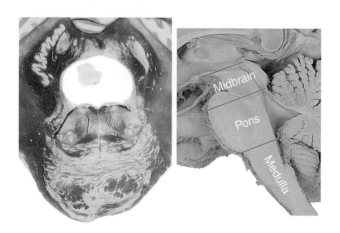

Pontine nuclei. A collective term for the many small nuclei in the *basal pons** that receive afferents from cerebral cortex (via the *internal capsule* and *cerebral peduncle*) and project to contralateral cerebellar cortex (via the *middle cerebellar peduncle*).

Pontocerebellar fibers. Projections from *pontine nuclei* that cross in the *basal pons**, traverse the *middle cerebellar peduncle*, and enter the contralateral cerebellar cortex, where they terminate as mossy fibers (as do all cerebellar afferents except those from the *inferior olivary nucleus*).

Postcentral gyrus. A vertically oriented convolution of the *parietal lobe** immediately posterior to the *central sulcus*. The postcentral gyrus is the site of primary somatosensory cortex.

Posterior cerebral artery. A prominent artery that arises from the bifurcation of the *basilar artery* at the level of the *midbrain*. The posterior cerebral artery forms the caudal part of the circle of Willis and supplies the rostral midbrain, much of the thalamus, the medial *occipital lobe,* and inferior and medial surfaces of the *temporal lobe*.

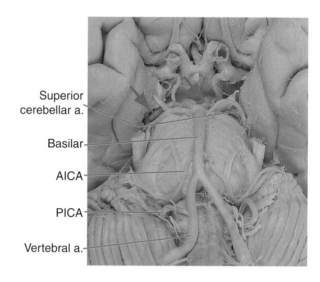

Superior cerebellar a.
Basilar
AICA
PICA
Vertebral a.

Posterior column. The entire contents of one *posterior funiculus* except for its share of the propriospinal tract (a thin shell of white matter around the gray matter).

Posterior column nuclei. *Nuclei gracilis* and *cuneatus*, the principal collections of second-order neurons receiving touch and position information from the body. Site of termination of *fasciculi gracilis* and *cuneatus* and origin of the contralateral *medial lemniscus*.

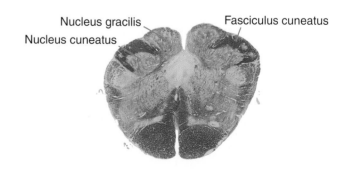

Nucleus gracilis   Fasciculus cuneatus
Nucleus cuneatus

Posterior commissure. Crossing fibers interconnecting the two sides of the rostral *midbrain* and *pretectal area*.

These crossing fibers are involved in the consensual pupillary light reflex and in coordinating vertical eye movements.

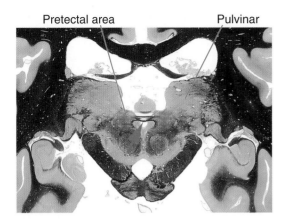

Pretectal area   Pulvinar

Posterior communicating artery. A short vessel connecting the *posterior cerebral artery* to the *internal carotid*, thereby forming one link in the circle of Willis. These arteries are often asymmetrical, with one being considerably larger than the other. Normally, pressures in the *internal carotid* and *posterior cerebral arteries* are balanced so that little or no blood flows around the circle, but if one vessel is occluded, the posterior communicating artery may allow anastomotic flow and thus prevent neurological damage.

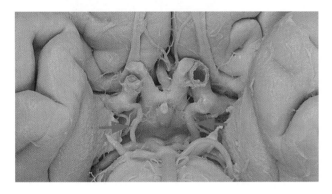

Posterior funiculus. One of the three major divisions of the spinal white matter, the others being the *anterior* and *lateral funiculi*. Principally occupied by ascending collaterals of large myelinated primary afferents carrying impulses from various kinds of mechanoreceptors. This is the first stage of the major pathway to cerebral cortex for low-threshold cutaneous, joint, and muscle receptor information.

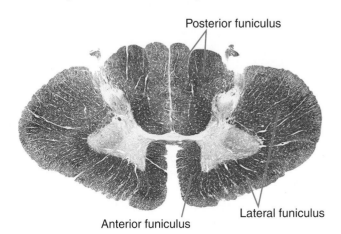

Posterior funiculus

Anterior funiculus

Lateral funiculus

Posterior horn. One of the three general divisions of the spinal gray matter, the others being the *anterior horn* and the *intermediate gray;* contains second-order sensory neurons of multiple types, and capped at all levels by the *substantia gelatinosa.*

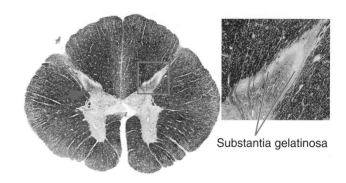

Substantia gelatinosa

Posterior inferior cerebellar artery. A long, circumferential branch of the *vertebral artery,* arising before the two vertebrals fuse to form the *basilar artery.* It supplies much of the inferior surface of the cerebellar hemisphere and vermis, en route sending shorter branches to the *choroid plexus* of the *fourth ventricle* and to much of the lateral *medulla;* commonly referred to by the acronym *PICA.*

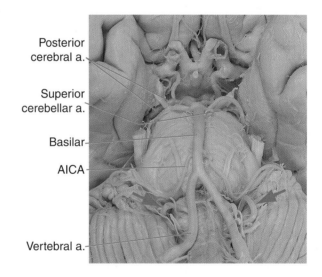

Posterior cerebral a.

Superior cerebellar a.

Basilar

AICA

Vertebral a.

Posterior root. See *dorsal root.*

Posterior spinocerebellar tract. Uncrossed fibers from *Clarke's nucleus,* carrying proprioceptive information from the arm to the ipsilateral half of the *cerebellar vermis* and intermediate zone via the *inferior cerebellar peduncle.*

Precentral gyrus. A vertically oriented convolution of the *frontal lobe** immediately anterior to the *central sulcus.* The precentral gyrus is the site of primary motor cortex.

Precuneus. The part of the *parietal lobe** on the medial surface of the hemisphere, excluding the posterior *paracentral lobule* (the medial extension of the *postcentral gyrus*).

Preoccipital notch. The midpoint of a shallow, curved indentation along the inferior margin of the lateral aspect of each cerebral hemisphere. The preoccipital notch serves as a landmark for synthesizing boundaries for the *parietal,* *occipital,* and *temporal lobes* on the lateral and medial surfaces of hemisphere.

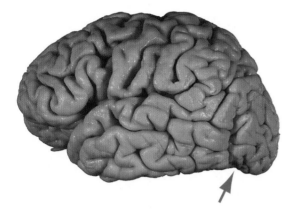

Preoptic region. The area in the walls of the *third ventricle* immediately anterior to the *optic chiasm;* technically a telencephalic region, but structurally and functionally continuous with the *hypothalamus** of the *diencephalon.*

Pretectal area. The region between the *superior colliculus* and caudal *thalamus.* The pretectal area receives afferents from the retina and visual association cortex. It projects efferents bilaterally to the *Edinger-Westphal nuclei,* crossing both in the *posterior commissure** and in the ventral *periaqueductal gray.* It is important in the pupillary light reflex.

Pulvinar. See *thalamus*.*

Putamen. The part of the *striatum** involved most prominently in the motor functions of the basal ganglia. The putamen receives afferents from cerebral cortex (primarily motor and somatosensory areas) and from the *substantia nigra* (compact part) and thalamic centromedian nucleus. It projects efferents to the *globus pallidus,* which in turn projects via the *thalamus* (VA, VL) to premotor and supplementary motor areas. The putamen forms the outer component of the *lenticular nucleus* (the *globus pallidus* is the inner part).

Pyramid. *Corticospinal* fibers from the ipsilateral *precentral gyrus* and adjacent areas of cerebral cortex, forming a prominent fiber bundle (roughly triangular in cross section, which gave rise to the name) on the ventral surface of the *medulla.*

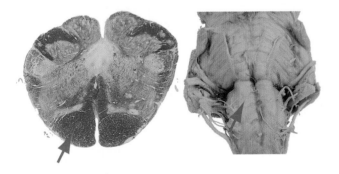

Pyramidal decussation. The site, located at the spinomedullary junction, at which most fibers in each *pyramid* cross the midline to form the contralateral *lateral corticospinal tract.*

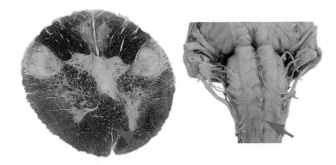

Raphe nuclei. A series of nuclei extending through the brainstem near the midline of the tegmentum, collectively providing the serotonergic innervation of the CNS.

Red nucleus. The site of termination of part of the *superior cerebellar peduncle,* and the site of origin of uncrossed fibers to the *inferior olivary nucleus* and of the crossed rubrospinal tract.

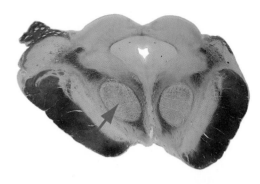

Reticular formation. The central region of the *brainstem,* forming the *tegmentum* of the *midbrain, pons,* and *medulla,* with a complex netlike fabric of nerve cell bodies and interwoven processes; its myriad multimodal afferents, profusely collateralizing efferents running upward and downward to every level of the CNS, and involvement in virtually every activity from visceral functions to consciousness make it a core integrating structure of the brain.

Reticular nucleus. See *thalamus*.*

Rhinal sulcus. A sulcus demarcating the lateral boundary of the *uncus* on the medial aspect of the *temporal lobe;* sometimes continuous with the *collateral sulcus* behind it.

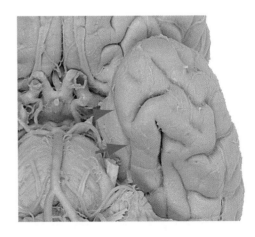

Septal nuclei. A component of the medial wall of the cerebral hemisphere just beneath the base of the largely glial *septum pellucidum.* The septal nuclei are continuous inferiorly with the *preoptic area* and *hypothalamus* and are reciprocally connected with the *hippocampus, amygdala, hypothalamus,* and other limbic structures via the *fornix, stria terminalis,* and other tracts. They also are the source of cholinergic input to the *hippocampus.*

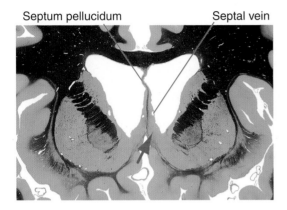

Septum pellucidum   Septal vein

Septal vein. A deep cerebral vein that runs posteriorly across the *septum pellucidum* to join the *thalamostriate* (terminal) *vein* and form the *internal cerebral vein.*

Septum pellucidum. A thin, chiefly glial, almost transparent, paired membrane separating the two *lateral ventricles,* grading inferiorly into the *septal nuclei*.* (In most brains, the two septa pellucida are so closely apposed as to appear as a single structure, and for simplicity they are so labeled in most of the illustrations in this book.)

Solitary tract. Primary afferents conveying visceral information from CN VII, IX, and X to the adjacent *nucleus of the solitary tract*,* which surrounds it.

Spinothalamic tract. Crossed fibers from neurons in the *posterior horn* of the spinal cord conveying pain and temperature information to the *thalamus* (VPL and other nuclei).

Straight sinus. A venous channel in the line of attachment between the falx cerebri and tentorium cerebelli. The straight sinus collects blood from the deep cerebral veins, which reaches it primarily through the *great vein.* The straight and *superior sagittal sinuses** then meet at the confluens of the sinuses and empty into the transverse sinuses.

Stria medullaris (of the thalamus). The site of attachment of the roof of the *third ventricle* and a route through which *septal* efferents reach the *habenula.*

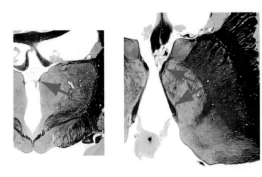

Stria terminalis. A slender, poorly myelinated tract following a long C-shaped course within the thalamostriate groove that separates the *caudate nucleus* from the *thalamus.* The stria terminalis plays a role analogous to that played by the *fornix* for the *hippocampus*—it conveys efferents from the *amygdala* to the *septal nuclei* and *hypothalamus.*

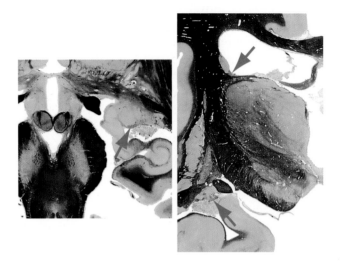

Striatum. An inclusive term for the *caudate nucleus, putamen,* and *nucleus accumbens.*

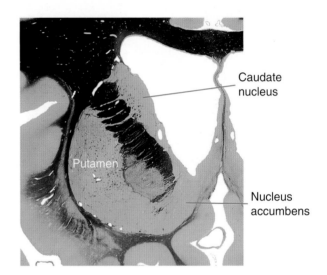

Caudate nucleus

Putamen

Nucleus accumbens

Stripe of Gennari. A sheet of myelinated fibers that run through one of the middle layers of primary visual cortex, giving it the distinctive appearance that gave rise to its alternate name, striate cortex. Named for the medical student who first described it in the 18th century.

Strumus (commonly misspelled "strumous"). A primitive telencephalic extension that, unlike structures such as the neocortex that have expanded greatly in primates, has remained constant in size and position. It is located rostral to the *lamina terminalis,* medial to *gyrus rectus,* and ventromedial to the *substantia innominata.* Only the anterior and ventral nuclear groups are developed in humans, and these are subdivided cytoarchitectonically into four discrete nuclei: the anteroventral, anterior ventral, and the subdivided anterior and ventral ventral anterior nuclei. The interconnections of the strumus are extensive and complex, but their importance cannot be underestimated. There are four major afferent pathways: a substantial input from a variably present limbic nucleus, the effluvium, traveling through the superior and inferior effluviostrumular tracts, and minor inputs from the trivium and nimbus in the *temporal lobe*. Because the strumus has no known efferent pathways, however, its functional importance has been difficult to justify anatomically. (The frequently mentioned strumulotrivionimboeffluviostrumular loop apparently does not exist.) The clinical importance of the strumus is based on the disorder subacute combined strumuloma. This is an idiopathic disease of exquisitely rare occurrence and indeterminate symptoms, which forms the basis for the identification of the strumus as the center controlling involuntary higher cortical functions.

Subcallosal fasciculus. A compact group of lightly staining myelinated fibers in the white matter of each cerebral hemisphere (visible mainly in the *frontal lobe*). The subcallosal fasciculus forms a pale, arched band subjacent to the *corpus callosum*. Traditionally considered to be an association bundle interconnecting the *frontal* and *occipital lobes* (hence its alternate name, *superior occipitofrontal fasciculus*), it may instead interconnect the *thalamus* and the *frontal* and *parietal lobes*.

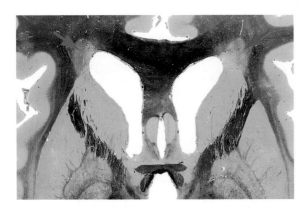

Subparietal sulcus. A variable sulcus on the medial surface of the hemisphere, separating the *precuneus* from the posterior part of the *cingulate gyrus*. The subparietal sulcus is roughly in line with the *cingulate sulcus*, and in about a third of hemispheres the two are continuous with each other (see Fig. 1–8A).

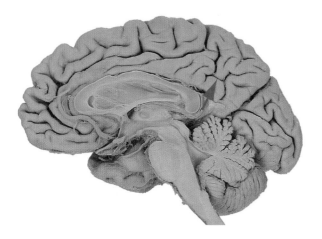

Substantia gelatinosa. A distinctive region of gray matter, surmounted by *Lissauer's tract,* that caps the *posterior horn* of the spinal cord at all levels. The substantia gelatinosa looks pale in myelin-stained material because its inputs are poorly myelinated or unmyelinated. It deals mostly with pain and temperature sensation.

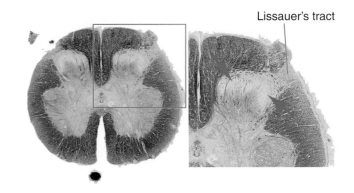

Lissauer's tract

Substantia innominata. Literally, "the substance with no name," a now seldom used term roughly synonymous with *basal forebrain*, left over from an era when the components of the *basal forebrain* were less well understood.

Substantia nigra. A large nucleus in the *midbrain*, interposed between the *red nucleus* and *cerebral peduncle*. The substantia nigra has two parts: a compact part, containing closely packed, pigmented (with neuromelanin) dopaminergic neurons that project to the *striatum*, and a reticular part, containing more loosely arranged neurons, receiving inputs from the *striatum* and projecting to the *thalamus*.

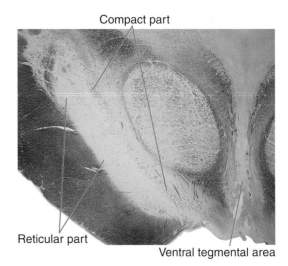

Compact part

Reticular part

Ventral tegmental area

Subthalamic fasciculus. Small bundles of fibers, much like the teeth of a comb, that cross the *internal capsule*. Fibers of the subthalamic fasciculus interconnect the *globus pallidus* and *subthalamic nucleus**, which face each other on either side of the *internal capsule*.

Subthalamic nucleus. A lens-shaped, biconvex mass of gray matter just medial and superior to the junction of the *internal capsule* and *cerebral peduncle*. The subthalamic nucleus is a major link in an indirect route through the basal ganglia: *striatum → globus pallidus (external segment) → subthalamic nucleus → globus pallidus (internal segment) → thalamus*. The *globus pallidus*–subthalamic nucleus connections travel in the *subthalamic fasciculus*.

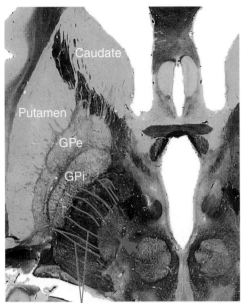

Subthalamic fasciculus

Sulcus limitans. A longitudinal groove in the embryonic neural tube that separates sensory nuclei from motor nuclei. In the adult brain, it persists as a groove in the floor of the *fourth ventricle* that separates motor nuclei of cranial nerves (medial to it) from sensory nuclei of cranial nerves.

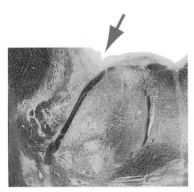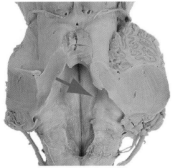

Superior brachium. See *brachium of the superior colliculus**.

Superior cerebellar artery. A branch of the *basilar artery** that arises just caudal to its bifurcation. Long circumferential branches supply the superior surface of the *cerebellum*, and shorter branches supply much of the rostral *pons* and caudal *midbrain*.

Superior cerebellar peduncle. The major efferent route from the *cerebellum*, containing projections from deep cerebellar nuclei on their way to the *red nucleus* and the *thalamus* (mainly VL). Sometimes referred to as the brachium conjunctivum (a "conjoined arm," named for its course through a decussation with its contralateral counterpart).

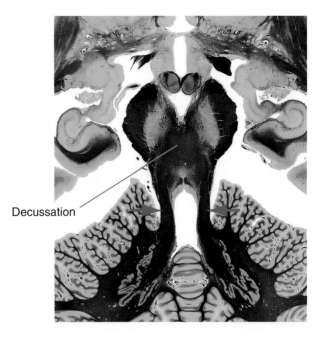

Decussation

Superior cistern. The enlarged, cerebrospinal fluid–filled subarachnoid cistern above the midbrain, also termed the quadrigeminal cistern and the cistern of the great cerebral vein. The superior cistern is an important radiological landmark, continuous anteriorly and posteriorly with the *transverse fissure* and laterally with thin, curved spaces that partially encircle the midbrain before joining its underlying interpeduncular cistern (see *interpeduncular fossa*). (The combination of the superior cistern and these sheetlike extensions is known as the *ambient cistern*.)

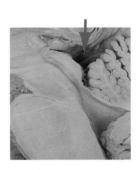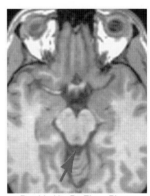

Provided by Dr. Elena Plante, University of Arizona

Superior colliculus. A large, rounded mass of gray matter in the roof of the rostral *midbrain*. The superior colliculus receives afferents from the retina and visual cortex (via the *brachium of the superior colliculus**), sends efferents to the pulvinar and other structures, and plays a role in visual attention and control of eye movements.

Superior frontal gyrus. The most superior of three longitudinally oriented gyri in the anterior part of the *frontal lobe**, continuing onto the medial surface of the hemisphere. The superior frontal gyrus includes supplementary motor cortex and part of premotor cortex.

Superior olivary nucleus. A complex of nuclei near the rostral end of the *facial nucleus* in the caudal *pons*. The superior olivary nucleus is the first site of convergence of fibers representing the two ears and is the source of many fibers of the *lateral lemniscus*. It is also the origin of the crossed olivocochlear bundle that runs centrifugally in the contralateral *vestibulocochlear nerve* and terminates in the organ of Corti, modulating hair cell activity.

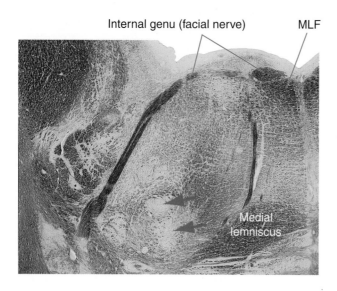

Internal genu (facial nerve)   MLF

Medial lemniscus

Superior parietal lobule. The upper part of the lateral surface of the *parietal lobe**, above the *intraparietal sulcus*. The superior parietal lobule contains somatosensory association cortex.

Superior sagittal sinus. A venous channel in the superior line of attachment of the falx cerebri, providing the major outflow pathway for superficial cerebral veins.

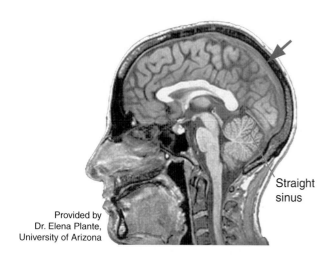

Straight sinus

Provided by
Dr. Elena Plante,
University of Arizona

Superior temporal gyrus. The uppermost gyrus of the *temporal lobe**, bordering on the *lateral sulcus*. The superior temporal gyrus includes primary auditory cortex (actually located in the wall of the lateral sulcus, in *transverse temporal gyri* crossing the top of the superior temporal gyrus), auditory association cortex, and (usually on the left) Wernicke's area. This is one example of a region of visibly different size and configuration in the two cerebral hemispheres, typically being more extensive in the left hemisphere.

Supramarginal gyrus. The part of the *inferior parietal lobule** usually surrounding the up-turned end of the *lateral sulcus*. Although variable in size and shape, the supramarginal gyrus is important in language function.

Tegmentum. A general anatomical term for the area anterior to the ventricular spaces of the *medulla, pons,* and *midbrain*. Tegmentum (Latin for "covering") is a useful umbrella term for all structures covering the basal components of the *brainstem (pyramids, basal pons, cerebral peduncles)* and includes the *reticular formation,* nuclei of cranial nerves, most ascending and descending tracts, the *red nuclei,* and *substantia nigra.*

Temporal lobe. The most inferior lobe of each cerebral hemisphere, inferior to the *lateral sulcus* and anterior to the *occipital lobe*. The temporal lobe includes auditory sensory and association cortex, part of posterior language cortex, visual and higher order association cortex, primary and association olfactory cortex, the *amygdala,* and the *hippocampus*. (The *parahippocampal gyrus,* a major part of the *limbic lobe,* also is commonly referred to as part of the medial temporal lobe.)

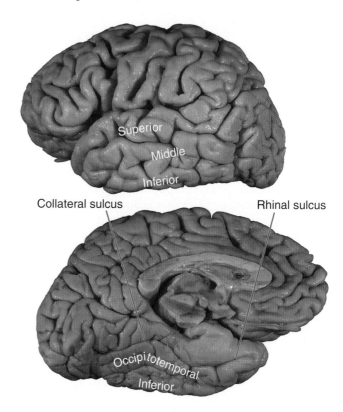

Superior
Middle
Inferior
Collateral sulcus   Rhinal sulcus
Occipitotemporal
Inferior

Terminal vein. A deep cerebral vein, also referred to as the *thalamostriate vein,* that travels with the *stria terminalis* in the groove between the *thalamus* and adjacent *caudate nucleus* and drains much of these two structures.

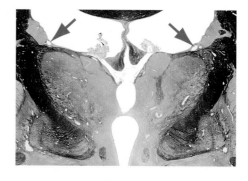

Thalamic fasciculus. Projections from the *cerebellum* (via the *superior cerebellar peduncle*) and basal ganglia (via the *ansa lenticularis* and *lenticular fasciculus*), gathered together beneath the ventral anterior and ventral lateral nuclei (VA/VL) of the *thalamus*.

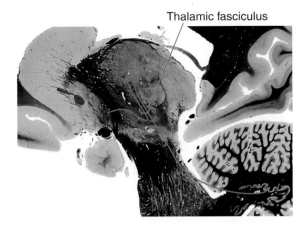

Thalamic fasciculus

Thalamostriate vein. A frequently used alternate name for the *terminal vein**, more useful because it says not only where the vessel is, but also what it does.

Thalamus. A collection of nuclei that collectively are the source of most extrinsic afferents to the cerebral cortex. Some thalamic nuclei (relay nuclei) receive distinct input bundles and project to discrete functional areas of the cerebral cortex. Others (association nuclei) are primarily interconnected with association cortex. Still others have diffuse cortical projections, and one has no projections to the cortex at all.

Anterior nucleus. The thalamic relay for part of the *limbic lobe*. Afferents from the *mammillary body* and other limbic structures, efferents to the *cingulate gyrus*.

Centromedian nucleus (CM). The largest intralaminar nucleus; afferents from the *globus pallidus*, efferents to the *striatum* (with branches projecting diffusely to widespread cortical areas).

Dorsomedial nucleus (DM). Interconnections with prefrontal association cortex and parts of the *limbic lobe*.

Lateral dorsal nucleus (LD). Efferents to the posterior part of the *cingulate gyrus;* in many ways an extension of the anterior nucleus.

Lateral geniculate nucleus (LGN). The thalamic relay for vision. Afferents from the retina via the *optic tract*, efferents to primary visual cortex above and below the *calcarine sulcus*.

Lateral posterior nucleus (LP). Interconnections, similar to those of the pulvinar, with posterior association cortex.

Medial geniculate nucleus (MGN). The thalamic relay for hearing. Afferents from the *inferior colliculus* via the *brachium of the inferior colliculus*, efferents to auditory cortex in the *transverse temporal gyri*.

Parafascicular nucleus (PF). An intralaminar nucleus with connections similar to those of the centromedian nucleus.

Pulvinar. The largest thalamic nucleus, interconnected with parietal-occipital-temporal association cortex.

Reticular nucleus. An unusual thalamic nucleus with no projections to the cortex. Afferents from the thalamus and cerebral cortex, GABAergic efferents back to the thalamus.

Ventral anterior nucleus (VA). A thalamic relay for the motor system. Afferents from the *cerebellum* and *globus pallidus*, efferents to motor areas of cortex.

Ventral lateral nucleus (VL). A thalamic relay for the motor system. Afferents from the *cerebellum* and *globus pallidus*, efferents to motor areas of cortex.

Ventral posterolateral nucleus (VPL). The thalamic relay for somatic sensation from the body. Afferents from the *medial lemniscus* and *spinothalamic tract*, efferents to somatosensory cortex in the *postcentral gyrus*.

Ventral posteromedial nucleus (VPM). The thalamic relay for somatic sensation from the head and for taste. Afferents from the trigeminal regions of the *medial lemniscus* and *spinothalamic tract* and from the *nucleus of the solitary tract;* efferents to somatosensory cortex in the *postcentral gyrus* and to gustatory cortex in and near the *insula*.

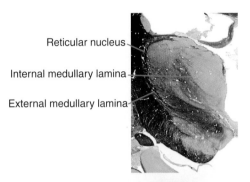

Reticular nucleus
Internal medullary lamina
External medullary lamina

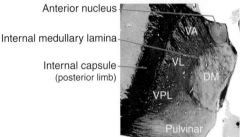

Anterior nucleus
Internal medullary lamina
Internal capsule (posterior limb)
VA
VL
DM
VPL
Pulvinar

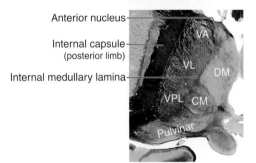

Anterior nucleus
Internal capsule (posterior limb)
Internal medullary lamina
VA
VL
DM
VPL
CM
Pulvinar

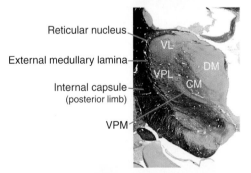

Reticular nucleus
External medullary lamina
Internal capsule (posterior limb)
VPM
VL
DM
VPL
CM

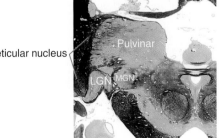

Reticular nucleus
Pulvinar
LGN
MGN

Third ventricle. The single, median, vertically oriented cavity of the *diencephalon*, separating the *thalamus* and *hypothalamus* of the two hemispheres. The third ventricle is confluent anteriorly with both *lateral ventricles* through the *interventricular foramina* and posteriorly with the *aqueduct*, and has four small outpocketings:

Infundibular recess. Leads into the hollow *infundibulum*.

Optic recess. Small recess just above and anterior to the *optic chiasm*.

Pineal recess. Leads into the stalk of the *pineal gland*.

Suprapineal recess. An outpocketing of the roof of the third ventricle just anterior to the *pineal gland*.

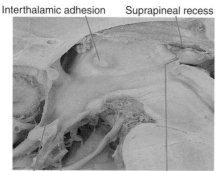

Transverse fissure. An extension of subarachnoid space, situated above the roof of the *third ventricle* and containing the *internal cerebral veins*. We use the term in a more extended sense in this book, to refer to the long slit intervening between the cerebral hemispheres and structures below them—the cleft normally occupied by the tentorium cerebelli, continuing into the *superior cistern* and from there into the subarachnoid space above the roof of the *third ventricle*.

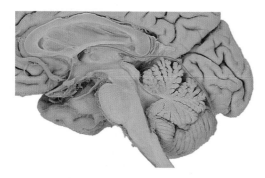

Transverse temporal (Heschl's) gyri. Gyri (often two in number) that run transversely across the lower bank of the *lateral sulcus*. The location of primary auditory cortex.

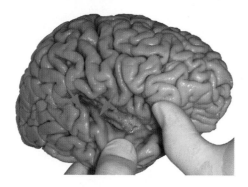

Trapezoid body. Auditory fibers from the *cochlear nuclei* to the *superior olivary nucleus* that cross the midline in a trapezoid-shaped area of the pontine *tegmentum*.

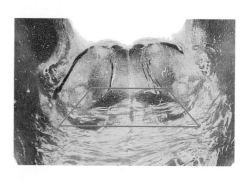

Triangular part (of the inferior frontal gyrus). The middle of the three parts of the *inferior frontal gyrus*, the most inferior of three longitudinally oriented gyri in the anterior part of the *frontal lobe**. Contains the anterior half of Broca's area.

Trigeminal nerve. The 5th cranial nerve, emerging anterolaterally from the *basal pons*. The trigeminal nerve conveys somatosensory (and some chemosensory) fibers from the ipsilateral half of the head, as well as efferents to ipsilateral muscles of mastication.

Motor root. Small, anterior root containing efferent fibers that distribute through the mandibular division of the nerve.

Sensory root. Massive, posterior root containing afferent fibers that arrive over all three divisions of the nerve.

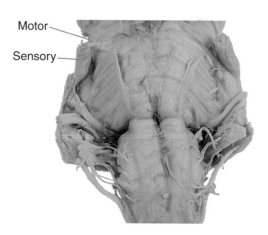

Trigeminal nuclei

Main sensory. Termination site of large-diameter afferents (the equivalent of a *posterior column nucleus* for the trigeminal system). Most of its efferents project to the contralateral VPM via the *medial lemniscus;* some, however, project to the ipsilateral VPM via the dorsal trigeminal tract.

Mesencephalic. The cell bodies of primary afferents from muscle spindles in muscles of mastication and from other oral mechanoreceptors.

Motor. Motor neurons for ipsilateral muscles of mastication.

Spinal. The termination site of the spinal *trigeminal tract*. The most caudal part of the nucleus (in the caudal *medulla*) resembles the spinal *posterior horn,* has a component similar to the *substantia gelatinosa,* and processes pain and temperature information. Its efferents project to VPM (and other thalamic nuclei) through the *spinothalamic tract.*

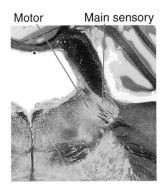

Motor   Main sensory   Spinal nucleus & tract

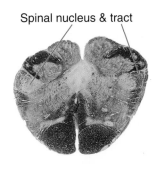

Trigeminal tracts

Mesencephalic. Processes of cell bodies in the adjacent mesencephalic *trigeminal nucleus* that send one branch to innervate mechanoreceptors in and around the mouth, and others to central termination sites such as the *trigeminal main sensory nucleus.*

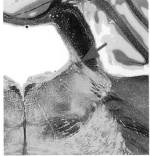

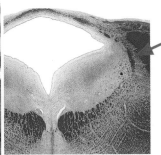

Spinal. Central processes of primary afferents from the ipsilateral side of the face, conveying information about pain and temperature (and some tactile information) to the *spinal trigeminal nucleus*.*

Trochlear nerve. The 4th cranial nerve, emerging as an already crossed small bundle from the posterior aspect of the *midbrain,* just caudal to the *inferior colliculus.* The trochlear nerve innervates the superior oblique muscle, which helps to intort the eyeball and turn it downward and laterally.

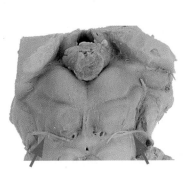

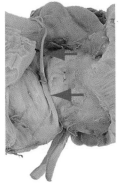

Trochlear nucleus. Motor neurons for the contralateral superior oblique muscle, located in the caudal *midbrain* just caudal to the *oculomotor nucleus.* Trochlear axons exit the paired nuclei, turn caudally in the overlying *periaqueductal gray,* arch posteriorly to decussate (similar to old-time ice tongs used to handle large blocks of ice), and leave the *brainstem* at the *pons-midbrain* junction.

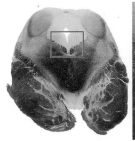

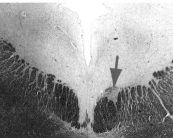

Tuber cinereum. A low mound of gray matter on the inferior aspect of the *hypothalamus,* bounded by the *optic chiasm, optic tracts,* and anterior edge of the *mammillary bodies.* The tuber cinereum contains the median eminence and the beginning of the *infundibulum* and is a region of great importance in hypothalamic hormonal regulation of the adenohypophysis.

Uncus. A medial protuberance from the anterior end of the *parahippocampal gyrus* caused by the underlying *amygdala* and anterior end of the *hippocampus.* The proximity of its surface to the adjacent *cerebral peduncle* can cause clinical problems during cerebral edema or as a result of space-occupying masses.

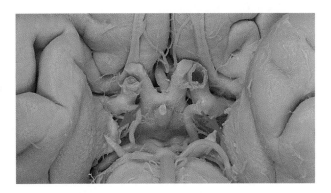

Vagal trigone. A small elevation in the floor of the caudal *fourth ventricle* with boundaries forming a narrow triangle just lateral to the *hypoglossal trigone.* Each vagal trigone is a fusiform swelling produced by the underlying *dorsal motor nucleus of the vagus.*

Vagus nerve. The 10th cranial nerve, emerging as a series of filaments from a groove dorsal to the *olive.* The vagus has diverse components: efferents to branchial arch muscles arise from *nucleus ambiguus* in the *medulla* and mediate swallowing and phonation; efferents to parasympathetic ganglia for thoracic and abdominal viscera arise from the *dorsal motor nucleus of the vagus* and *nucleus ambiguus* in the *medulla;* afferent fibers mediate general visceral sensation, taste from the epiglottis, and cutaneous sensation in and near the outer ear.

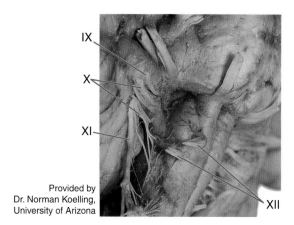

Provided by
Dr. Norman Koelling,
University of Arizona

Vein of Galen. See *great vein*.

Venous angle. The point at which the newly formed *internal cerebral vein* turns sharply caudally as it leaves the *interventricular foramen*. This is an important radiological landmark indicating the location of the genu of the *internal capsule* and the anterior end of the *thalamus*.

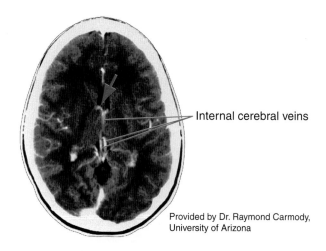

Internal cerebral veins

Provided by Dr. Raymond Carmody,
University of Arizona

Ventral amygdalofugal pathway. A massive but loosely organized fiber bundle running transversely in the *basal forebrain*. It interconnects the *amygdala* with the *hypothalamus, septal nuclei, thalamus,* and even the *brainstem,* and is thus an important pathway of the limbic system.

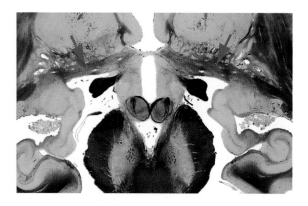

Ventral anterior nucleus (VA). See *thalamus*.

Ventral lateral nucleus (VL). See *thalamus*.

Ventral pallidum. A limbic extension of the *globus pallidus,* located beneath the *anterior commissure,* with inputs from the *ventral striatum*. The ventral pallidum is part of a basal ganglia circuit similar to that involved in motor functions, but in this case has limbic inputs (*amygdala, hippocampus → ventral striatum →* ventral pallidum) and outputs (via the dorsomedial nucleus of the *thalamus*) to prefrontal and *orbital* cortex.

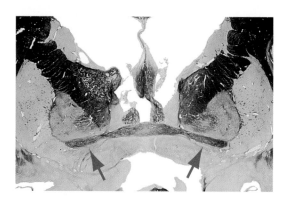

Ventral posterolateral nucleus (VPL). See *thalamus*.

Ventral posteromedial nucleus (VPM). See *thalamus*.

Ventral root. The anterior (motor) root of a spinal nerve, coalescing from a variable number of unevenly spaced rootlets that depart the spinal cord along its anterolateral sulcus.

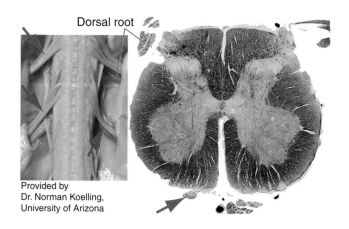

Dorsal root

Provided by
Dr. Norman Koelling,
University of Arizona

Ventral striatum. The primarily limbic subdivision of the *striatum,* comprising *nucleus accumbens* and adjacent parts of the *caudate nucleus* and *putamen*.

Ventral tegmental area. An unpaired region of the *midbrain* medial to the compact part of the *substantia nigra*, containing dopaminergic neurons that project to various limbic and neocortical areas.

Vermis. Midline, sinuous (*vermis* is Latin for "worm") zone of the *cerebellum** between the two cerebellar hemispheres. The vermis includes a representation of the trunk conveyed by the spinocerebellar tracts; its outputs, primarily through the *fastigial nucleus*, reach the *vestibular nuclei* and *reticular formation*.

Vertebral artery. One of the two major arteries that supply each side of the CNS (see also *internal carotid artery*). The vertebral artery originates as the first branch of the subclavian, runs cranially through foramina in cervical vertebrae, enters the base of the skull through the foramen magnum, and ascends along the *medulla*. At the pontomedullary junction, it unites with its contralateral counterpart to form the *basilar artery*. The vertebral artery and its *posterior inferior cerebellar* branch (PICA) supply blood to the *medulla* and inferior part of the *cerebellum*, and it supplies the cervical spinal cord via the posterior and *anterior spinal arteries*.

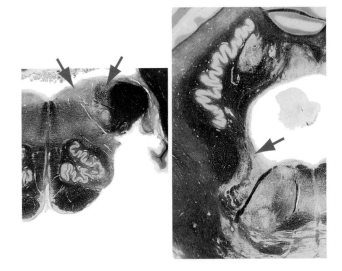

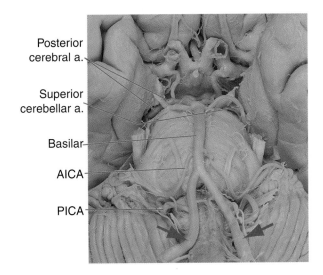

Vestibulocochlear nerve. The 8th cranial nerve, emerging anterolaterally from the *brainstem* in the cerebellopontine angle. It has vestibular and cochlear divisions innervating hair cells in vestibular organs (semicircular canals and maculae of the utricle and saccule) and the auditory spiral organ of Corti in the cochlear duct, respectively.

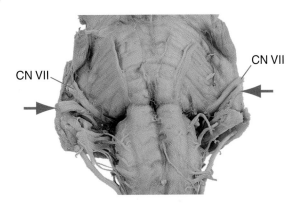

Vestibular nuclei. Four elaborately subdivided secondary sensory nuclei of the vestibular division of the 8th cranial nerve in the floor of the *fourth ventricle*, extending through much of the *medulla* and into the caudal *pons*. They reach their greatest extent near the pontomedullary junction, medial to the *inferior cerebellar peduncle*. Collectively, the vestibular nuclei project to the nuclei of extraocular muscles (mostly via the *medial longitudinal fasciculus*), the *cerebellum*, the *reticular formation*, and the spinal cord:

   Inferior. Peppered with small bundles of vestibular primary afferents that run through it.

   Lateral. Origin of the lateral vestibulospinal tract to ipsilateral extensor motor neurons.

   Medial. Origin of the medial vestibulospinal tract, projecting bilaterally to cervical motor neurons.

   Superior. Ascending and descending connections with nuclei of extraocular muscles (other vestibular nuclei also share in this).

Zona incerta. A small sheet of gray matter interposed between the *subthalamic nucleus* and *thalamus*, enveloped by efferent fibers of the *globus pallidus*. The zona incerta has widespread connections, including direct inputs to cerebral cortex, but its function is largely unknown.

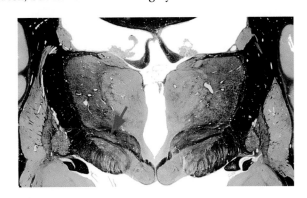

Index†

---

†Page numbers in **bold** type indicate particularly clear illustrations of a given structure. Page numbers in *italics* indicate a discussion of the structure, either in conjunction with a diagram or in the glossary. Page numbers in ***bold and italics*** indicate a discussion with an illustration—typically but not always a glossary entry.